Diagnostic Ultrasound

Diagnostic Ultrasound

Edited by

DONALD L. KING, M.D.

Associate Professor of Radiology,
Columbia University,
College of Physicians and Surgeons;
Director, Division of Ultrasound,
Presbyterian Hospital,
Columbia-Presbyterian Medical Center,
New York, New York

With 172 illustrations, including three 4-color plates

THE C. V. MOSBY COMPANY

Saint Louis 1974

COVER ILLUSTRATION. Stop-action cross-section of the left ventricle, demonstrating mitral stenosis. The cross-section was made through the long axis of the ventricle during diastole. The fused anterior and posterior mitral leaflets are seen ballooning into the left ventricle. Thickened posterior chordae tendineae are shown connecting the posterior leaflet to the posterior papillary muscle. (From Radiology **103:**387, 1972.)

Printed in the United States of America

Distributed in Great Britain by Henry Kimpton, London

Library of Congress Cataloging in Publication Data

Main entry under title:

Diagnostic ultrasound.

"Based on a series of lectures given at the College of Physicians and Surgeons, Columbia University, in the spring of 1973."

1. Diagnosis, Ultrasonic. I. King, Donald L., 1934- ed. II. Columbia University. College of Physicians and Surgeons. [DNLM: 1. Ultrasonics—Diagnostic use. WB141 K52d]
RC78.7.U4D5 616.07'54 74-12352
ISBN 0-8016-2665-X

GW/CB/B 9 8 7 6 5 4 3 2 1

Contributors

DONALD W. BAKER, B.S.
Technical Director, Center for Bioengineering, University of Washington

GILBERT BAUM, M.D.
Associate Professor of Ophthalmology and Director, Ultrasound Laboratory, Albert Einstein College of Medicine

D. JACKSON COLEMAN, M.D.
Associate Professor of Ophthalmology, Columbia University College of Physicians and Surgeons; Director, Ultrasound Laboratory, E. S. Harkness Eye Institute, Columbia-Presbyterian Medical Center

IAN DONALD, M.D., F.R.C.S.(Glasg.), F.R.C.O.G.
Regius Professor of Midwifery, University of Glasgow; Chief Consultant in Obstetrics, Queen Mother's Hospital; Chief Consultant in Gynaecology, Western Infirmary, Glasgow

RAYMOND GRAMIAK, M.D.
Professor of Diagnostic Radiology, University of Rochester; Radiologist, Strong Memorial Hospital

JOSEPH H. HOLMES, M.D.
Professor of Medicine and Radiology, University of Colorado School of Medicine; Director, Diagnostic Ultrasound, University of Colorado Medical Center

STEVE L. JOHNSON, M.D.
Assistant Professor of Medicine and Bioengineering, University of Washington School of Medicine; Director, Ultrasound Laboratory, University Hospital

DONALD L. KING, M.D.
Associate Professor of Radiology, Columbia University, College of Physicians and Surgeons; Director, Division of Ultrasound, Presbyterian Hospital, Columbia-Presbyterian Medical Center

MORRIS N. KOTLER, M.B., BCH., M.R.C.P.(Edin.)
Assistant Professor of Medicine, University of Pennsylvania; Chief of Cardiology (University of Pennsylvania Division), Veterans Administration Hospital, Philadelphia

PADMAKAR P. LELE, M.D., D.Phil.(Oxon.)
Professor of Experimental Medicine, Massachusetts Institute of Technology; Consultant in Radiology, Massachusetts General Hospital

GEORGE R. LEOPOLD, M.D.

Associate Professor of Radiology, University of California School of Medicine, San Diego; Head, Division of Ultrasound, University Hospital of San Diego County

WILLIAM M. McKINNEY, M.D.

Associate Professor of Neurology and Director, Sonic Laboratory, Bowman Gray School of Medicine

LAJOS I. Von MICSKY, M.D.

Assistant Professor of Obstetrics and Gynecology, Columbia University College of Physicians and Surgeons, Chief, Ultrasonic Division, St. Luke's Hospital Center

Acknowledgement and dedication

The conduct of medical research and the preparation of scientific papers, such as those appearing in this text, require many, many long hours of work beyond the ordinary. For that effort I thank the contributors to this book. Those hours take many of the evenings and week-ends of the researcher and of necessity call for many sacrifices by his wife and children. So they too, in no small measure, have contributed to the production of this book, to medical research, and to the improvement of medical care. Their contribution is often unsung and unrecognized and therefore it is to them that this book is dedicated with grateful appreciation.

Preface

Diagnostic ultrasound has emerged in the past decade as a highly effective and practical tool of great clinical value. Applied by a variety of techniques in different medical disciplines, it often provides diagnostic information not otherwise available without risk or discomfort to the patient. As a consequence ultrasound has become a permanent part of the diagnostic armamentarium and an essential ingredient of high-quality medical care.

This text is based on a series of lectures given at the College of Physicians and Surgeons, Columbia University, in the spring of 1973. Its purpose is to provide a comprehensive survey of the field of diagnostic ultrasound. It is part of a continuing effort by the individuals concerned to inform the medical community of the principles and applications of diagnostic ultrasound and to encourage its appropriate use. It not only reviews accepted, routine applications of diagnostic ultrasound in detail, but also presents several chapters on new or emerging techniques and applications. Hopefully, therefore, it will be useful to individuals already active in the field as well as those just beginning, or seeking an overview.

Lectures and texts cannot provide the student with an exceedingly important aspect of diagnostic ultrasound. They can only hope to impart an awareness of it. That aspect is the high degree of skillful operator interaction required for successful performance of ultrasound examinations. Ultrasound examinations require a "closed-loop" type of evaluation. Performance of an examination must be constantly modified and adapted to the patient and his problem on the basis of information gained during the examination.

Generally, ultrasonic information is not optimally recorded unless it is anticipated, actively elicited, and deliberately depicted. These examinations are not easy to perform and their clinical value is almost completely dependent upon the skill of the examiner. Those beginning in ultrasound are therefore urged not only to learn the appropriate body of knowledge but also to acquire an adequate amount of supervised experience developing the art of diagnostic ultrasound.

Donald L. King

Contents

Diagnostic Ultrasound

1 Diagnostic ultrasound: historical perspective

JOSEPH H. HOLMES, M.D.

In contrast to the early acceptance and rapid application of x-rays to medical diagnosis, the development of diagnostic ultrasound has been comparatively slow and beset with technologic difficulties. Progress has depended upon the development of efficient ultrasound transducers, powerful amplifiers, and complex electronic display devices, in a sense paralleling the development of modern electronic technology. Early investigators using ultrasound for diagnostic purposes depended heavily upon equipment and techniques previously developed for industrial or military purposes. Almost uniformly these proved inadequate for medical application. Only after the design of equipment specifically for medical diagnosis was progress rapid and the clinical value of diagnostic ultrasound proved. At present, ultrasonic techniques have assumed in many instances a preferred role in medical diagnosis and have become an essential ingredient of quality medical care.[1]

The first attempts at locating submerged objects with ultrasound probably came after the sinking of the Titanic in 1912. During World War I Langevin and associates[2] sought to utilize ultrasound for the detection of submarines. Improved technology led to the development and widespread military and civilian use of sonar (*so*und *n*avigation *a*nd *r*anging). Simultaneously, the industrial materials flaw detector[3-5] was developed. During the same period of time, just prior to World War II, Dussik[6] attempted the first application of ultrasound to medical diagnosis. He sought to visualize the cerebral ventricles by measuring attenuation of an ultrasound beam transmitted through the head. Unfortunately, variations in attenuation caused by the skull proved to be more significant than variations caused by the ventricular system, and the technique was abandoned.

Diagnostic ultrasound received its greatest stimulus from the World War II development of sonar and radar. The combination of advanced radar circuitry with sonar technology greatly improved ultrasonic instrument performance. Utilizing available industrial and war surplus equipment, several investigators began simultaneously to explore the medical applications of reflected ultrasound and to design and develop ultrasound instruments specifically for medical diagnosis. Among the earliest and most prominent of these were Douglass Howry and John Wild, the pioneering developers of ultrasonic imaging beginning in the late 1940's. In the early 1950's Leksell and Edler discovered and developed, respectively, the techniques of echoencephalography and echocardiography. Subsequently, many others undertook the investigation of ultrasonic techniques for medical application. Outstanding among them were Baum, who developed two-dimensional imaging of the eye, and Donald, who developed the first contact compound scanner and pioneered its application in the field of obstetrics and gynecology.

Douglass Howry is credited with being one of the truly far-seeing pioneers of diagnostic ultrasound. He was awarded a Certificate of Recognition of the American Institute of Ultrasound in Medicine in 1956, the Gold Medal Award for Outstanding Research of the American Medical Association in 1957, the Medal of Honor of the Radiological Society of North America in 1957, as well as the University of Colorado Recognition Award for Outstanding Research.[7] Howry (Fig. 1-1) began his efforts at ultrasonic visualization of soft tissues in 1947, while an intern at the Denver General Hospital, shortly after graduation from the University of Colorado School of Medicine.[8] During 1948 and 1949 he collaborated with Dr. W. Roderic Bliss, an engineer, in the construction of a successful pulse-echo system. The system utilized surplus Navy sonar equipment, a radar amplifier, a Heathkit oscilloscope, and a high-fidelity recorder power supply. During the fall of 1950, while a resident in radiology at the Denver Veterans Administration Hospital, he and Dr. Bliss produced their first cross-sectional ultrasonic images. During 1951 Howry developed the principle of compound scanning—the combination of circular, angular, or linear scanning patterns—to improve image quality. The scans were made with the transducer immersed in water, the latter transmitting the sound waves to the object being examined. Initially a laundry tub was used for this purpose. Later they used a metal cattle watering trough with the transducer running along hardwood rails attached to the side of the tank. At this time significant improvement in image quality was also achieved by the use of a lithium sulfate monohydrate transducer, grown in a tank specially con-

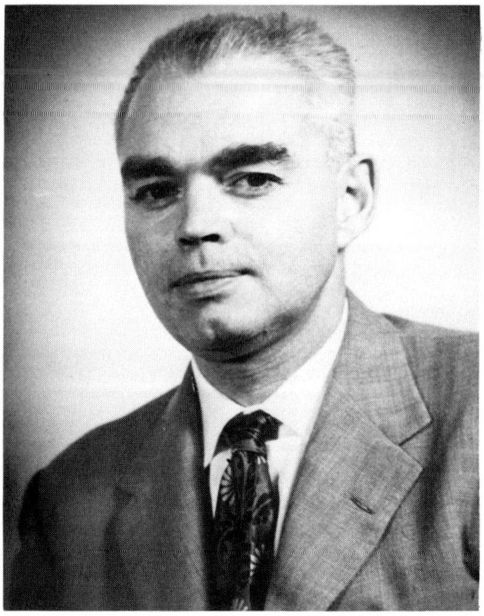

Fig. 1-1. Dr. Douglass H. Howry (1920-1969). Dr. Howry pioneered the compound scanning concept for ultrasonic imaging of the soft tissues. (Courtesy Mrs. Douglass Howry.)

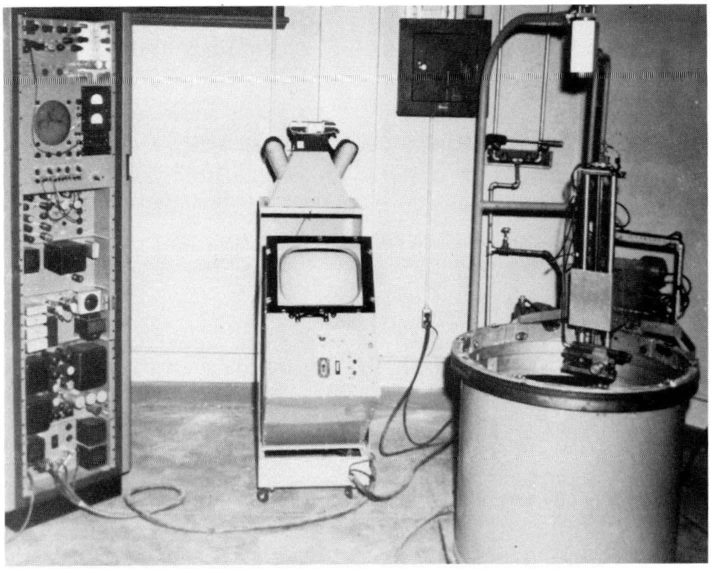

Fig. 1-2. Circular water-path scanner developed by Dr. Howry at the University of Colorado. On the right is the scanning tank. The display system with Polaroid camera is shown in the center. The electronic circuits are mounted in the rack to the left. (From Howry, D. H.: Radiol. Clin. North Am. **3**:433-452, 1965.)

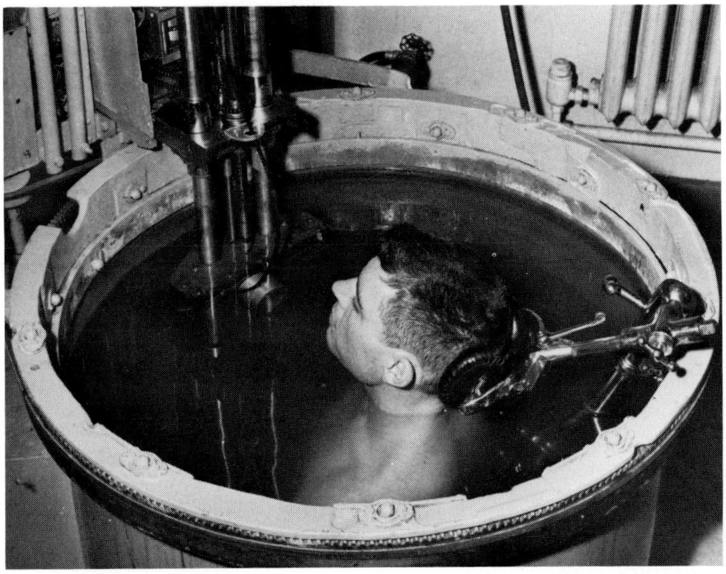

Fig. 1-3. Scanning position for transverse cross-section of the neck. The 2½-inch focused transducer is seen just below the water level. The transducer carriage travels around the tank on the outside track.

structed for this purpose. In 1952 the first publication by Howry and Bliss appeared in the *Journal of Laboratory and Clinical Medicine.*[9]

By 1954 the third generation of Howry's "Somascope" (Fig. 1-2) was constructed under the supervision of Drs. Howry and Holmes.[10,11] The scanning tank (right) was originally a B-29 gun turret. The transducer carriage was mounted on a metal ring, immersed in water, and rotated 360 degrees around the tank. During rotation of the carriage around the tank the 2½-inch focused transducer moved back and forth across the carriage in a 4-inch linear scan. The combined linear and circular motions produced a compound scan in a plane of cross-section parallel to the surface of the water. The patient under examination sat in the tank holding lead weights to maintain his position (Fig. 1-3). The echoes received were displayed as intensity-modulated dots in their appropriate orientation on the large screen and photographed by the camera mounted above it. A long persistence phosphor screen was used and provided a form of gray scale to record variations in echo intensity. One of the most successful images made with this apparatus,[12] a cross-section of the neck, is shown in Fig. 1-4. In this illustration can be seen the outlines of the neck muscles, the carotid arteries and jugular veins, the larynx, and the vocal cords.

Additional examples of the outstanding performance obtained with this apparatus, in many instances yet to be surpassed, are presented in Howry's review article.[8]

By the 1960's a series of studies on animals was also carried out to verify the anatomic accuracy of the ultrasonic pictures.[13] The animals were scanned in the water tank, overdosed with anesthesia, the bodies then frozen, and comparable anatomic cross-sections obtained. Fig. 1-5 shows a transverse cross-section of a dog urinary bladder. The echo pattern of the spine and lumbodorsal muscle groups is seen at the top. The circular structure (center) is the distended urinary bladder, while the flank folds and penis are at the bottom. The group of echoes within the bladder arises from the intravesicle catheter. Upon release of the catheter and drainage of the bladder, the circular outline of the bladder collapses. Fig. 1-6 shows a transverse cross-section of a cat liver in which an abscess was produced by injection of a suspension of *Escherichia coli* and turpentine. The spine and dorsal muscle groups are outlined at the top. The circular ring of echoes to the right arises from the stomach. Left of this, within the otherwise echo-free liver, are multiple irregular echoes produced by the hepatic abscess (arrow). The location of these echoes corresponded to the site of the abscess at autopsy.

Although excellent results were obtained with the circular water-path scanner, seri-

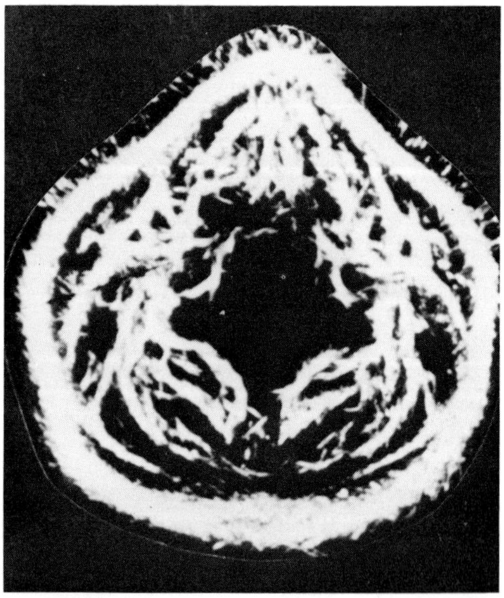

Fig. 1-4. Transverse scan of the neck. The black central area represents the cervical vertebra. Posteriorly (at bottom) can be seen the outlines of the various muscle groups. Anterolaterally on either side are two small circular structures, the carotid artery and jugular vein. Anteriorly (top) are echoes representing the larynx and vocal cords. (From Howry, D. H.: Radiol. Clin. North Am. **3:**433-452, 1965.)

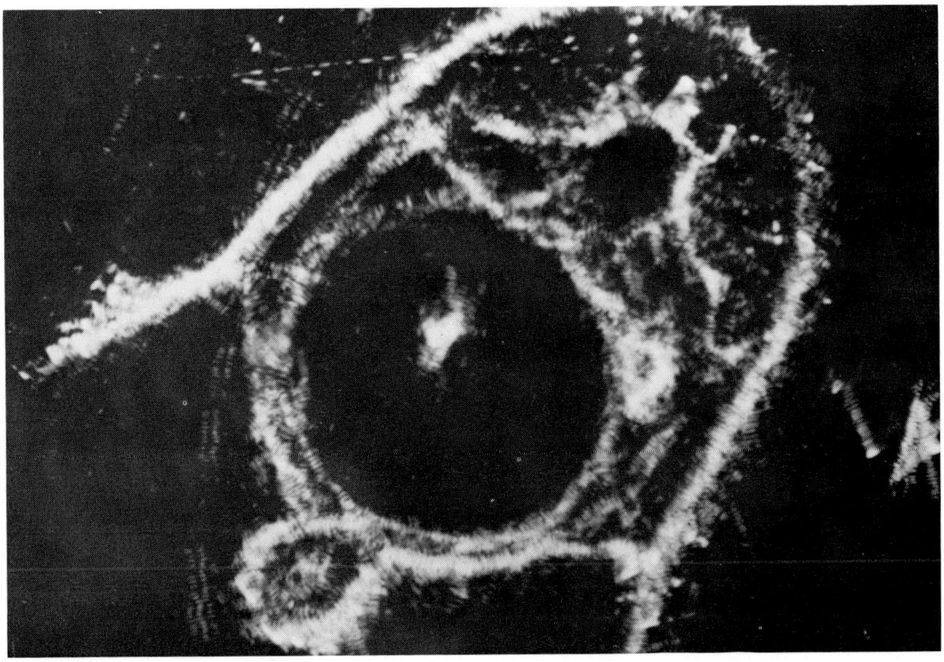

Fig. 1-5. Transverse cross-section of dog urinary bladder. (From Holmes, J. H.: Am. J. Dig. Dis. **8**:12, 1963.)

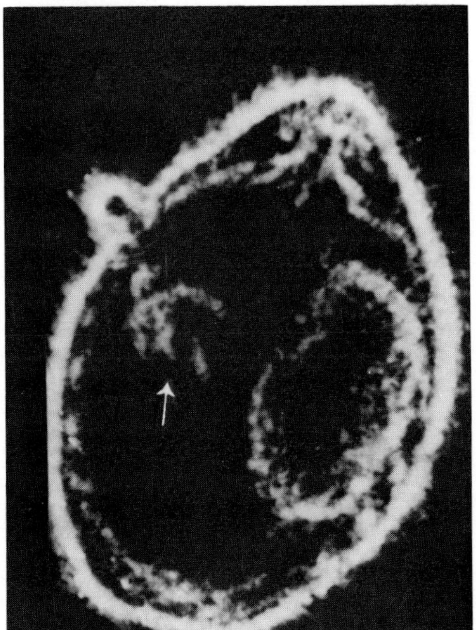

Fig. 1-6. Transverse cross-section of cat liver following creation of hepatic abscess (arrow). (From Holmes, J. H., and Howry, D. H.: Am. J. Dig. Dis. **8**:12-32, 1963.)

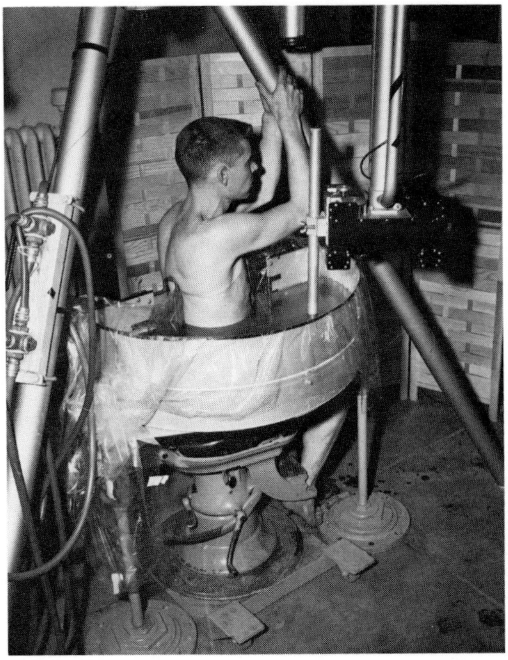

Fig. 1-7. Semicircular water-path scanner. (From Holmes, J. H., and Howry, D. H.: Am. J. Dig. Dis. **8**:12-32, 1963.)

ously ill patients could not be examined with it, and the technique was too cumbersome for routine clinical use. These difficulties were partly circumvented by construction of a modified water-path scanner (Fig. 1-7), using a semicircular tank with a rectangular window cut into its flat surface. The tank was lined with heavy plastic and the patient positioned against the plastic in a sitting position. A modified dental chair was used that could be easily raised or lowered to obtain serial cross-sections at multiple levels. The transducer carriage was suspended from an overhead tripod and rotated through a 140-degree path. Excellent images could be obtained with this system (Fig. 1-8); however it also was cumbersome for use on very sick patients and pregnant women. Therefore, in 1960 design of a contact scanner was begun.[14]

The instrument, completed in 1962, is shown in Fig. 1-9. The scanning carriage was suspended from an overhead framework. The vertical, horizontal, and angular movements of the carriage were hand-controlled. The motor-driven transducer inside the carriage moved in a sector scan 30 degrees to each side of perpendicular. A plastic shoe in contact with the skin prevented the transducer from digging into the patient. A typical cross-section obtained with this instrument is shown in Fig. 1-10. Utilizing this scanner, extensive obstetric and gynecologic studies were initiated by Thompson[15] and Gottesfeld.[16] Subsequently, a completely hand-operated con-

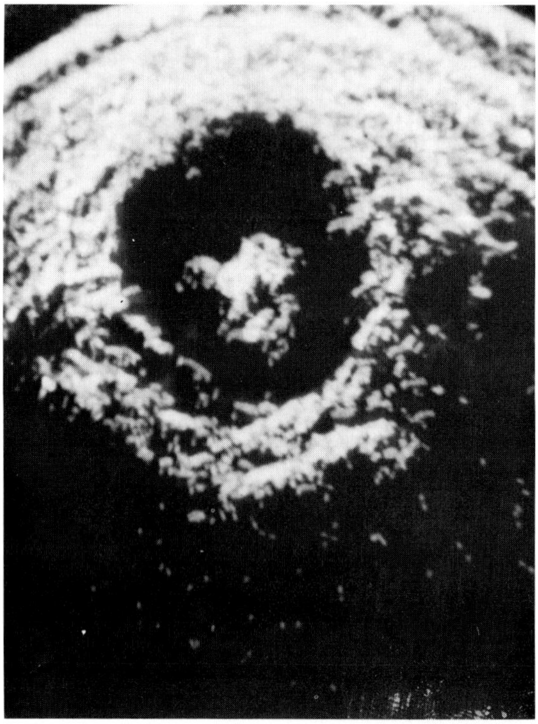

Fig. 1-8. Transverse cross-section of the kidney obtained with the semicircular water-path scanner. Skin surface is at the top. The renal cortex appears echo-free. Centrally are echoes from the vessels and collecting system.

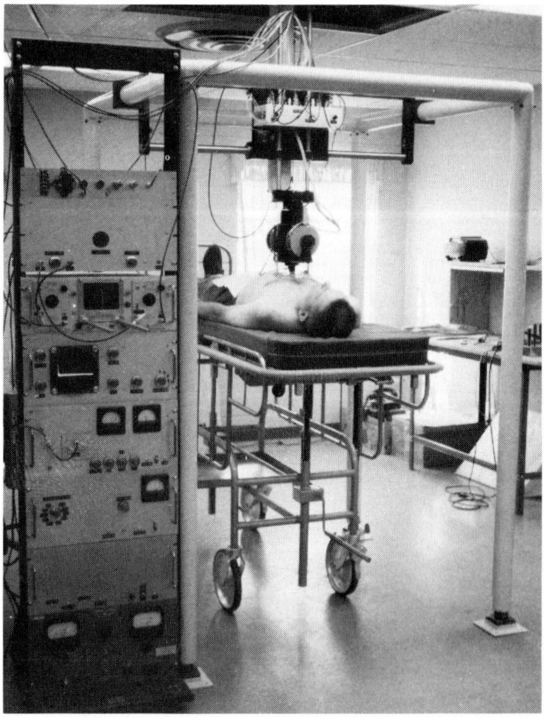

Fig. 1-9. Compound contact scanner developed at the University of Colorado, 1960-1962. The electronics and display oscilloscopes are in the rack at the left.

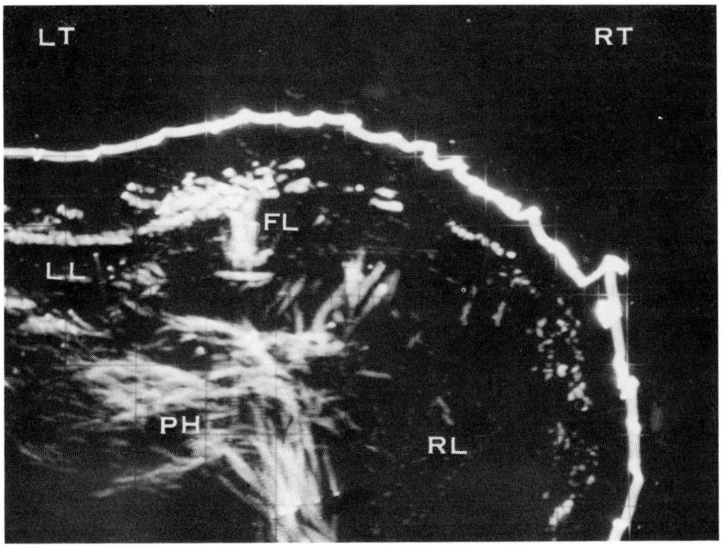

Fig. 1-10. Transverse cross-section of the liver made by the compound contact scanner, viewed looking toward the feet. Note echoes from the porta hepatis *(PH)* and falciform ligament *(FL)*. *LL,* Left lobe; *RL,* right lobe; *RT;* right; *LT,* left.

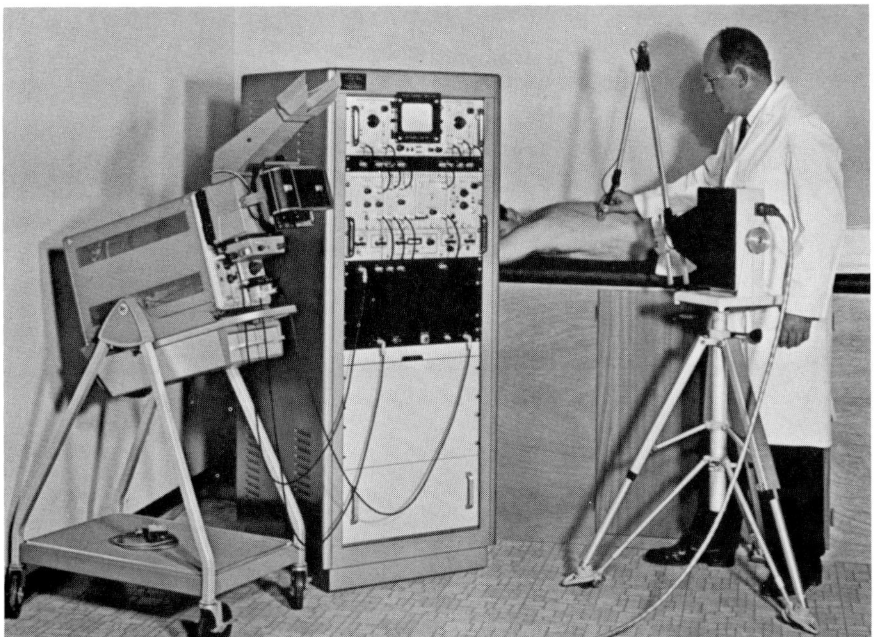

Fig. 1-11. First commercial ultrasonic scanner manufactured in the United States of America. The pivot-arm scanner is mounted on a tripod at the right. The electronics and display oscilloscope are in the rack and cart at the left. The three-jointed arm scanner remains a widely utilized design concept. (Courtesy Picker Corp.)

tact scanner (Fig. 1-11) was designed by William L. Wright, an engineer working with the University of Colorado research group. It became the first commercial scanner marketed in the United States. The design concepts incorporated in this scanner remain in widespread use today.

John J. Wild (Fig. 1-12) was also one of the earliest pioneers in the development of diagnostic ultrasound. He is credited with demonstrating that ultrasound could detect differences between normal tissues, benign tumors, and malignant cancers.[17] He began his investigations in 1949 with the cooperation of the Naval Air Station, Wold-Chamberlain Field, Minneapolis, Minnesota. He and his co-workers utilized equipment modified from a naval ultrasonic trainer. His first tissue studies were done on pieces of intestine and showed that different echo patterns could be obtained from each of the different layers of the specimen.[18] Other studies revealed the ability of ultrasonic echo pattern to differentiate cerebral neoplasms from surrounding normal brain tissue.[19]

At this time Dr. John Reid, an engineer, began work with Dr. Wild on the development of a two-dimensional scanning system.[20,21] Fig. 1-13 is their first published example of an ultrasonographic cross-section of the breast.[22,23] The one-dimensional A-mode records of the normal breast and breast with tumor are shown in *A*, while in *B* are the corresponding two-dimensional cross-sections.

Fig. 1-14 shows a close-up view of the transducer designed by Dr. Wild for scanning the breasts. A sloping plastic chamber

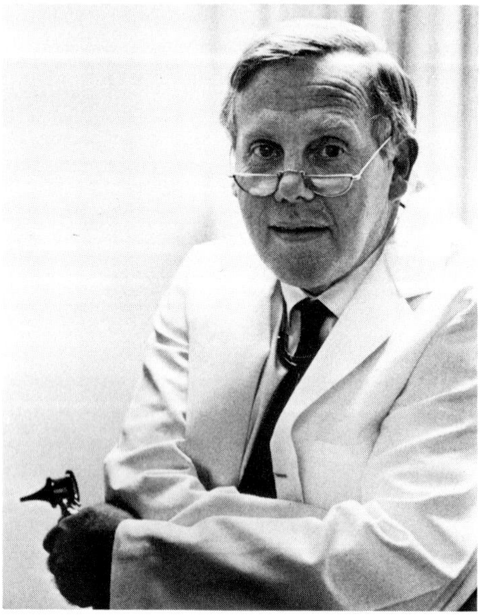

Fig. 1-12. Dr. John J. Wild. Dr. Wild's early investigations demonstrated the ability of ultrasound to differentiate different types of tissue. (Courtesy Dr. John J. Wild).

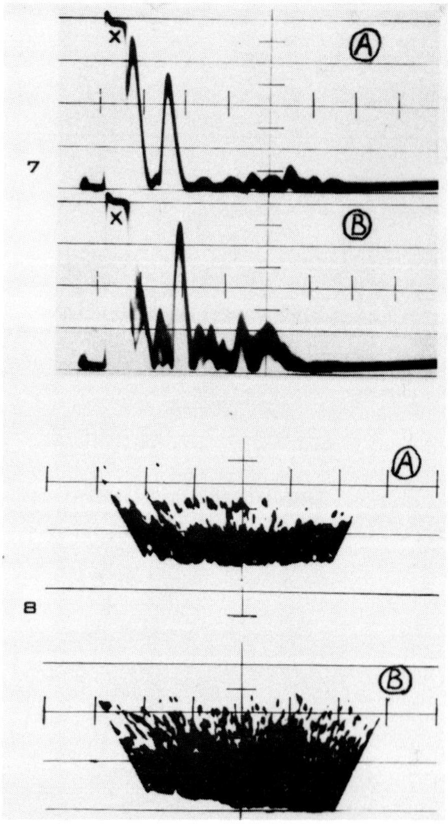

Fig. 1-13. Reproductions of the early one-dimensional and two-dimensional scans of the breast by Wild and Reid. *A*, The normal scan, *B*, the tumor of the breast. (From Wild, J. J., and Reid, J. M.: Am. J. Pathol. **28**:839-861, 1952.)

with its smaller end covered with a rubber diaphragm is applied directly over the breast and sonic contact achieved by use of aqueous jelly. The transducer moves back and forth within the plastic chamber to provide the scanning motion. By 1956, after studying a series of seventy-seven patients with suspected breast abnormalities, Wild and Reid reported a 90% accuracy in the diagnosis of benign versus malignant lesions.[24] While his success at diagnosis of breast cancer awaits confirmation, Wild's greatest contribution, the demonstration that ultrasound could differentiate between normal and malignant tissue, has served as a constant stimulus for the improvement of ultrasonic techniques and instrumentation.

Ian Donald is largely responsible for the development of the contact scanning concept and for pioneering the extensive application of ultrasonic imaging in obstetrics and gynecology. In 1954, while in London, he met Dr. Wild and learned of his early work in diagnostic ultrasound. Donald began his own investigations with ultrasound shortly thereafter in Glasgow. His initial experiments utilized an ultrasonic metal flaw detector. With this he examined excised uterine fibromyomata and ovarian tumors and found that the echo patterns reflected from the specimens demonstrated distinct differences. With this encouragement he began clinical evaluation of patients. The ultrasonic flaw detector available to him at that time could only operate successfully through a water-filled tank at some distance from the patient's skin. The tank used was a flexible latex rubber bucket. The difficulties presented by this arrangement led to his consideration of various alternatives and ultimately to the development of the contact scanner.

In 1955, Mr. Tom Brown, an engineer at the Research and Development Department, Kelvin and Hughes, Ltd., began his long association with Professor Donald. During the next 2 years they designed and constructed a prototype hand-operated, two-dimensional contact scanner.[25] The principle of contact scanning is now almost universally used clinically for ultrasonic imaging of the pelvis and abdomen. The primary advantage of contact scanning

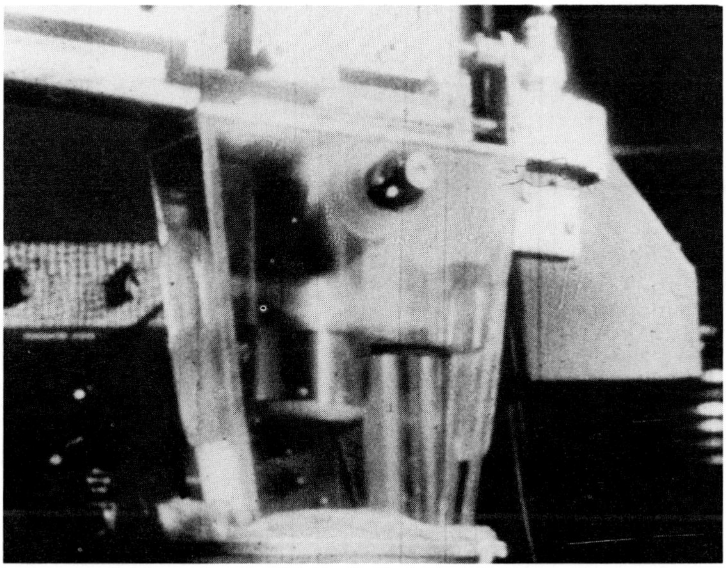

Fig. 1-14. Close-up photograph of Wild and Reid's early breast scanner.

is elimination of the sound-transmitting water tank and its inconvenience. In contact scanning the transducer probe is placed in direct contact with the patient's skin. Acoustic coupling is achieved by use of an oil or jelly. An example of an early contact scan obtained by Donald is shown in Fig. 1-15. The first results obtained with this new scanner were published in 1958.[26]

Because the appearance of a hydatidi-

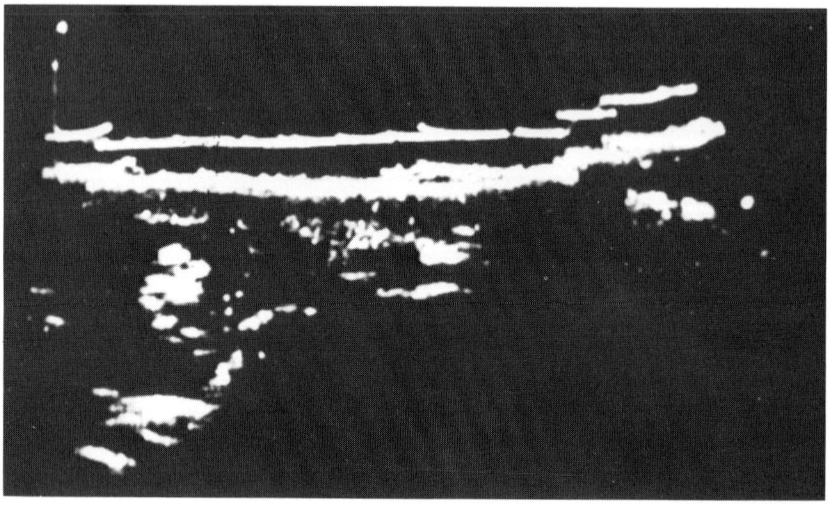

Fig. 1-15. An early ultrasonic cross-section made by Donald. In this longitudinal cross-section cephalad is to the right, caudad to the left. At the left is a cystic cavity containing strong echoes arising from a 12- to 14-week fetus. (From Brown, T. G.: Direct contact ultrasonic scanning techniques for the visualization of abdominal masses, Proceedings of the Second International Conference on Medical Electronics, Paris, June 24-27, 1959, London, 1959, Iliffe & Sons, Ltd., pp. 358-366.)

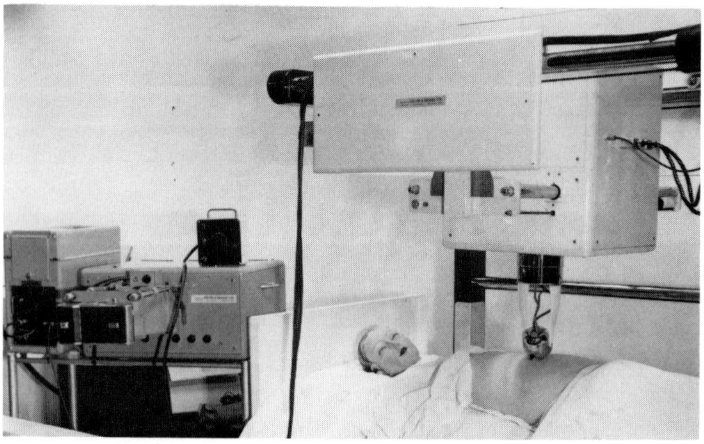

Fig. 1-16. Automatic contact scanner developed by Donald and Brown to operate at constant speed, pressure, and angle of sector scan. Automatic scanning was expected to compensate for errors arising from variations in scanning technique but eventually proved impractical. (Courtesy Dr. Ian Donald.)

form mole could be simulated by "overscanning" with the hand-operated instrument, a second automatic scanner was built[27] (Fig. 1-16). In order to obtain comparable images at different times without variation caused by scanning technique, the second scanner operated at constant speed, pressure, and angle of sector scan. This instrument contributed greatly to the development of optimum technique in the next few years, but it was ultimately to prove too slow and expensive for clinical use. Hand scanning became more reliable and reproducible and was eventually accepted for clinical application. In addition to establishing the ultrasonographic criteria for diagnosis of hydatidiform mole[27] (Fig. 1-17), Donald and his co-workers contributed greatly to the development of fetal cephalometry and study of the "blighted" ovum.

Gilbert Baum of New York pioneered in the development of two-dimensional ultrasonic imaging of the eye and orbit. Although other investigators had earlier utilized unidimensional A-mode techniques for examination of the eye, Baum was the first to produce the graphic cross-sectional image. He worked in conjunction with Ivan Greenwood, an engineer at General Precision, Inc. They constructed a sophisticated scanning apparatus using a water-path coupling system.[28] The patient placed his face in a swimmer's mask built into the side of a saline-filled plastic tank (Fig. 1-18). The 15-MHz transducer, positioned in front of the eye, oscillated through approximately a 30-degree sector scan in a horizontal or transverse plane. With this apparatus Baum was able to produce the first cross-sectional ultrasonic images of the eye showing retinal detachment, intraocular tumors, and foreign bodies. Subsequently, he reported the first ultrasonic visualization of orbital tumors and foreign bodies.[29] An example of an early ultrasonogram of the eye is shown in Fig. 1-19. Ultrasonic imaging of the eye and orbit has proved to be invaluable in the presence of opaque media and suspected retrobulbar abnormalities.

Inge Edler of Lund is recognized as the pioneering developer of ultrasound cardiography,[30] or echocardiography. In 1953, working with Dr. Hellmuth Hertz,[31] a physicist, Edler discovered that echoes from the moving heart could be received and displayed on an ultrasonic flaw detector (Fig. 1-20). Technical improvements followed with the development of the time-motion mode of display[32] and simultaneous recording of the electrocardiogram (Fig.

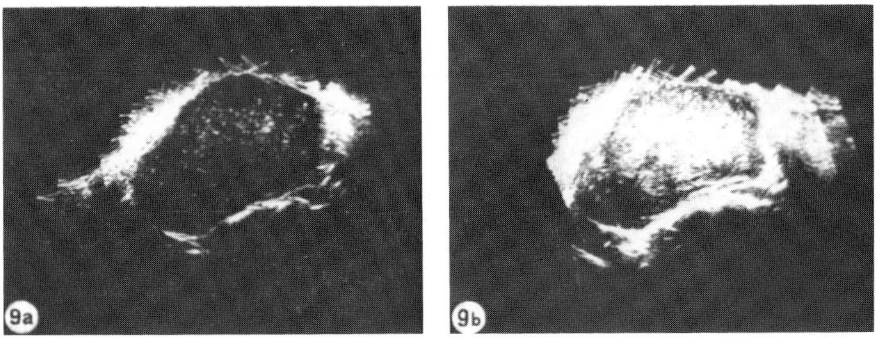

Fig. 1-17. Longitudinal cross-section (cephalad, right) of an enlarged uterus containing a hydatidiform mole. On the left, at low sensitivity, a few molar echoes are seen. High transonicity is demonstrated by the persistently strong far wall echoes. On the right, at high sensitivity, many echoes from the vesicular tissue are seen. (From Donald, I., and Brown, T.: Br. J. Radiol. **34:**543, 1961.)

1-21). By 1955 Edler reported the ability to diagnose mitral stenosis, thrombosis in the left atrium in mitral stenosis, as well as pericardial effusion.[33] Further technical improvement resulted from the use of barium titanate transducers in 1956. This development permitted recording of not only stenotic mitral valve motion but also the more rapid motion of the normal mitral leaflet. In 1959 Edler and co-workers demonstrated the anatomic source of the cardiac echo patterns using needles at the autopsy table.[34] In the following years he and other investigators have so greatly broadened the application of echocardiography that it has now become an essential technique for cardiac diagnosis.

Lars Leksell of Lund discovered that echoes could be recorded from the midline structures of the brain through the intact skull and launched the technique of echoencephalography. His research efforts with pulse-echo ultrasound began in 1953 with an ultrasonic flaw detector. It was not until 1954, using an improved instrument borrowed from Dr. Edler, that he was able to demonstrate the midline echo of the brain on a child. Shortly thereafter, on another unconscious child, he demonstrated displacement of the midline echo by a large frontal hematoma. He first reported his results in 1955.[35] Subsequent reports in 1956[36] and 1958[37] presented the technique and additional results and discussed the sources of the midline echo (Fig. 1-22). In the following years many others verified his findings, improved the technique, and confirmed its usefulness and accuracy as a method for detecting and localizing supratentorial space-occupying lesions.

Through the efforts of these early investigators and others working with them and after them, diagnostic ultrasound has evolved into a highly useful tool of diverse clinical application. The progress achieved over the past 25 years has been the result

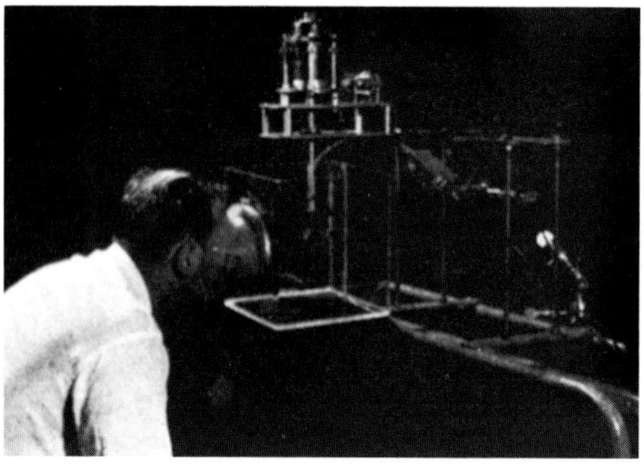

Fig. 1-18. Early apparatus developed by Baum for ophthalmic imaging with ultrasound. (From Baum, G., and Greenwood, I.: Arch. Ophthal. **60:**263-279, 1958.)

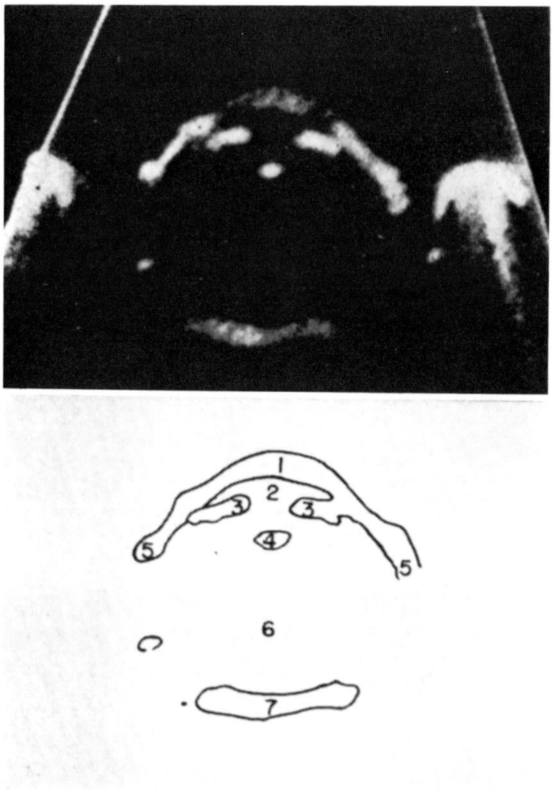

Fig. 1-19. Reproduction of the first two-dimensional ultrasonogram of the eye made by Baum. *1,* Cornea; *2,* anterior chamber; *3,* iris; *4,* lens; *5,* anterior sclera; *6,* vitreous; *7,* posterior sclera. (From Baum, G., and Greenwood, I.: Arch. Ophthal. **60:**263-279, 1958.)

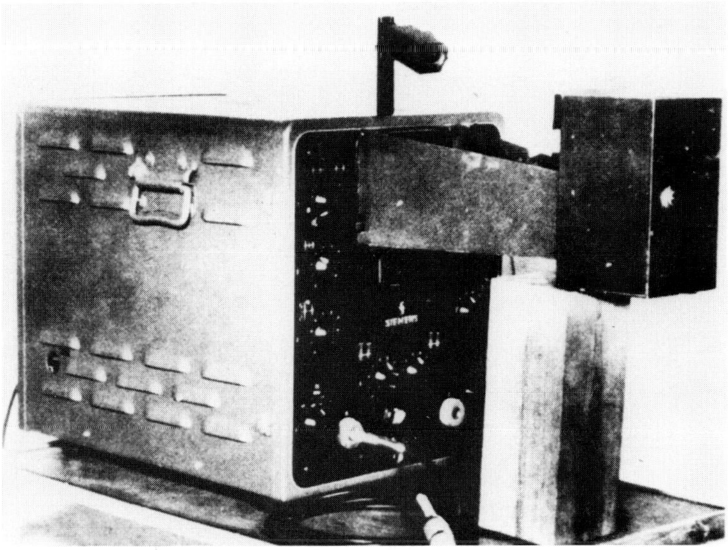

Fig. 1-20. Ultrasonic flaw detector adapted for use as an echocardiograph by Edler and Hertz. (From Hertz, C. H.: Ultrasound Med. Biol. **1**[1]:6, 1973. Reprinted with permission of Pergamon Press, Inc.)

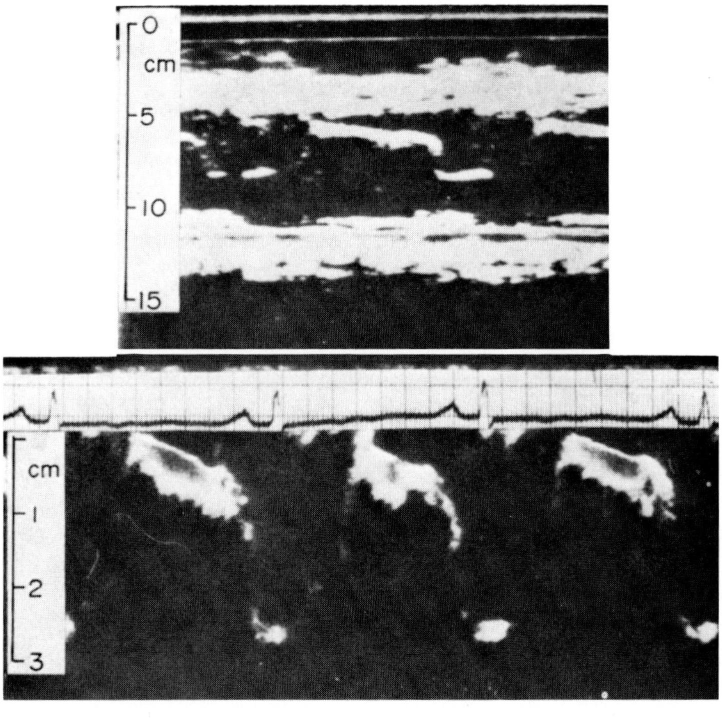

Fig. 1-21. Early time-motion echocardiogram showing the first successful recording of the mitral valve in mitral stenosis. (From Hertz, C. H.: Ultrasound Med. Biol. **1**[1]:6, 1973. Reprinted with permission of Pergamon Press, Inc.)

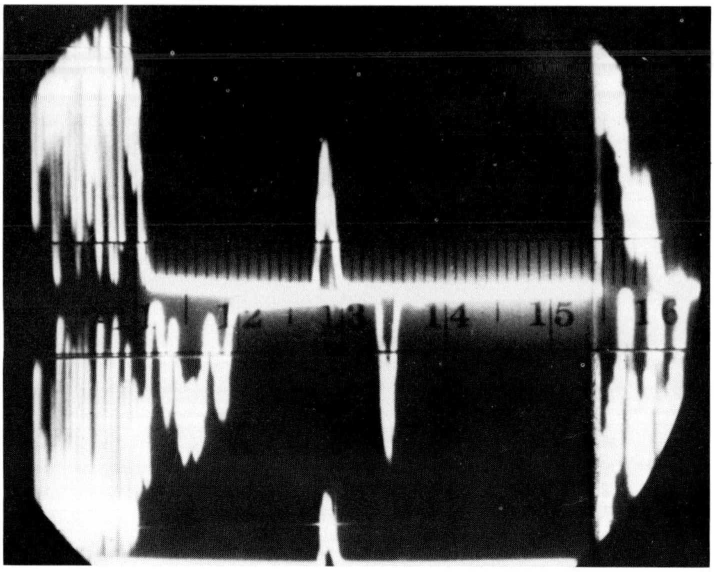

Fig. 1-22. Representative example of midline echoencephalogram showing a left to right shift of the posterior midline structures.

of close cooperation of physicians and engineers working as a team. Continuation of this effort and further study of the interaction of ultrasound with tissue should yield new and improved methods and applications of diagnostic ultrasound.

REFERENCES

1. Lele, P. P.: Applications of ultrasound in medicine, N. Engl. J. Med. **286:**1317-1318, 1972.
2. Langevin, M. P.: Les ondes ultrasonores, Rev. Gen. Elect. **23:**626-634, 1928.
3. Sokolov, S. Y.: Means for indicating flaws in materials, U. S. Patent 2,164,125, 1937.
4. Firestone, F. A.: Flaw detecting device and measuring instrument, U. S. Patent 2,280,226, 1940.
5. Firestone, F. A.: Supersonic reflectoscope, an instrument for inspecting the interior of solid parts by means of sound waves, J. Acoust. Soc. Am. **17:**287, 1945.
6. Dussik, K. T.: Über die möglichkeit hochfrequente mechanische schwingungen als diagnostisches hilfsmittel zu verwerten, Z. Neurol. Psychiatr. **174:**153-168, 1942.
7. Dedication: Douglass Howry, J. Clin. Ultrasound **1:**2-4, 1973.
8. Howry, D. H.: A brief atlas of diagnostic ultrasonic radiologic results, Radiol. Clin. North Am. **3:**433-452, 1965.
9. Howry, D. H., and Bliss, W. R.: Ultrasonic visualization of soft tissue structures of the body, J. Lab. Clin. Med. **40:**579-592, 1952.
10. Howry, D. H., Stott, D. A., and Bliss, W. R.: The ultrasonic visualization of carcinoma of the breast and other soft tissue structures, Cancer **7:**354-358, 1954.
11. Holmes, J. H., and others: The ultrasonic visualization of soft tissue structures in the body, Trans. Am. Clin. Climat. Assoc. **66:**208-225, 1954.
12. Howry, D. H.: Techniques used in ultrasonic visualization of soft tissues. In Kelly, E., editor: Ultrasound in biology and medicine, Publ. No. 3, American Institute of Biological Sciences, Baltimore, 1957, Waverly Press, Inc.
13. Holmes, J. H., and Howry, D. H.: Ultrasonic diagnosis of abdominal diseases, Am. J. Dig. Dis. **8:**12-32, 1963.
14. Holmes, J. H., and others: Ultrasonic contact scanner for diagnostic application, Am. J. Med. Electron. **4:**147-152, 1965.
15. Thompson, H. E., and others: Ultrasound as a diagnostic aid in diseases of the pelvis, Am. J. Obstet. Gynecol. **98:**472-480, 1967.
16. Gottesfeld, K. R., and others: Ultrasonic placentography—a new method for placental localization, Am. J. Obstet. Gynecol. **96:**538-547, 1966.
17. Wild, J. J., and Neal, D.: Use of high frequency ultrasonic waves for detecting changes in texture in living tissue, Lancet **1:**655-657, 1951.

18. Wild, J. J.: Use of ultrasonic pulses for measurement of biological tissues and detection of tissue density changes, Surgery **27**:183-188, 1950.
19. French, L. A., Wild, J. J., and Neal, B.: Detection of cerebral tumors by ultrasonic pulses: pilot studies on postmortem material, Cancer **3**:705-708, 1950.
20. Wild, J. J., and Reid, J. M.: Application of echo-ranging techniques to the determination of structure of biological tissues, Science **115**:226-230, 1952.
21. Reid, J. M., and Wild, J. J.: Ultrasonic ranging for cancer diagnosis, Electronics **25**:136-138, 1952.
22. Wild, J. J., and Reid, J. M.: Further pilot echographic studies on the histological structures of tumors of the living intact human breast, Am. J. Pathol. **28**:839-861, 1952.
23. Wild, J. J., and Reid, J. M.: Echographic visualization of lesions of the living, intact human breast, Cancer Res. **14**:277-283, 1954.
24. Wild, J. J., and Reid, J. M.: Diagnostic use of ultrasound, Br. J. Phys. Med. **19**:248-257, 1956.
25. Brown, T. G.: Direct contact ultrasonic scanning techniques for the visualization of abdominal masses. In Smyth, C. N., editor: Proceedings of the Second International Conference on Medical Electronics, Paris, June 24-27, 1959, London, 1959, Iliffe & Sons, Ltd., pp. 358-366.
26. Donald, I., MacVicar, J., and Brown, T. G.: Investigation of abdominal masses by pulsed ultrasound, Lancet **1**:1188-1195, 1958.
27. MacVicar, J., and Donald, I.: Sonar in the diagnosis of early pregnancy and its complications, J. Obstet. Gynaecol. Br. Commonw. **70**:387-395, 1963.
28. Baum, G., and Greenwood, I.: The application of ultrasonic locating techniques to ophthalmology, Arch. Ophthal. **60**:263-279, 1958.
29. Baum, G., and Greenwood, I.: Ultrasonography —an aid in orbital tumor diagnosis, Arch. Ophthal. **64**:180-194, 1960.
30. Edler, I., and Hertz, C. H.: The use of the ultrasonic reflectoscope for the continuous recording of movements of heart walls, Kungl. Fysiog. Sallsk. Lund Forh. **24**:1-19, 1954.
31. Hertz, C. H.: The interaction of physicians, physicists and industry in the development of echocardiography, Ultrasound Med. Biol. **1**:3-11, 1973.
32. Hertz, C. H., and Edler, I.: Die registrierung von herzwanbewegungen mit hilfe des ultraschall-impulsverfahrens, Acustica **6**:361, 1956.
33. Edler, I.: The diagnostic use of ultrasound in heart disease, Acta Med. Scand., Suppl. 308, pp. 32-36, 1955.
34. Edler, I.: Ultrasound cardiography, Acta Med. Scand., Suppl. 370, 1961.
35. Leksell, L.: Behandling av akuta skallskador och deras foljdtillstand. Kirurgisk behandling, Nord. Med. **15**:1444, 1955.
36. Leksell, L.: Echoencephalography: detection of intracranial complications following head injury, Acta Chir. Scand. **110**:301-315, 1955-1956.
37. Leksell, L.: Echoencephalography: midline echo from the pineal body as an index of pineal displacement, Acta Chir. Scand. **115**:255-259, 1958.

2 Physical and technical principles

DONALD W. BAKER, B.S.

Ultrasonic energy can be shaped into a beam and caused to interact with various tissues of the body. Recording these interactions with special electronic instruments may produce meaningful information contributing to the diagnosis and treatment of many of man's ailments.

The ultrasonic examination of a patient is basically different from most diagnostic procedures.[1,2] In the x-ray department, the radiologist or technologist prepares the patient and sets up the instrument; if the proper adjustments are made, a useful picture will be produced automatically. In the nuclear medicine laboratory the technician sets up the scanner, aligns the patient, and injects the bolus of isotope; the machine does the rest. In both of these techniques there is little interaction among operator, instrument, and patient once the actual procedure starts.

The final result of all ultrasonic procedures, good or bad, depends on the knowledge and the ability of the operator to use the instrument in an interactive way on the subject. The operator must be able to interpret the dynamic echo patterns as the procedure progresses in order to control the direction of the ultrasonic beam to secure the desired result. The information patterns produced must be optimized by movement of the transducer and manipulation of the instrument controls to achieve a scan or image that coincides with established standards and techniques. In all these applications there are appropriate acoustic or dynamic landmarks that serve as references in generating images that must be learned and understood.

This interactive process must become second nature if the physician or technologist is to be really effective. This means that the operator of the equipment should have an almost intuitive understanding of all the elements of this complex interactive detection and measurement system.

One approach to understanding the function and the role of the technical aspects of these procedures is based on the processes depicted in Fig. 2-1. There are three principal components involved in these interactive procedures: the physician or technologist, the instrument, and the patient. The instrument serves as a coupler or converter to transform acoustic information from the subject to another form interpretable by a qualified operator. The machine is not automatic; therefore, the results that it presents to the user depend on its design and how it is operated.

The basic instrument has two principal interfaces. First, the electroacoustic interface, called the transducer, converts electric signals into acoustic pulses or beams, which are coupled into the tissue of the patient. These same transducers serve as receivers to detect the reflected pulses from within the subject. Second, an audiovisual electronic interface converts the detected or processed echo signals, which pass through the electronics of the instrument, into a form that the technologist can evaluate. This interface may be the screen of an oscilloscope, a chart recorder, a camera, or a speaker.

The most basic ultrasonic instrument transmits a short burst of high-frequency sound into the patient via the transducer. The time required for a pulse to travel out to an interface, reflect, and return can be used to measure depth or range as in radar. In tissue, it takes approximately 13 μsec for the sound to travel out and back for each centimeter of depth.

There are four principal modes of operation used in ultrasonic procedures. These are as follows, in order of instrument complexity.

A mode. Information is shown on an oscilloscope screen in the form of echo amplitude plotted versus depth.[2] It is used in neurology for determinations of midline position, in ophthalmology, for foreign body localization, and in conjunction with

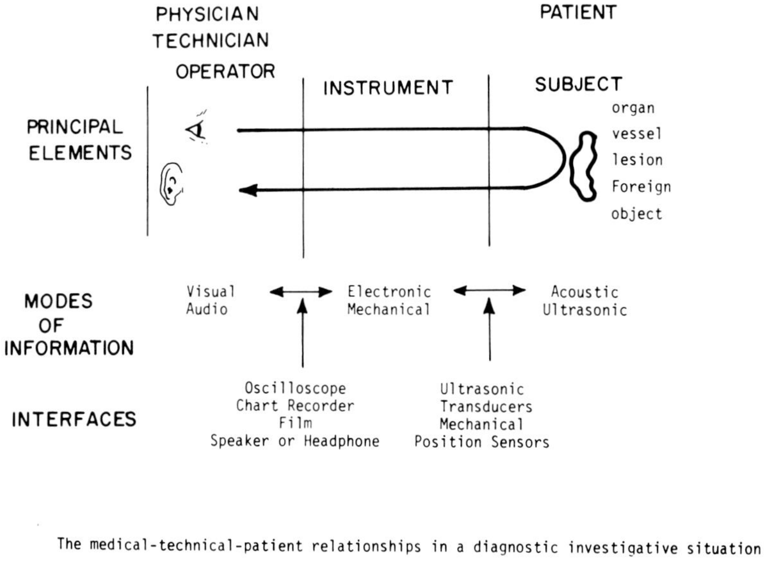

Fig. 2-1. Electronics, acoustics, and mechanics are used to transform information in a physical form within the subject into a form that the operator or physician can interpret. The optimal instrument permits the most efficient transfer of information through the two interfaces.

T-M–mode display to locate heart valves and to help in separating cystic from solid masses.

T-M mode. An echo range displacement (depth) versus time type of display is added to the basic A-mode instrument for the purpose of recording and measuring heart valve displacements and velocities. It is sometimes used to evaluate motion of other interfaces, such as aortic aneurysms.[1]

B mode. This is the most complex instrument configuration at the present time. It permits scanning of the abdomen or other relatively stationary structures to produce cross-sectional images.[2] The scanning is performed using a specially designed instrumented arm to which the ultrasonic transducer is attached. The joints of the arm are fitted with angle-sensing electromechanical transducers whose outputs are used along with the echo signals to produce an image on an oscilloscope. These images can show outlines and some internal structures of the liver, kidney, spleen, aorta, vena cava, solid or cystic tumor mass, and many others. The display has geometric meaning and can be calibrated, photographed, and interpreted in a variety of ways.

Doppler. This mode of operation requires another set of electronics or a separate instrument since it involves different principles from pulse echo methods.[3] The concept involves the detection of the Doppler shift in either continuous wave or pulsed echo modes. These signals are derived from backscattered ultrasound emanating from moving blood or moving interfaces, valves, vessel walls, and the like. With these devices it is possible to investigate blood flow in many vessels.

Only continuous wave Dopplers are currently available for clinical use. They have either an audible output, which the physician must learn to evaluate, or analog signals that can be recorded. Pulse Dopplers that will provide depth information as well as flow velocity are still in the stage of development and evaluation.

Before going into the details of each of these modes, it will be necessary to touch upon the fundamentals of ultrasound and then, with some basic understanding in hand, build up a description of the instrument, eventually leading to its applications.

ULTRASOUND: DEFINITION AND CHARACTERISTICS

Ultrasound is the name given to a class of mechanical pressure waves that can be propagated through liquids, solids, and, to some extent, gases.[4] In addition to their mechanical characteristics, the principal distinction of these waves is that their frequency of oscillation lies above 20,000 cycles per second (cps), or 20*K* hertz ($K = 1{,}000$). The uses of ultrasound are far reaching. They appear in many fields of endeavor and at frequencies from 20 kHz to 10 MHz (1×10^7 cps).

We are concerned with waves in the band extending from 1 MHz (1×10^6 cps) to 20 MHz (2×10^7 cps) and having average intensities less than 100 milliwatts per square centimeter (mw/cm^2).

In these discussions we will work with simple models to develop a basic understanding only of the physical effects of interest, because the subject of sound wave propagation in layered heterogeneous substances such as tissue is actually very complex. To begin we shall assume a transducer shaped in the form of a disk that is mechanically vibrating in a piston or thickness mode. This element is immersed in water, and disk-like planar pressure waves are being coupled into the fluid from both the front and the back surfaces. We will be concerned with the waves from only one surface traveling away from the element in one direction. These waves, as shown edge on in Fig. 2-2, *A*, will travel at a velocity of approximately $C = 1{,}490$ meters/sec in water and up to 1,550 meters/sec in blood and tissue. The velocity de-

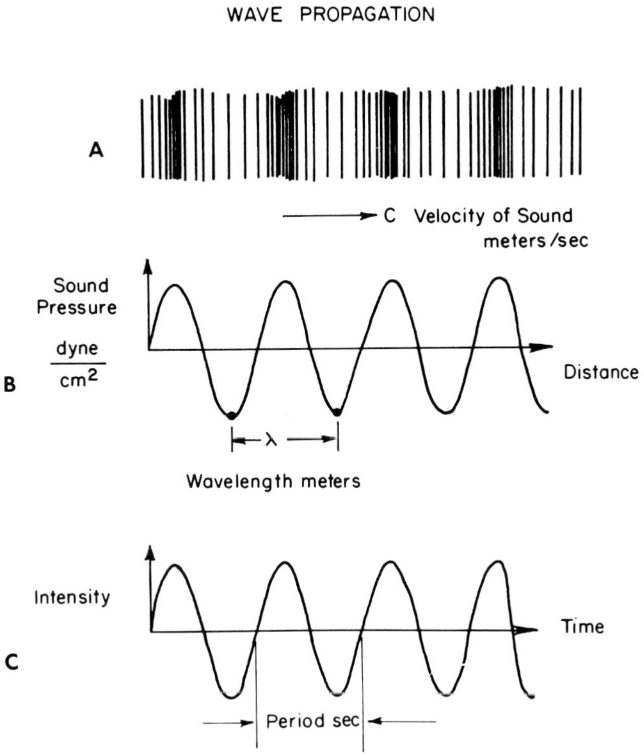

Fig. 2-2. Ultrasonic waves consist of sinusoidal compressions and rarefactions propagating along the sound beam axis within the fluid.

pends on the temperature and characteristics of the propagating medium. The magnitude of these effects is negligible in terms of the current level of accuracy of medical instruments. The sound pressure measured along the path of the sound beam will be sinusoidal and will have a wavelength, lambda (λ), that is defined mathematically by:

$$\lambda = \frac{c}{f}$$

where

c = velocity of sound in medium (cm/sec)
f = frequency of wave (cps)

A fixed test point in the sound beam would monitor a sinusoidal fluctuation in intensity (pressure) as a function of time (Fig. 2-2, C). The period (τ) in seconds can be measured and, when divided into 1, gives the frequency of the wave:

$$f = \frac{1}{\tau}$$

As the beam moves through the fluid medium, a number of things happen to it. A large fraction of the input energy or intensity is absorbed by the fluid and converted to thermal or heat energy. This leads to an attenuation of the signal. The attenuation is usually of an exponential nature and depends on the properties of the medium and the frequency of the wave.[4] Mathematically this is expressed as:

$$I = I_0 \epsilon^{-\alpha \chi}$$

where

I_0 = initial intensity (w/cm^2)
α = attenuation coefficient (nepers)
χ = distance (cm)
ϵ = 2.71828

The attenuation coefficient varies with different tissues and is also a function of the ultrasound frequency. A typical value for soft tissue at a frequency of 1 MHz is 0.2 nepers/cm.

The neper, a unit of attenuation, is defined as:

$$N = ln \frac{I_1}{I_2}$$

the logarithm to the base ϵ of the two scaler quantities I_1, intensity at point 1, and I_2, the intensity at point 2.

These equations are useful in basic scientific applications of ultrasound and are of help to the instrument designer. A more convenient shorthand way of referring to attenuation uses the decibel notation.

DECIBEL NOTATION

The amplitude or intensity of ultrasonic echoes received from within the body can have values ranging over 10,000 to 1. These same echoes may be as small as 1.0×10^{-6} of the input signal level from the transmitting transducer. The wide range of these signals is best shown using a logarithmic scale; however, such a scale is nonlinear and inconvenient to use.

A system of notation has been devised that was originally based on the logarithmic response characteristics of the human ear.[4] The perceived increase in loudness of a sound is proportional to the $\log_{10}$ of the ratio of the sound powers (acoustic watts).

$$\text{Loudness change (bel)} = \log_{10} \frac{P_2}{P_1}$$

where

P_1 = original power level (watts)
P_2 = new power level (watts)

A curve of this type of response is shown in Fig. 2-3, *A*. When the power is plotted to the logarithmic base 10 on the abscissa versus perceived loudness on a linear scale on the ordinate, the result is a linear relationship, as seen in Fig. 2-3, *B*.

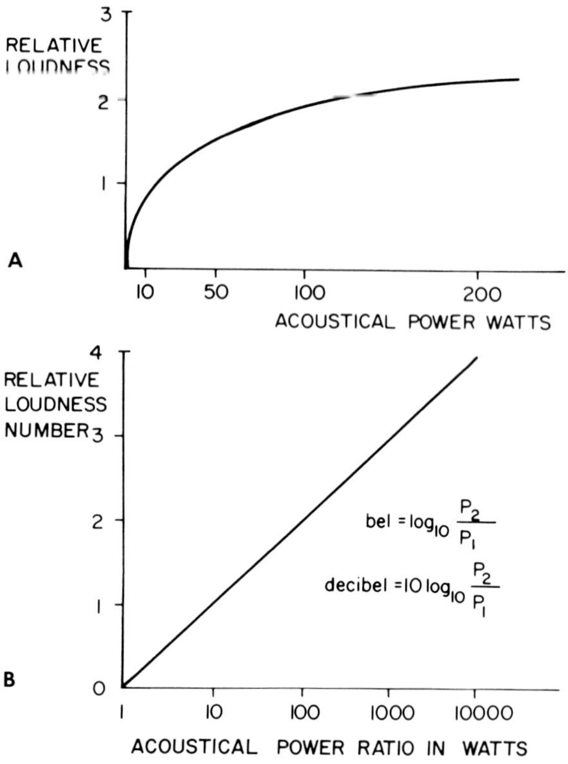

Fig. 2-3. Decibel notation is used to describe the wide range of sound field intensities that are encountered in the biologic applications of ultrasound.

The relative loudness number is equal to the $\log_{10}$ of the acoustic power ratio.

The unit of loudness in the example is the bel. It turns out to be an inconveniently large unit for most applications, so a smaller unit called the decibel (dB) was defined; it is given by

$$\text{Decibel} = 10 \log_{10} \frac{P_2}{P_1}$$

In ultrasonics and also in electronics, measurements in units of power (acoustic watts or electric watts) are not that convenient, so still another form of this definition was derived and is in common use.

Since electric power is defined as:

$$P = \frac{E^2}{R}$$

TABLE 1. The wide dynamic range of the decibel notation

RATIO	LOG OF RATIO	DECIBEL FOR POWER RATIO	DECIBEL FOR CURRENT OR VOLTAGE RATIO
1	0	0	0
10	1	10	20
100	2	20	40
1,000	3	30	60
10,000	4	40	80
100,000	5	50	100
1,000,000	6	60	120

we can substitute this form in the decibel equation:

$$dB = 10 \log \frac{\frac{E_2^2}{R}}{\frac{E_1^2}{R}}$$

With further manipulation and assuming that the resistance is a constant before and after the electric power level change will give:

$$dB = 10 \log \frac{E_2^2}{E_1^2}$$

or

$$dB = 20 \log \frac{E_2}{E_1}$$

In ultrasonics E_1 and E_2 can be the excitation voltage applied to a transducer or the output voltage from a receiving transducer. Both E_1 and E_2 are proportional to the sound intensity I.

A handy chart is shown in Table 1, with common ratios and the decibel power and decibel voltage values.

SOURCES OF ECHOES

Sudden changes in the acoustic properties of tissue occurring at boundaries of organs and at other interfaces are the source of echoes used for developing images of tissue structure. The principal acoustic property of the tissue, called acoustic impedance, can change very

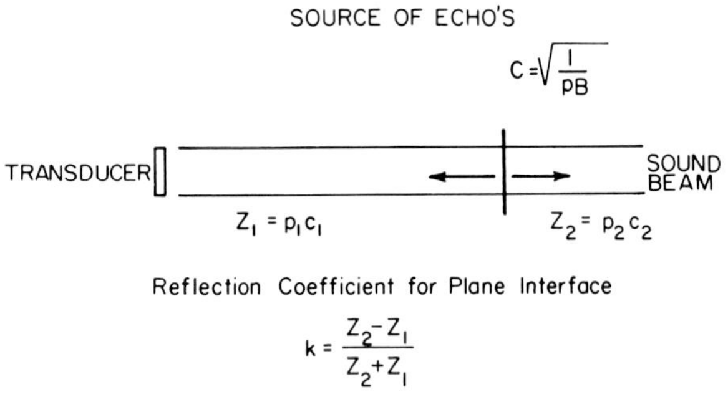

Fig. 2-4. Echoes are produced at boundaries between tissues of different acoustic properties.

abruptly at some interfaces and very gradually at others. The impedance *(z)* of a typical sample of tissue can be defined as the product of the density (ρ) times the velocity of sound in that sample *(c)*.

$$z = \rho c$$

An acoustic interface might occur at the juncture of the vessel wall and the blood. The echo amplitude at this interface will be proportional to the change in the impedance as the sound pulse passes from one tissue to the next. These concepts may be more clearly understood by referring to Fig. 2-4. In the figure the sound beam is depicted as a tube or cylinder of sound in the direction that the transducer is pointing. The sound beam intercepts an interface such that the impedance proximal to the interface is defined as $\rho_1 c_1$. The impedance distal to the interface is $\rho_2 c_2$. A reflection coefficient *(k)*, can be defined for the interface.

$$k = \frac{Z_2 - Z_1}{Z_2 + Z_1}$$

Since $\Delta Z = Z_2 - Z_1$ is small:

$$k \approx \frac{\Delta Z}{2Z}$$

$$\text{Reflection loss (dB)} = -20 \log_{10} k$$

Examples of reflection losses for different interfaces are:

Muscle-blood	−38 to −44 dB or 1%
Fat-muscle	−26 to −30 dB or 15%
Tissue-bone	−3 to −6 dB or 50% to 70%

At any interface a certain portion of the energy is reflected and the remaining energy passes through the interface and on through the tissue to the next interface. In the example of the muscle-blood interface, 1% of the impinging energy is reflected back toward the transmitting transducer and 99% of the energy passes on through. In the case of the tissue-bone interface, 50% to 70% of the impinging energy is reflected back to the transducer and only 30% to 50% actually passes through. This last example explains why it is difficult to pass the sound beam through bone. The amount of reflection that occurs at the bone interface is dependent among other things on the age of the subject. Sound will pass through the bones of young children up to the age 6 to 10 very readily; the amount of attenuation increases rapidly after that age.

The shape of an echo from a particular interface will depend on how abruptly the acoustic impedance changes, the orientation of the sound beam to the interface, whether it is a smooth or a rough and irregular interface, and whether the interface is near or far from the transducer. The smoother the interface, the more the magnitude of the reflection will depend on the angle between the interface and the sound beam. Maximum reflections will occur when the interface is 90 degrees to the beam. As the interface takes on a more irregular or roughened shape, the angular dependence will decrease. Thus echoes received from interfaces that are in the far field of the transducer will have a specular characteristic. If the smooth interface is positioned in the near field of the transducer, it may produce echoes as if it were irregular or roughened because of the irregular intensity pattern of the near field. Because the sound beam may not be spatially coherent (disk-like plane waves) along its full length, it can be difficult to interpret the degree of specularity on the basis of the echo pattern as a function of the angle between the beam and the interface. Fig. 2-5, *A*, shows how the specular reflection characteristics of ultrasound resemble those of coherent laser light. From Snell's law, the angle of incidence is equal to the angle of reflectance. In Fig. 2-5, *B*, one can see the effect of this specular reflection characteristic when the sound beam is pointed in the direction of a blood vessel. The maximum echo return will be from the outer near wall and the inner far wall. The best way to completely image a vessel cross-section is to move the transducer back and forth to develop as many echoes from the vessel wall interfaces as possible when the beam is normal to it. This procedure for moving the transducer in a sector scan as well as moving it back and forth in an arc is called compound scanning. It is a basic characteristic type of motion required in all pulse echo imaging.

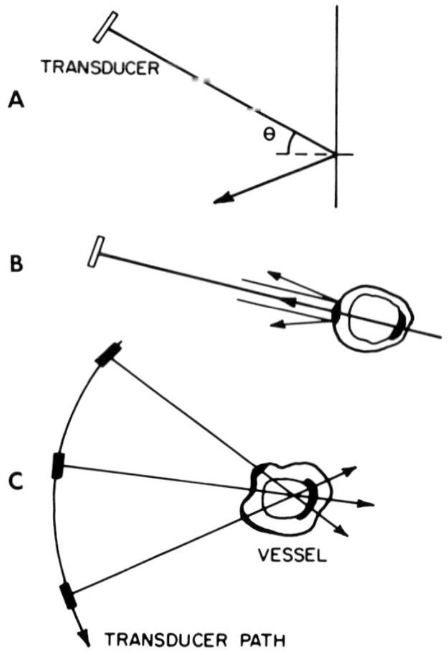

Fig. 2-5. The image of a blood vessel cross-section is a good example of the specular reflection characteristics of ultrasound.

SCATTERING

The next most important interaction between the sound beam and the tissue and blood is the mechanism of scattering. This phenomenon is used primarily in Doppler devices. Acoustic scattering is much like optic scattering, and the analogous effect is easily observed by passing a light beam through a cloud of smoke or fog. The backscattered light from the particles in the air makes the light beam visible. The forward scattering from the light beam causes the cloud to glow as well as to defocus the narrow beam of the light. Similar effects occur when ultrasound is passed through blood. The primary scatterer in the body is the red blood cell, which has a dimension of about 8 to 10 μ. This compares to wavelengths as short as 100 μ at 15 MHz to as long as 750 μ at 2 MHz. Scattering under these circumstances is referred to as "Rayleigh-like" because the wavelength-to-particle size ratio is large. The effect of this type of scattering is that each red cell will absorb a certain amount of ultrasonic energy and reradiate it to all directions. Aggregates of cells as they would occur in blood flow have this same property. This means that a vessel can be sonically irradiated by a transmitting beam and that the resulting scattering can be detected from any angle as long as the receiving beam is pointing at the scattering region.

In an echo system, if an interface is highly irregular and the irregularities are of small dimensions, the interface can tend to act as a scatterer. Because many of the interfaces that are encountered in biologic tissue have irregular and diffused surfaces, there is a gray area of understanding between reflection and scattering. This fact is demonstrated by Doppler devices that are able to pick up "Doppler" signals from moving interfaces, even though the interface may not be normal to the beam, for example, heart valves. As they move through the sound beam, scattering will occur that can be detected as a Doppler shifted signal because of the velocity of the valve leaflet. These same reflections or scattered signals would not produce an image in a conventional pulse echo system. However, they would produce signals in a Doppler system. This will be discussed in more detail later.

TRANSDUCERS

A transducing element is required to convert electric signals to acoustic signals and vice versa. The most common transducers are fabricated of manmade ceramic materials that have been processed to have piezoelectric characteristics. The piezoelectric characteristic means that when a voltage is supplied to the transducer element it will either compress or expand according to the polarity of the potential. Conversely, when the material is compressed or expanded, a potential will be developed according to the magnitude and direction of the deformation. While the details of piezoelectricity are rather complex, simple models can be used to convey an understanding of the operation of the transducers.

From elementary physics we know that like charges will repel and unlike charges will attract. The magnitude of the force of attraction or repulsion is proportional to the product of the charges *(Q)* divided by the square of the distance between them. Positive and negative charges coupled together and spaced a certain distance apart are called dipoles. Dipoles can occur naturally in quartz crystals, which are piezoelectric, and can be formed in manmade ceramic materials, for example, lead zirconate titanate. When a charge of polarity opposite to that at one end of the dipole is brought near, an attraction causing a turning or torquing moment will be induced into the dipole (Fig. 2-6, *A*).

In the ceramic material of the transducer one can model a series of dipoles as shown in Fig. 2-6, *B*. The actual alignment of these dipoles depends on the specific crystal lattice structure. In the model they are shown lined up in the same direction. On the surfaces of the ceramic material are applied electrodes. When an electric charge is applied to the electrodes from an external voltage source, a force will be exerted on the dipoles according to the charge. In the example with the plus charges on the right and the negative charges on the left, the dipoles will be forced to rotate in a counterclockwise direction. The displacement will be extremely small. However, the result of the displacement will be to cause the ceramic material to expand to the right and left in

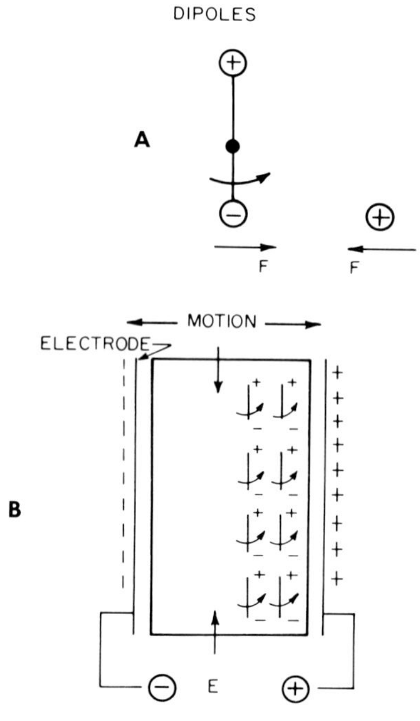

Fig. 2-6. A piezoelectric crystal is composed of electric dipoles. The external electric field causes a movement of the dipoles and corresponding change in dimension of material.

the example. The length of the sample will shorten at the same time. If the charges are reversed, there will be a compression of the material and a lengthening along the other axis. Conversely, in a reciprocal fashion, when the material is compressed, the dipoles will be displaced an amount sufficient to produce a charge on the surface of the material at the electrodes that can be detected and amplified. When an alternating charge is applied to the electrodes, the material will alternately compress and expand according to the frequency of the applied voltage.

Ceramic materials have other important characteristics in addition to their piezoelectric properties. Three examples will be used: quartz, barium titanate, and lead zirconate titanate. Each of these, when fabricated into a transducer, exhibits the properties of an electric capacitor. The magnitude of the capacitance in microfarads is proportional to the dielectric constant of the material times the area of the material divided by its thickness. Its construction is similar to a capacitor in that the electrodes on each side of the material are separated by a space occupied by the ceramic material. The size and spacing between the planes of the electrodes determine the area and the thickness of the transducer. The dielectric constant is determined from the electric properties of the ceramic material itself. Table 2 shows some other properties of the ceramic elements.

It is important to understand the meaning of Curie temperature related to the manufacture and use of transducers. First, heat is never used to sterilize these trans-

TABLE 2. Characteristics of several ceramic elements

MATERIAL	CURIE TEMPERATURE	Q	DIELECTRIC CONSTANT (K)	COUPLING COEFFICIENT (KT)
Quartz	550° C	Very high	4.5	0.09
Barium titanate	100° C	400-700	1,700	0.38
Lead zirconate titanate	300° C	90-500	1,450	0.51

ducers, for if it were, it would certainly destroy many of them. In order to polarize and make piezoelectric a man-made ceramic material, it is necessary to heat the element above a certain temperature, called the Curie temperature. Once this temperature has been reached and exceeded, an electric potential of a specific value is applied to the electrodes. The high temperature permits the dipoles to move freely, and they will align themselves in the electric field produced by the electrodes. The material is then cooled to room temperature while maintaining the high voltage, and as a result, when the voltage is removed, it will have piezoelectric or polarized characteristics. If the piece of ceramic material is heated back up to the Curie temperature, the polarized characteristics will relax and the material will simply become a piece of ceramic without piezoelectric properties.

Obviously, heat will damage the transducer, particularly if it exceeds the Curie temperature. The dielectric constant *(K)* is shown in Table 2 for the three materials. Notice the difference between them. The coupling coefficient (KT) is important because it indicates how much of the electric energy can be converted to acoustic energy in the ideal transducer. Both barium titanate and lead zirconate titanate are approximately five to six times more efficient than quartz. Because of the very low dielectric constant of quartz and its low coupling constant, it is seldom used for ultrasonic transducers in modern equipment.

Transducer frequency characteristics

A transducer can be made to vibrate or ring at a certain frequency and in a manner much like that of the cymbals used in the symphony orchestra when they are struck by a hammer. The frequency at which the transducer rings depends on its mechanical properties and its shape. For example, a flat bar of ceramic material can have three different resonant frequencies. It can have one frequency in the thickness mode when it compresses and expands; it can have another resonance in the length mode as it lengthens and shortens; and it can have still another in the width mode. If the piece of material is a disk, it can have a thickness and a radial mode when the diameter of the disk becomes larger and smaller. A transducer can be excited by sinusoidal voltages applied to appropriate electrodes to cause it to vibrate in any of these modes. When this occurs, a small portion of the electric energy is coupled into the other modes so that the crystal will actually vibrate in the principal mode on which it is being driven and at the same time vibrate in the other modes.

The manufacturers of these ceramic materials provide what is called a frequency constant for each mode of vibration. This constant can be used in a formula along with the dimensions of the element for that mode to calculate what the natural vibration frequency will be. In ultrasonic transducers for medical applications we are primarily concerned with the thickness mode. For barium titanate the resonant frequency is equal to a constant equal to 101 divided by the thickness *(T)* when measured in inches. The same equation for lead zirconate titanate is equal to 78 divided by the thickness *(T)* in inches. These two equations tell us that barium titanate will be thicker for the same resonant frequency than the lead zirconate titanate.

When a fast rise time electric transient is applied to either of these materials, they will tend to ring or vibrate at this frequency. The magnitude of the vibration will gradually decay away to zero in a damped manner. If a sinusoidal voltage is applied to the element, it can be caused to vibrate at frequencies other than the resonant frequency, but at lower amplitude. As the driving frequency approaches the natural resonant frequency, the magnitude of the excursion will continue to increase until internal limiting factors such as friction and heat loss restrict the amplitude of the vibration. If these internal friction losses did not exist, the crystal would literally fracture and blow apart. This would be analogous to the sympathetic vibration that can be induced into crystal glassware by high frequency pure tones that may cause them to fracture.

Transducer Q

The vibration in every ceramic material is to some extent dependent upon how it is mounted or damped. This effect is observed by shock exciting the crystal with a voltage spike and watching the ringing reduce slowly to zero. This occurs since for each cycle of vibration of the crystal—compression and expansion—a certain amount of the energy in the crystal is lost because of heat. The more energy that is lost per cycle, the sooner the vibration will dampen out. This characteristic is sometimes described as the *Q* of the transducer. When defined this way, the *Q* is equal to the ratio of the energy stored to the energy lost per cycle of vibration. A high *Q* transducer would lose very little energy from internal losses per cycle and would ring for a long time. A low *Q* transducer would dissipate a lot of energy per cycle and the vibrations would dampen out very quickly. The duration or length of the shock-excited acoustic pulse that can be generated by the transducer element will be determined by the *Q* of the transducer. This will ultimately determine the resolution of the ultrasonic echo-ranging system. The *Q* may be defined in another way. The equation is:

$$Q = \frac{f_0}{\Delta f}$$

where

f_0 = natural resonant frequency of the ceramic material
Δf = 3-dB bandwidth of the crystal

Fig. 2-7 shows a plot of the relative acoustic output versus frequency for a low and a high *Q* material. The high *Q* material will vibrate only over a very narrow band of frequencies, whereas the low *Q* material will vibrate over a wide band of frequency. To determine the 3-dB bandwidth, the peak magnitude of this vibration or output is given the 0-dB reference and then, following the curve down until the −3-dB point on each side of the 0-dB peak is reached, the span Δf of the frequency between the points is noted. The *Q* can then be computed according to the formula. The *Q* value for some typical materials, unmounted, are given in the following list:

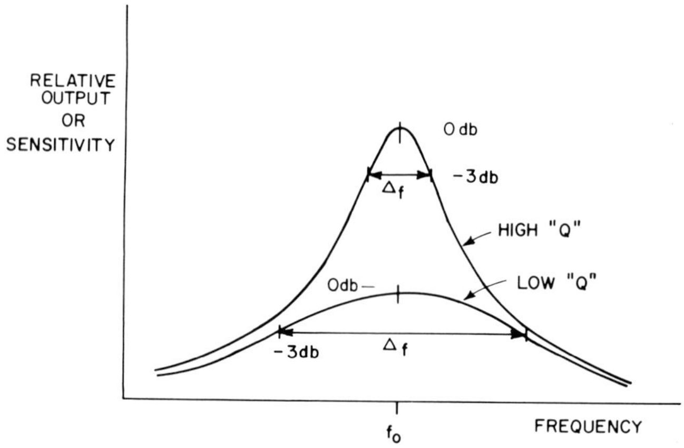

Fig. 2-7. The transducer Q affects its bandwidth and damping characteristics.

Barium titanate $Q \approx 400$ to 750
Lead zirconate titanate, type 5 $Q \approx 500$
Lead zirconate titanate, type 2 or 4 $Q \approx 70$-90

The high Q materials are the most efficient for generating acoustic signals, but they are limited because of their narrow bandwidth. The low Q materials are more efficient as receivers and have a wide bandwidth. Generally the same ceramic element is used for transmitter and receiver, since the bandwidth is the deciding factor.

Vibration modes

Piezoelectric ceramic elements can be manufactured to oscillate in a variety of modes. The compression or thickness mode is most frequently used in ultrasonic instruments; however, any ceramic element is capable of vibrating in other modes. Fig. 2-8 shows a variety of transducer configurations that are all being excited in the same direction of polarization. When electric energy is coupled into the ceramic element in the direction of primary polarization, small amounts of energy are always coupled into the other modes of vibration.

In Fig. 2-8 are shown different configurations of ceramic elements, their corresponding natural resonance equations, and the calculations of resonance for some typical dimensions. Generally, some small component of all of these modes is present in every piece of ceramic material. The instrument is designed to excite the crystal in a primary mode, and the receiving amplifiers are tuned only in the frequency band of the primary mode. The type of mechanical mounting, and thus the damping or Q of the transducer, will also determine the extent and presence of other modes.

Transducers that are fabricated so that the ceramic element has an air backing have the greatest number of modes of vibration. Air-back transducers are used primarily for continuous wave Doppler

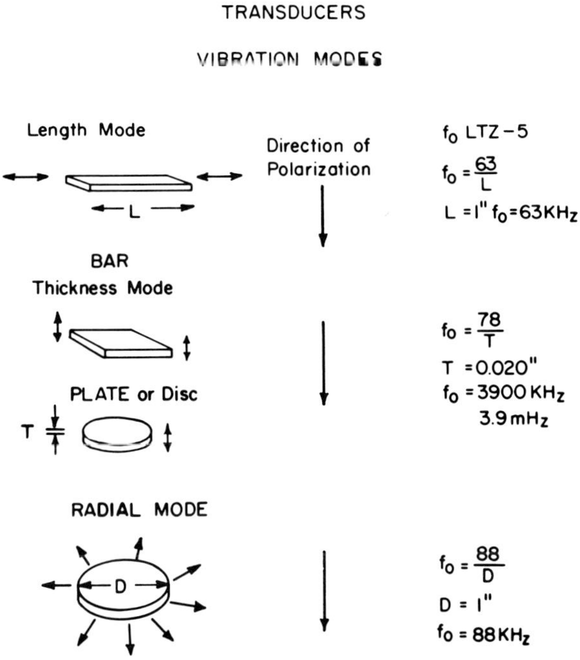

Fig. 2-8. Ceramic crystal elements can be driven to vibrate in a variety of modes.

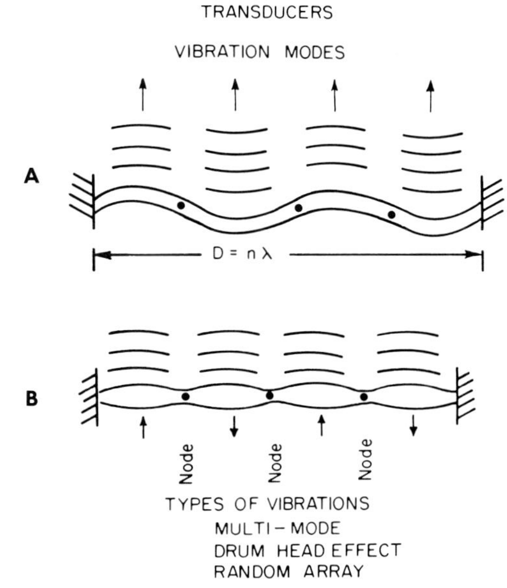

Fig. 2-9. Thin plate-like transducers usually vibrate in a compression mode as in **B**. Other modes are possible, however, as shown in **A**.

devices and for high sensitivity pulse Doppler devices.

Fig. 2-9 shows a cross-section view of the edge of a thin plate of ceramic material intended to be vibrating in the thickness mode. Depending on the thickness of the ceramic material, other modes may be excited as shown. Since the nature of the vibration mode depends on the mounting of the transducer, it is not always easy to predict which will be the typical mode. The example in Fig. 2-9, *B*, is the most likely situation, with regions of adjacent compression and expansion separated by nodes.

Sound field generation

The sound beam from a typical transducer can be divided into two components: the near field, or Fresnel region, and the far field, called the Fraunhofer region. A detailed investigation of the formation of the sound field will give greater insight into the difference between these two regions. In Fig. 2-10, *A*, we see a model of an ideal transducer consisting of a line of five point sources. As these waves progress outward from the source, we find that the points of maximum value of the sound fields add along a certain direction. This principle of addition, or superposition, is called Huygens' principle. We can see from the example that the beam is the result of the superposition of the sound field from the various vibrating regions or elements of the transducer. Restated, the line of sources adds in phase to produce coherent waves moving in a direction nor-

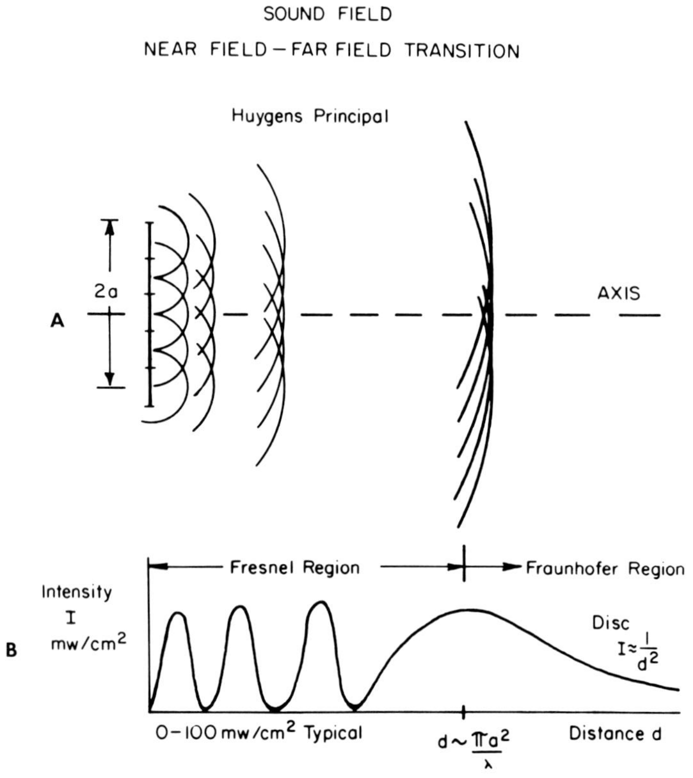

Fig. 2-10. The processes involved in generating the sound field beam are easily modeled using a series of point sources for the transducer and applying the Huygens principle of superposition.

mal to the surface of the transducer. The resulting beam projects outward in both directions from both the front and the back faces. The energy from the back face is usually coupled to a damping material or air space and is lost.

The sound field intensity pattern in the near field is quite different from that in the far field. If a test probe is moved along the axis of the beam from the face of the ceramic element outward, we can find large variations in amplitude that oscillate between peak values and zero. At some point along the beam, as set by the wavelength and the diameter of the elements, we will reach the point of the last maximum in these variations. From this point on, the sound field intensity will decrease at a rate governed by the inverse square law. The transition point between near and far fields is approximately at the point of the last maxima, shown in Fig. 2-10, *B*. Fig. 2-11 shows a photograph of the sound field from a flat transducer. It illustrates the transition from near field to far field. By following a line along the axis of the transducer and observing the brightness of the photograph, one gets the impression of the variations in sound field intensity. Fig. 2-12 shows a chart that can be used to determine the transition point between near and far field for a transducer if the diameter of the element and the transmitting frequency are known.

Beam shaping and focusing

As ultrasonic techniques become more sophisticated, there is an increasing need for transducers that have narrow collimated sound beams. The narrow beam permits more precise aiming of the transducer when detecting small interfaces. It also will increase the sensitivity in the focal region compared to a standard transducer. Simply reducing the size of the transducer element for a given frequency does not in itself produce a narrow collimated beam over a wide range of depths. In fact, the smaller the transducer, the more divergent the beam becomes. One of the best methods for shaping the beam into a narrow diameter to minimize the divergence effects is to affix to the face of the element a plastic lens of the correct curvature to produce a focusing effect at the desired depth. These lenses are usually molded in place to have a spherical focus. The focal point is approximately at the diameter of the

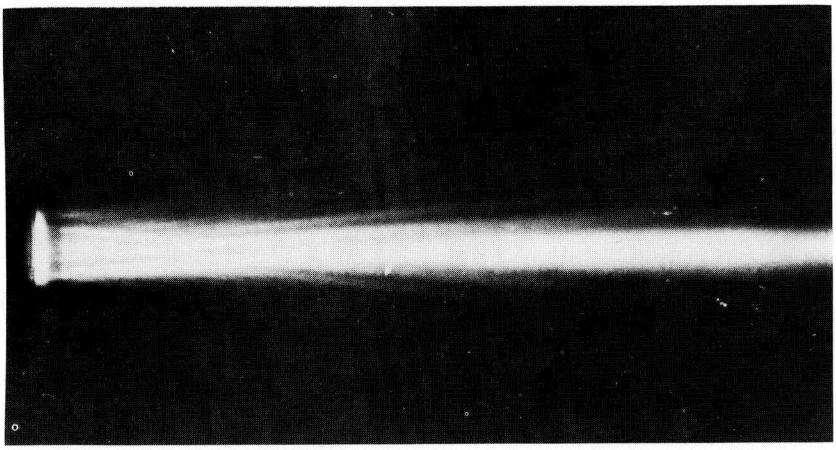

Fig. 2-11. The ray-like characteristics of the near field or Fresnel region are apparent in the schlieren photograph. The smooth characteristics of the far field, the Fraunhofer region, are also readily apparent.

curvature of the lens face. The net effect of the lens is to move the transition point between near and far fields closer to the transducer face and to reduce the beam width accordingly. Fig. 2-13 shows a Schlieren photograph of a focused transducer. Because the lens produces a more directive beam, the user will find that these transducers are sometimes more difficult to aim because of their extreme angle

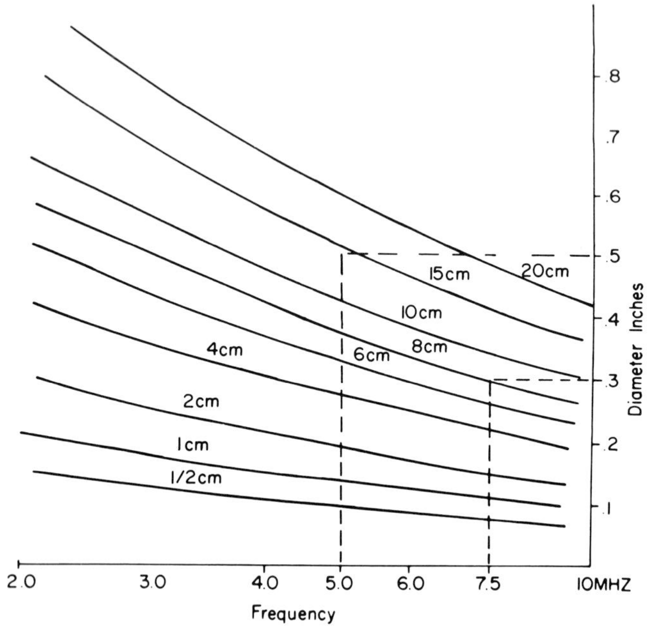

Fig. 2-12. The transition point between the near and the far field for a variety of transducer diameters and operating frequencies is easily determined.

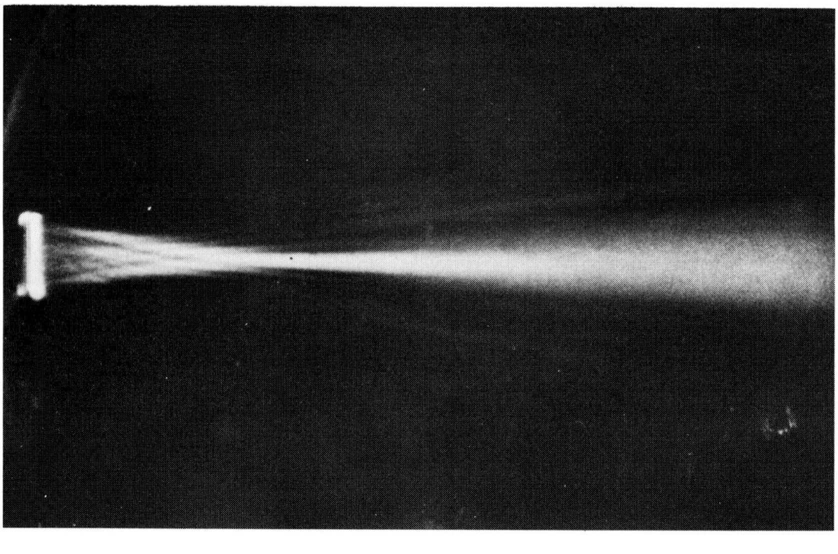

Fig. 2-13. Plastic lenses can be affixed to the front face of the transducer in order to focus the beam down to a narrow cross-section.

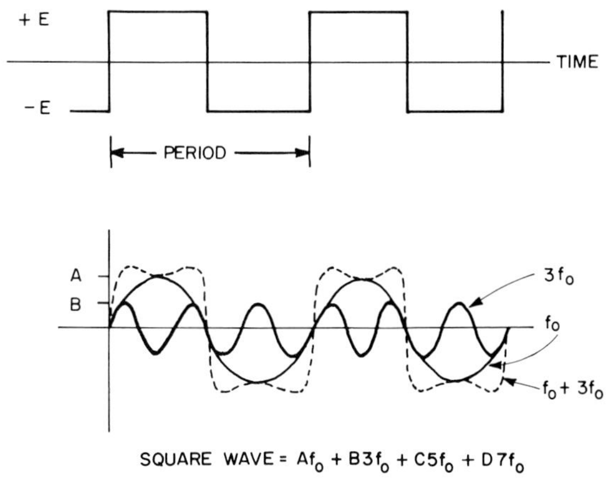

Fig. 2-14. Simple Fourier analysis concepts are easily understood by adding sine waves together to form square waves.

sensitivity. Focused transducers also have characteristics similar to those for optic lens systems. That is, there is a certain narrow focused region that has a depth of field analogous to that in cameras. The sensitivity is maximum within this region, falling off in the near field and the far field. The beam width also increases outside this region, as can be observed in the figures.

RESOLUTION AND BANDWIDTH

The resolution of a pulse echo ultrasound system depends on the bandwidth of the overall system. In order to understand the relationship between resolution and bandwidth, it is necessary to have an idea of the concepts of Fourier analysis. Many of the signals in the electronics of the ultrasonic instrument exist in the form of voltage, or current pulses that repeat at the pulse repetition frequency. These pulses can be displayed on the screen of an oscilloscope and observed. When shown in this manner, they are depicted as voltage fluctuations or variations as a function of time. That is, the voltage of the pulse varies in a very definite manner as time goes on. This type of observation is sometimes referred to as being in the time domain.

Another approach to understanding these pulses is to observe their equivalent frequency characteristics. For example, the pulse repetition frequency of a pulse echo system might be 1,000 pulses per second; however, the pulses are very short—they are not simple sine waves. Instead, they are made up of many related frequencies or harmonics. There are mathematic techniques for decomposing these pulses into all of the frequency components required to reproduce them. A graphic example of these components is shown in Fig. 2-14 for a square wave. A square wave form is one in which the voltage is on for the same amount of time it is off. It has a square appearance when shown on the cathode ray tube display. The figure shows a square wave being built up from the fundamental frequency and its first harmonic.

The lowest frequency is called the fundamental frequency and corresponds to the pulse repetition frequency of the pulse. Multiples of the fundamental frequencies are added together to reconstruct a wave form identical to the pulse. Thinking in terms of fundamentals and harmonics, as required to represent these signals, is to consider them in their frequency domain. The pulses that exist in ultrasonic equipment are generally not square waves but waves that are "on" for a very brief period of time and "off" for some long time. For example, a pulse might be on for 1 μsec and off for 1,000 μsec. The pulse repetition frequency of such a pulse would be 1 divided by the interval between the pulses, which is 1/1,000 μsec. This is equal to a repetition frequency of 1,000 pulses per second. The fundamental frequency would be 1,000. However, since the pulse is extremely short, most of the energy in the frequency spectrum will be centered around a frequency corresponding to the number 1 divided by the duration of the pulse. If the pulse has a duration of 1 μsec (1×10^{-6} second), this corresponds to a frequency of 1 MHz. Therefore, the spectrum to represent this kind of pulse will have frequencies extending from 1,000 Hz (cycles) to a megahertz and higher. The amplitude of the low-frequency components in this case would be low, while those of the high-frequency terms, 1 MHz and above, will be higher. The crystal will be caused to oscillate at its natural or fundamental frequency, when it is excited by a very short, high-voltage spike, of 1 μsec or less in duration. The duration of the resulting burst will depend on the damping characteristics of the transducer. Thus only a few cycles may actually be propagated.

In order to appreciate the bandwidth of these short bursts, or spikes, we must refer to our Fourier analysis. A feeling for the frequencies that exist in a short burst of ultrasound can be arrived at by referring to Fig. 2-15. We will assume that we are going to transmit a short burst of sine waves, 1 or 2 cycles. The generation of this burst can be represented by multiplying an ideal gate (rectangular pulse) shown on the top line with a continuous sine wave on the next line. The ideal gate has a value of 0 up until the instant it assumes the value of 1. It has a duration of τ, which might be equal to 1 μsec, and then it returns to 0. The product of these two waves will be 0 except for the time interval τ in which the ideal gate has a value of 1. The third line shows the output. From the Fourier or frequency domain point of view, the sine wave contains only one frequency while the gate waveform contains all of the Fourier harmonics required to reproduce its shape. For a 1 μsec pulse there would be frequencies of 1 MHz or higher, plus low-frequency components in the pulse repetition rate range. Therefore, to pass the gated burst, it would be necessary to

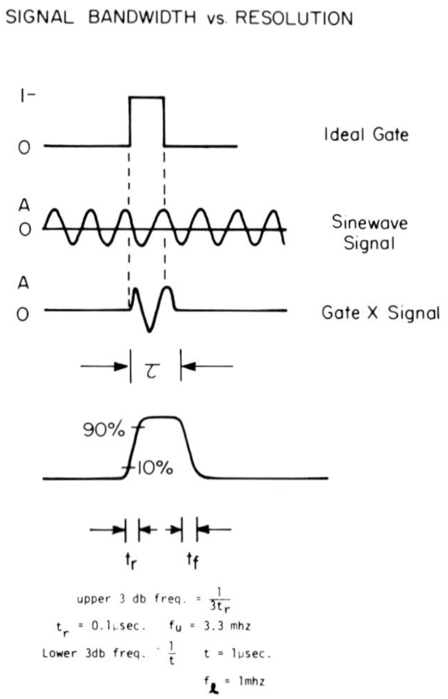

Fig. 2-15. The frequency spectrum of a short sinusoidal burst can be analyzed by considering the spectrum of the two waves that, when multiplied together, produce the burst.

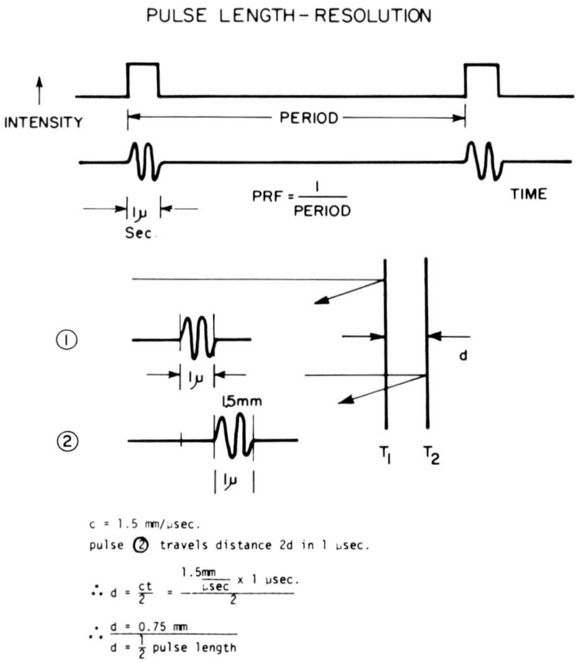

Fig. 2-16. The ability to resolve two closely spaced parallel interfaces is determined by the duration of the transmitted burst length.

amplify or transmit all frequencies present, including the sine wave signal. When such a signal is applied to the transmitting element, it will pass only those frequencies that are within its passband. The passband is determined by its Q—that is, the higher the Q, the narrower the passband; the lower the Q, the wider the passband. So to transmit short pulses it is necessary to have transducers of low Q and wide bandwidth.

After developing the capability to transmit very short pulses, it is necessary to determine how closely two parallel interfaces can be spaced and still be detected. Fig. 2-16 shows the derivation of the range resolution specifications. We will assume that ideal short bursts at 2.25 MHz are transmitted at a certain repetition rate. In the example shown, the bursts are 1 μsec in duration. The spacing between each burst is of no consequence when discussing resolution. When a pulse of 1 μsec is propagated through a fluid medium, it will form an acoustic packet whose length can be computed if we know the velocity of sound in that medium. Since sound travels at approximately 1.5 mm/μsec in tissue, pulses 1 μsec long will be 1.5 mm in length.

The simple way to evaluate the resolution is to consider two interfaces, $T1$ and $T2$, that are spaced by a distance, d. Echoes will be received from $T1$, shown as ①, and from $T2$, shown as ②. As d is decreased, the echo from $T2$ will move closer to the end of the echo from $T1$. When the leading edge of echo ② just touches the trailing edge of echo ①, d is at its smallest valve without the echoes overlapping. When this situation occurs d corresponds to 1 μsec, or 1.5 mm. Pulse ② travels through a distance $2d$ to $T2$ and back and will have traveled 1.5 mm. The spacing of the two interfaces is then 0.75 mm. The optimal resolution for a system transmitting 1-μsec long pulses is therefore demonstrated to be half the transmitted burst length. Since the actual real instrument is unable to transmit these ideal rectangular bursts, we find that in general as the bandwidth decreases, the transmitted pulses are degraded (stretched) and the resolution is decreased.

Fig. 2-17 shows the echo envelopes that might be received from four different but parallel interfaces using a range of bandwidths or Q's. As the Q of the transducer is increased, the echo pattern will run together as shown until echoes from nearby interfaces are smoothed together. In general, any loss of resolution in a pulse echo system can be resolved in terms of the decrease in bandwidth of either the transmitted signal, the transmitting element, the receiving element, or the receiving amplifier.

BASIC ECHO SYSTEM

The simplest pulse echo system is very much like a simple radar. The depth or

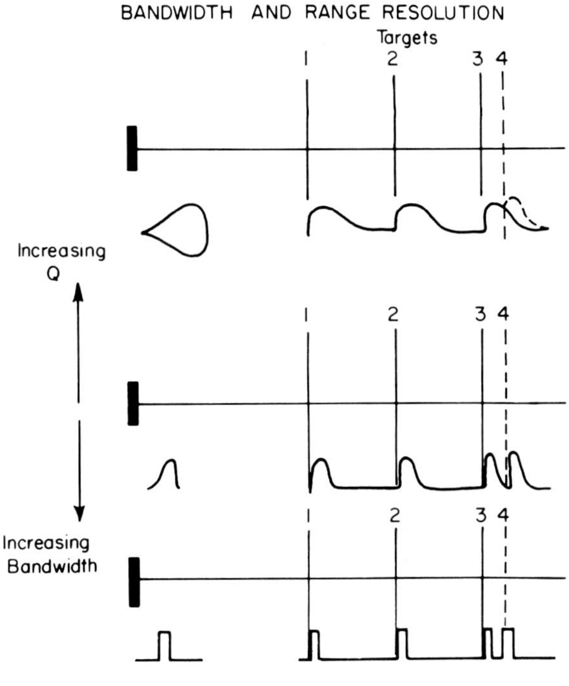

Fig. 2-17. The resolution of a pulse-echo system is dependent on the bandwidth of the transducers and receiving amplifiers.

range of an interface can be determined by measuring the round trip transit time of an acoustic pulse from the transmitter to the interface and return to the receiver. One of the simplest ways to measure the transit time electronically is to use the face of a cathode ray tube (CRT) as the indicator for the received echo. A line or trace is displayed on the cathode ray tube so that the left end corresponds to the emission time of the transmitted burst. The trace, which is formed by a spot moving rapidly to the right, can be calibrated to indicate the depth by knowing the spot velocity in centimeters per microsecond. From the velocity of sound in the medium, it is possible to calculate a range constant (microseconds per centimeter of depth). The range constant is in turn multiplied by the trace velocity to give the depth calibration in centimeters per centimeter of cathode ray tube deflection. The received echo is amplified and used to deflect the cathode ray tube trace. The time interval from the trace beginning to the deflection pip corresponds to depth.

A block diagram of the essential components of the basic pulse echo device is shown in Fig. 2-18. Among these is an oscillator that establishes the pulse repetition frequency and a linear power amplifier, or spike generator, that excites the transmitting element through a decoupling circuit. The decoupler permits the trans-

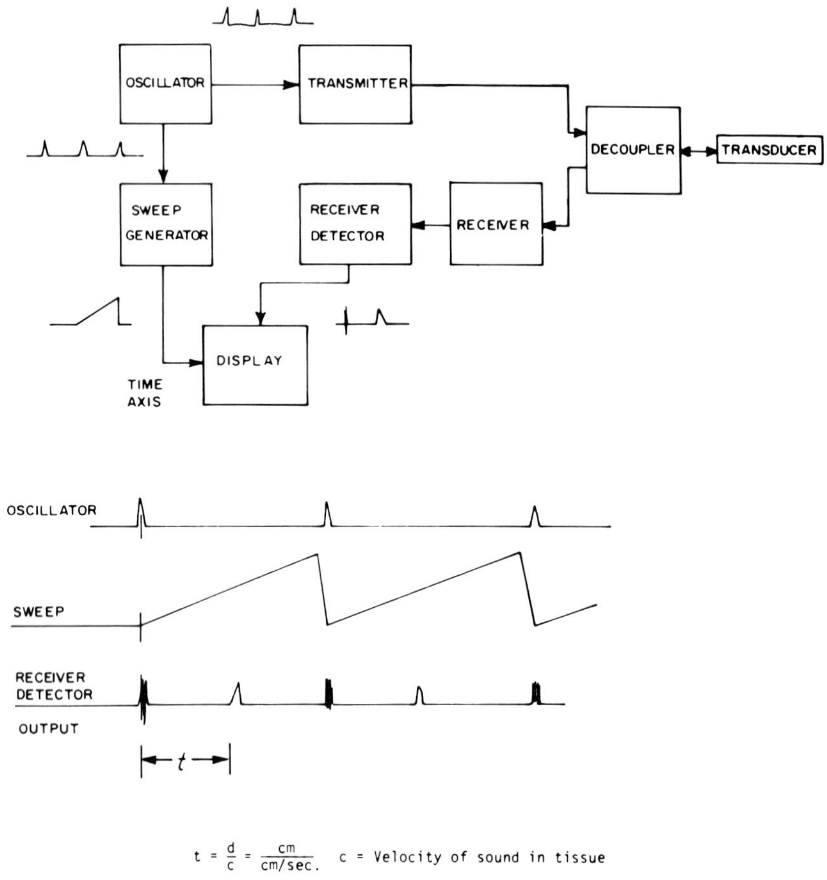

Fig. 2-18. Basic pulse-echo system.

ducer to be used both as transmitter and as receiver. The oscillator also triggers a time base sweep generator that is used to produce the time base trace on the cathode ray tube display.

Line 2 of the wave form shows the time base sweep. It is calibrated to move the trace across the face of the oscilloscope at a fixed rate. The received pulses are sent via the decoupler into the receiving amplifier for amplification and detection, and then they are presented on the display. The cathode ray tube beam is deflected in the Y direction at an instant τ corresponding to the transit time from the transducer face out to the interface and back.

Line 3 of the illustration shows the A-scan presentation of a single echo for each sweep. From the velocity of sound in tissue it is possible to calculate the range calibration coefficient, which is approximately 13.2 μsec/cm in depth. The cathode ray tube display on the unit is calibrated in units of depth by controlling the slope (volts per second) of the sweep generator. For example, if the display has ten 1 cm graduations across the face of the scope, then the sweep can be calibrated so that every centimeter on the scope face corresponds to 13.5 μsec. The slope of the sweep is adjusted so that the spot is moved 1 cm in 13 μsec.

The pulse repetition frequency (PRF) of the system is usually based on several criteria. The minimum pulse repetition frequency that can be used is determined by the velocity of the interfaces. If, for example, it were necessary to determine the velocity of the mitral valve, it is possible to use Fourier concepts to determine the minimum necessary sample or pulse repetition frequency (PRF). Plotting the mitral valve displacement versus time will give a waveform that is a function of time. A Fourier analysis of the resulting function determines the highest frequency component of the spectrum. It could typically be on the order of 100 Hz. Basic sampling theory states that in order to accurately measure this type of signal, the sample rate, in this case the PRF, must be twice the highest frequency present. Therefore, if the highest frequency present is 100 Hz, then the PRF or sample rate must be 200 Hz.

The upper limit of the PRF is determined by the decay time of natural reverberation echoes that occur within the body and the maximum tissue depth of interest. For example, at a depth of 20 cm, based on 13.5 μsec/cm of depth, the period of the PRF would be 264 μsec. This corresponds to a PRF of 3,787 Hz. Such a high repetition frequency cannot be used for this depth because of the multiple interfaces that exist in the path of the beam. The acoustic pulses will reverberate between these various interfaces such that echoes would be received during a given PRF period that may actually have been generated during the previous period. This causes confusion and ambiguity in interpreting the echo pattern. To ensure that this problem does not occur, the actual PRF chosen is usually somewhere between 1,000 and 2,000 Hz. At these PRF rates the cathode ray tube will also provide a bright display, whereas if a lower PRF rate were used the display would be somewhat dim even though all the echo information is present.

FUNCTION OF INSTRUMENT CONTROLS

The pulse echo instrument is the principal interface between the operator and the patient. The process of locating, detecting, and evaluating echo patterns depends on a close interaction between the operator, the equipment, and the subject. The positioning of the transducer is based on the display results that the operator can observe and interpret. The signals that appear on the display depend upon the settings of the various controls on the instrument, as well as on the direction in which the transducer is pointed. The decisions to move the transducer are based on these interactive judgments. The basic pulse echo system can be expanded to a slightly more detailed block diagram shown in Fig. 2-19. The control functions indicated in various blocks are the principal knob adjustments that the operator will use to modify the display.

Signals detected from the transducer are amplified in the receiver, detected, amplified further by the video amplifier, and then presented to the cathode ray tube display. Almost all of the controls with which the operator is concerned have to do with this amplifying and detecting sequence. The first of these is the receiver and time-compensated gain functions. The receiver is used to amplify weak echoes up to the point at which they will be displayed. This amplifier must be capable of compensating for the attenuation of the echo, which becomes more pronounced with increasing depth. The compensation is accomplished with a time-compensated gain unit coupled to the receiving amplifier. Without compensation, the echoes will fall in amplitude, as shown in Fig. 2-20. The rate of falloff of the echo amplitude depends on the transmitted frequency, attenuation characteristics of the tissue, and transducer design, that is, focused versus nonfocused.

Basically, the time-compensated gain unit is designed to increase the echo amplitude for increasing depths in an amount offseting the depth dependent attenuation. The result is that the echoes from far targets have the same amplitude (deflection) as echoes from near targets. However, since the attenuation properties of

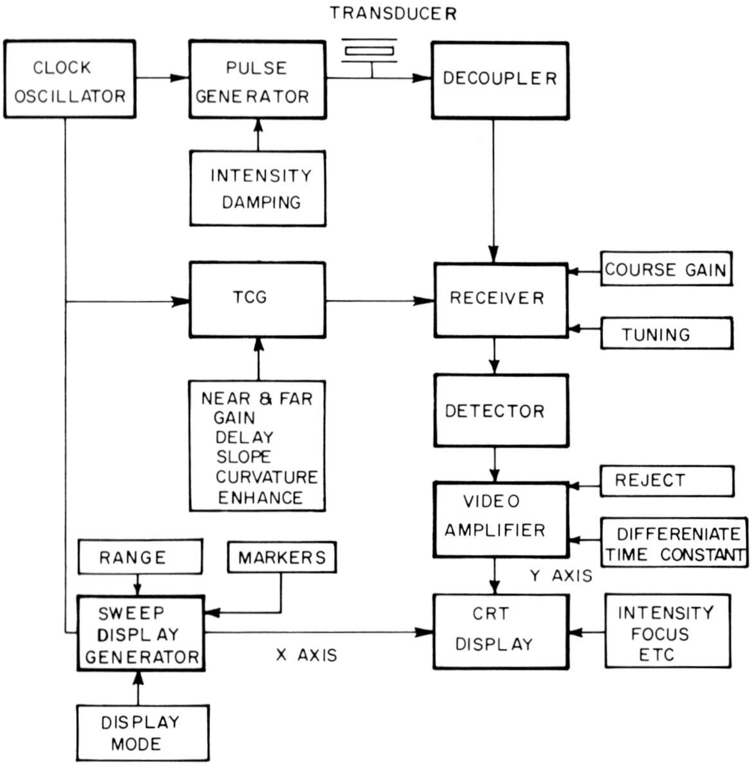

Fig. 2-19. The important control functions of a basic pulse echo system modify the operation of the principal functional elements.

tissue are not necessarily well behaved and known in advance, it is necessary to offer a variety of time-compensated gain functions that the operator can modify to optimize the display. Fig. 2-21 shows an idealized time-compensated gain function that includes features available in a variety of instruments; however, they may not all appear on any one instrument. These will be discussed in sequence.

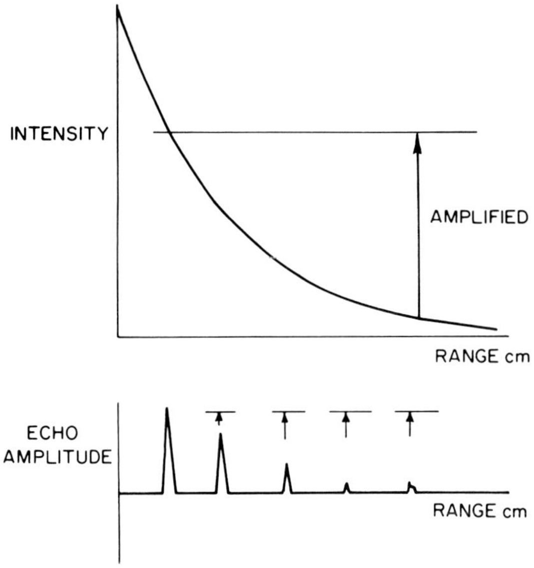

Fig. 2-20. Echoes from distant interfaces need to be amplified more than near echoes in order to produce equal amplitudes on the A-scan display.

1. **Overall coarse gain.** The coarse gain control sets the overall gain of the receiver, independent of range. It is used for the initial gain setting.

2. **Near gain.** Near gain, for the first few centimeters, is controlled separately and is used primarily to attenuate large amplitude echoes and artifacts near the transducer. The depth over which the near gain is functional is controlled by the delay.

3. **Delay.** The delay setting can be used to determine when the time-compensated gain function actually begins.

4. **Slope.** The gain function can start gradually or abruptly, depending upon the initial slope, set by the slope adjustment.

5. **Curvature.** Since the echo amplitude falls exponentially with range, it is necessary to increase the gain exponentially if it is to effect the attenuation. The curvature

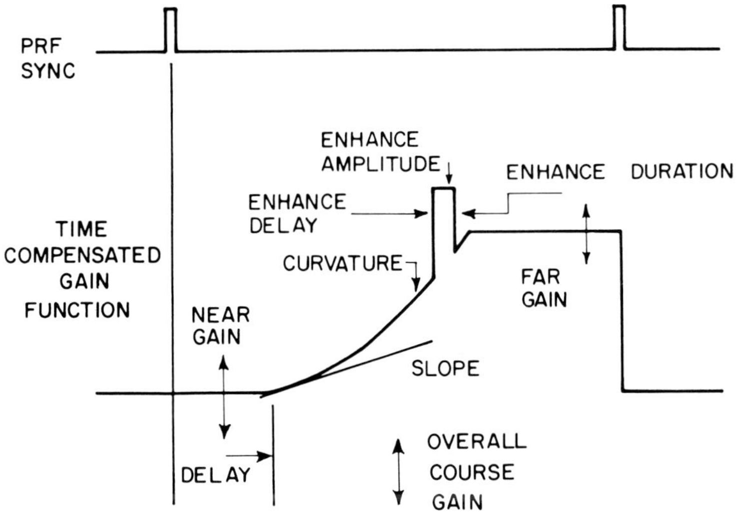

Fig. 2-21. Mastering the time-compensated gain function is a very important step in learning to use pulse-echo techniques.

control varies the rate of change of the gain function. It might be set to be flat or to increase exponentially, or it may actually fall in some cases, depending on what the operator chooses.

6. **Far gain.** The far gain is similar to the near gain. It is an independent control that allows very distant echoes to be enhanced or suppressed.

7. **Enhancement.** Some units provide an additional characteristic that allows enhancing a specific echo or group of echoes. This is shown as a rectangular pulse riding on top of the gain function, and it provides additional amplification at the depth set by the operator. The enhancement delay would control the onset of the enhancement. The amplitude of the pulse indicates the amount of additional gain for that particular echo, and the duration of the enhancement would correspond to the depth over which the enhancement function is operating. With these controls the operator can ordinarily modify the echo pattern to almost any desired configuration.

Once the radio frequency (RF) echoes have been amplified to the desired level, they are detected to follow the echo envelope and then further amplified for display on the cathode ray tube. Fig. 2-22 shows a very simple diagram of a receiver and detector. The signal from the receiving transducer is coupled through an amplifier of gain A, in which the RF signal from the crystal is amplified. This is the amplifier whose gain will be modified according to the time-compensated gain function. Following the RF amplifier receiver is a video detector and filter that is designed to follow the envelope of the echoes. This envelope is shown on the bottom line in

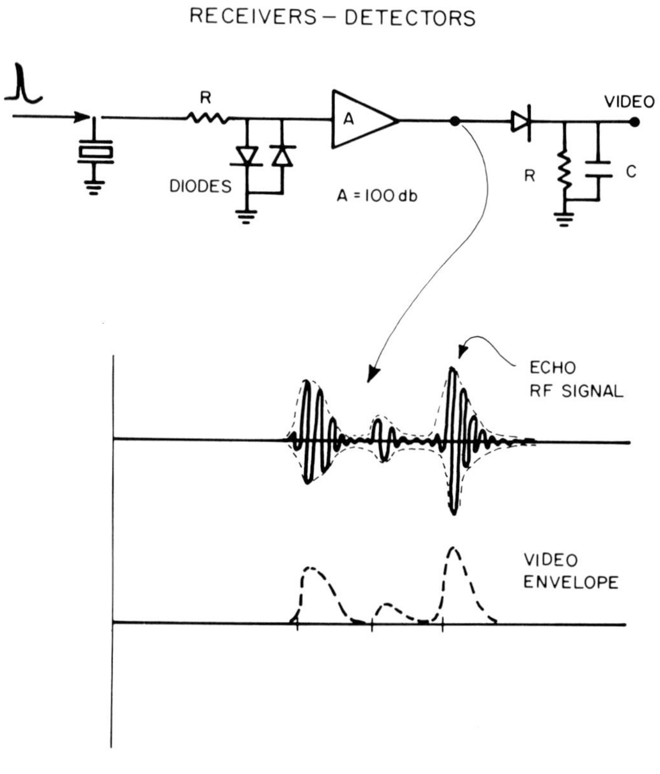

Fig. 2-22. Most pulse-echo systems display the envelope of the radio frequency echo signals.

the example. Some instruments permit modification of the detected video envelope in order to enhance certain echo features. An example that demonstrates video processing of an echo is shown in Fig. 2-23. In this case the sound beam was pointed at a hypothetical valve leaflet, and the echoes from it are analyzed. If the system has high resolution (wide bandwidth), there will be a discrete echo from the near and the far wall of the valve, particularly if there is any calcification present. If the system has low resolution and narrow bandwidth, one large echo would occur from the entire valve leaflet. Often it is possible to modify the echo envelope from the low-resolution system to give the appearance of higher resolution.

VIDEO PROCESSING

The video signal may be differentiated electronically to give the waveform shown on line 3 in Fig. 2-23, in which the amplitude of A corresponds to the slope of point A and the amplitude B corresponds to the slope of point B. Positive slopes produce positive pulses and negative slopes negative pulses. If the positive portion of the differentiated signal is applied to the display, the leading edge of the echo will be

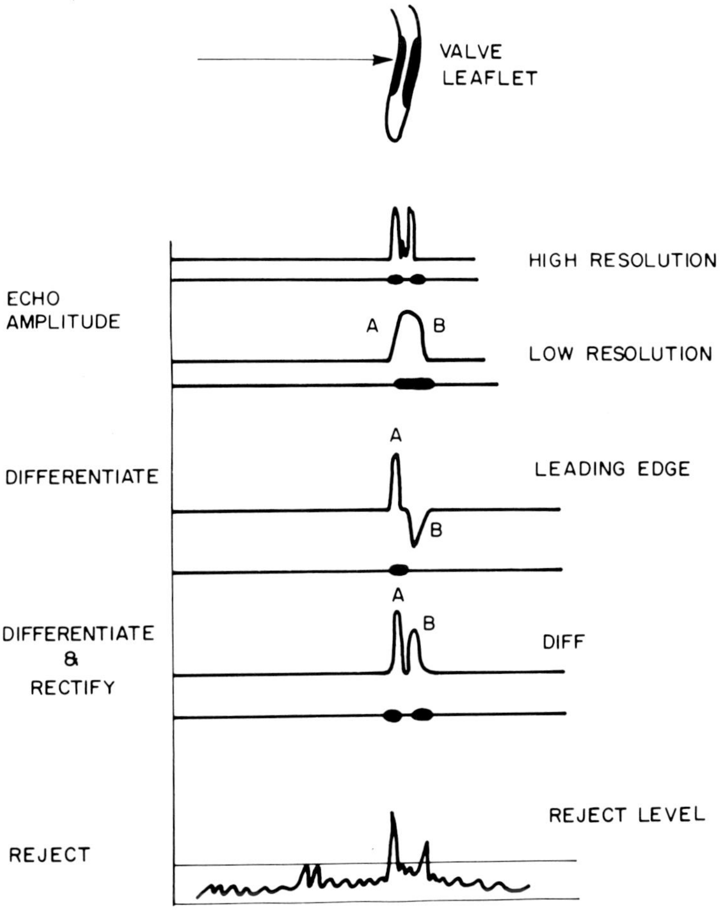

Fig. 2-23. The detected video signals from the pulse-echo receiver can be processed to enhance the quality of the displayed images.

enhanced. This type of differentiation processing is sometimes called leading edge display. The differentiated video can be further detected or rectified such that the waveform at point B is folded over the baseline so that A and B are now on the same side of the baseline. The effect will be to produce a double echo indicating both edges of the valve to give the appearance of a high-resolution system. One additional step that can be made in processing the video is to add a reject level. The purpose of the reject level is to display only those large amplitude echoes that rise above a certain threshold. Small weak echoes would not be displayed. The setting of the reject level knob controls the level of the threshold. This control has to be used carefully since small, weak echoes that could be important might also be obscured.

There are other controls shown in Fig. 2-19 that can modify the display in addition to those just discussed. The pulse generator, which is used to excite the transducer, may have an intensity or damping control. This has the effect of controlling the amount of energy applied to the transmitting element. For near (short-range) interfaces, which produce large echoes, it is sometimes convenient to reduce the transmitter amplitude in order to prevent overdriving the receiver. Receivers can usually be tuned for use with a variety of transducers. These may function anywhere from 1 MHz to as high as 10 to 12 MHz. Some receivers have continuous tuning similar to a radio, while others have bands over which they operate. The cathode ray tube display contains the usual controls for effecting the brightness of the display, the focusing, and the like.

The sweep display generator is used principally to determine the horizontal size of the display shown on the cathode ray tube.

DISPLAY MODES

There are three types of display modes currently in use. They are called the A mode, the B mode, and the T-M mode

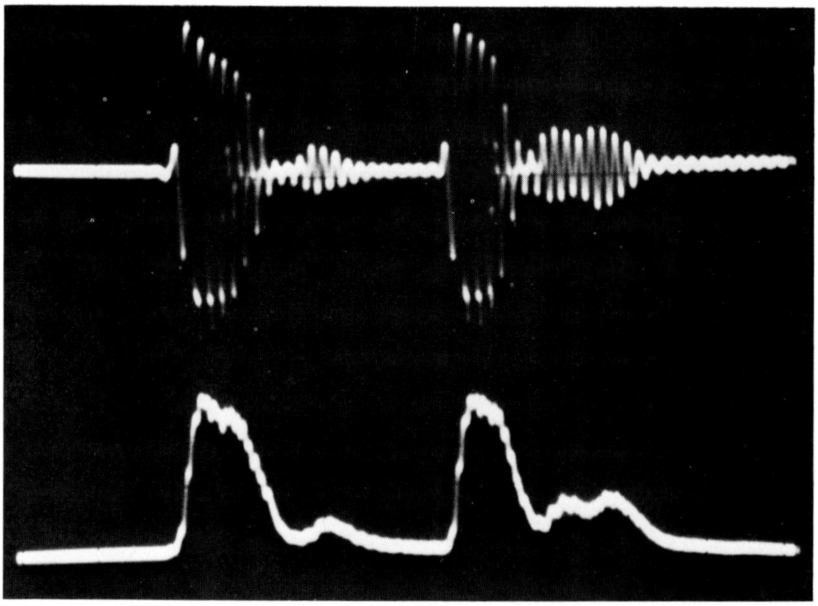

Fig. 2-24. The detected video signal should correspond closely to the envelope of the raw echo pulses.

(sometimes called the M mode). The A mode is the most basic display and is most commonly used for midline position measurement. In the A mode the detected echo amplitude is displayed versus depth. The depth calibration on the horizontal axis of the display would ordinarily be marked in centimeters, and on many instruments small marker pips are added to the trace in order to identify 2-mm, 5-mm, and 1-cm graduations on the horizontal axis. On most units there are controls that can be used to alter the marker sequence or to turn them on or off. The range or depth displayed on the cathode ray tube on the horizontal axis can also be adjusted such that a range from 0 to 5 cm, or 0 to 20 cm, depending on the instrument, can be displayed. The range markers shift as the scale depth is changed. Some devices have a delay function on the horizontal display such that the origin of the trace on the left side of the scope corresponds for example to a depth of 10 cm instead of beginning at zero depth. This feature is usually adjustable at the operator's wish. Fig. 2-24 shows a typical A-scan display. The upper trace is the undetected radio frequency and the lower trace the detected signals. Many instruments show the A-scan display simultaneously on a separate oscilloscope while the instrument is used for either the B-mode or the T-M–mode application.

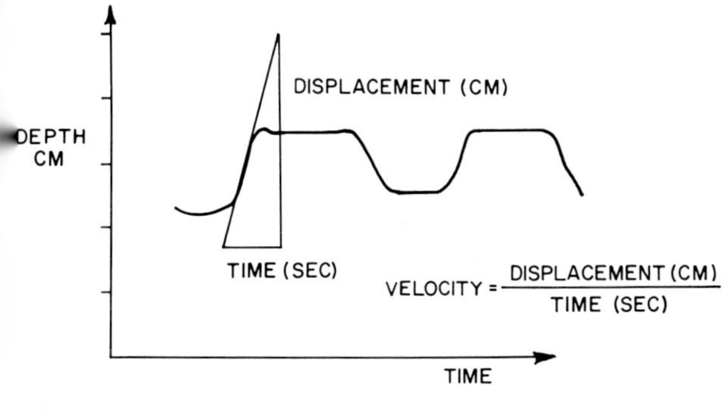

Fig. 2-25. The initial opening velocity of the valve is easily computed from the depth versus time wave form.

T-M–mode display

In cardiology it is often necessary to know the opening and closing velocity of the mitral valve to determine the degree of mitral stenosis. While pulse echo devices do not read out velocity directly, it is possible to develop a display from which velocity measurements can be calculated. The basic concept is to plot or store on a cathode ray tube the range or depth of the echoes as a function of time. The path of motion of an interface can be easily followed, and lines tangent to the path of motion can be drawn at any selected site. These tangent lines can be used to determine the slope of the displacement that is equal to the velocity (Fig. 2-25). By using these simple graphic techniques the velocity of an interface can easily be determined.

The T-M–mode display is generated from the A-scan echo information. Fig. 2-26 shows the development of the T-M–mode display. The transducer in the example is positioned to detect the motion of the leaflets of the mitral valve. In the middle of the illustration is the detected A-scan display and below that is the T-M–mode display. Two sweeps (ramp functions) are used to generate the T-M–mode display. The fast sweep running horizontally in the illustration gives the depth information. This same fast sweep is moved slowly up the face of the cathode ray tube by a slow sweep to give the time axis. The A-scan echoes are used to intensity-modulate the z axis of the fast sweep, as shown on the bottom line. Bright spots will appear where echoes of large amplitude occur. As the trace moves up the scope, the path of the motion of the echoes will be inscribed on the screen. Markers are introduced at 0.5-second intervals on the time base and at 1-cm intervals on the depth axis. Fig. 2-26, *A*, shows a diagrammatic normal mitral valve displacement.

B-mode scanning

Two-dimensional images of sections of the abdomen or other structures can be

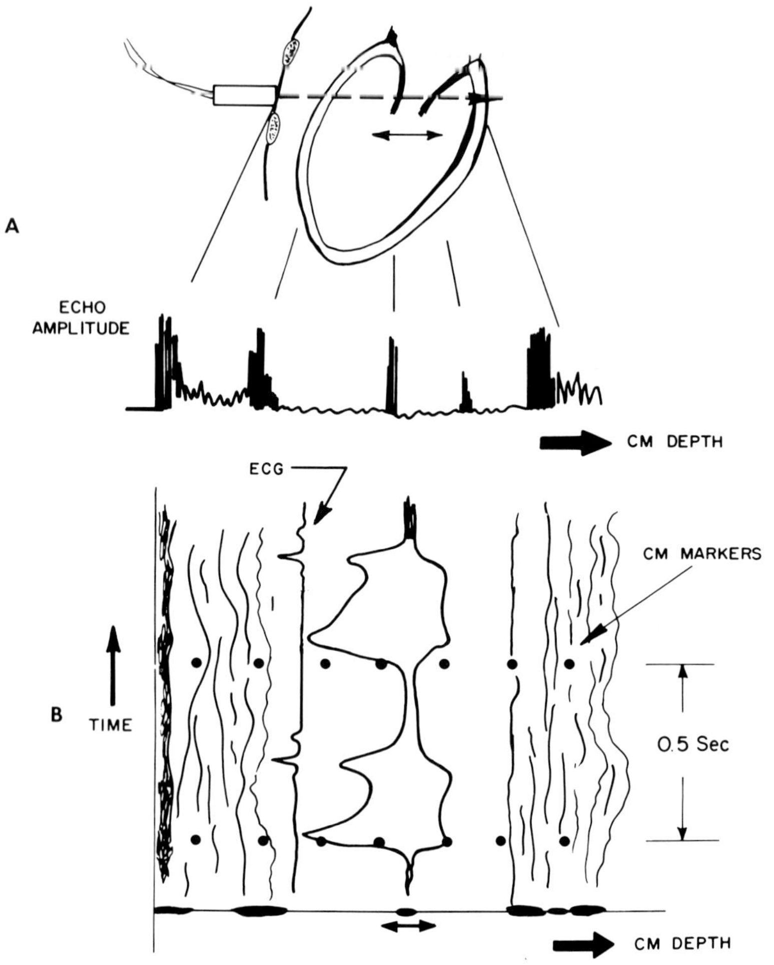

Fig. 2-26. The displacement of echoes can be written out on the cathode ray tube using the T-M–mode display concept.

made if pulse-echo equipment is coupled to a scanning arm mechanism. The scanning sequence and display is called B mode. The beam-like characteristics of the sound field make it possible to selectively pass the transducer over a region of interest to develop images. Two different methods are used to couple the transducer to the skin and to position it for the scan. The original method involved attaching the transducer to a motor-driven scanning mechanism and the transducer was coupled through a water bath to the subject. The water bath was usually contained within a plastic bag that was placed against the subject. Previous water bath scanners even involved immersing the subject in a tank. The most popular method currently in use involves contact scanning in which the transducer is placed directly on the skin and the acoustic coupling is maintained using either an oil or a gel. In both forms it is necessary to move the transducer through a type of compound scan.

The specular reflection characteristics of various tissues structures make it necessary that all tissue interfaces be insonated from as many angles as possible in order

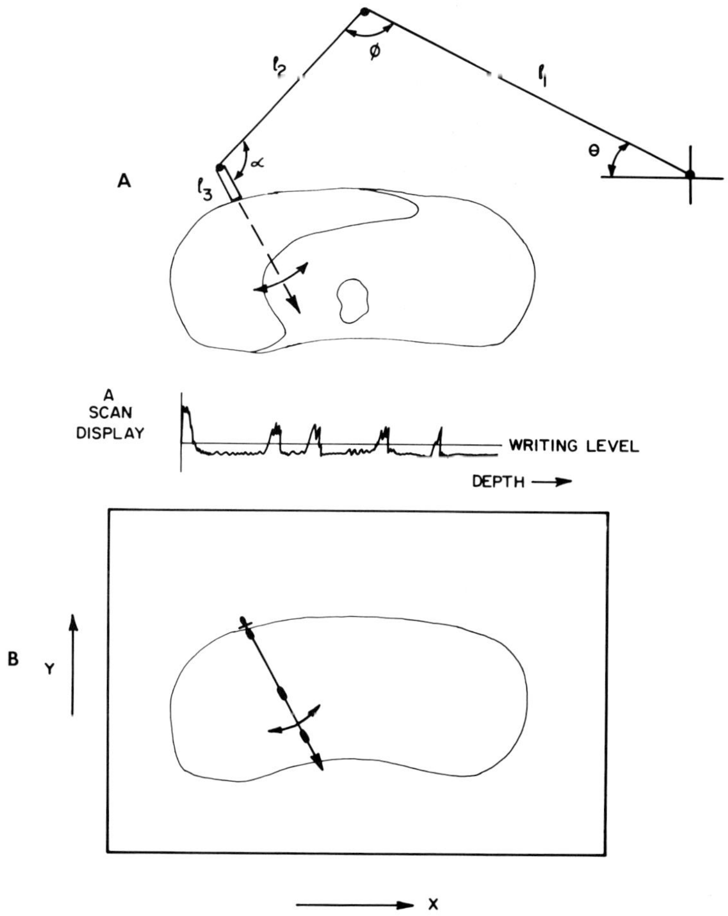

Fig. 2-27. A scan arm in **A** is used to map the transducer position and beam direction into the face of the cathode ray tube in **B**. The echo amplitude intensity modulates the trace in **B**.

to completely outline their margins. A variety of scanning techniques have been worked out. However, the most common involves a combination sector or pi scan while translating the transducer back and forth. The mechanical water bath scanners use a system of levers and gears driven by an electric motor to make the transducer sector scan and translate simultaneously. In the contact scanner the operator must move the transducer in a similar fashion. In the latter procedure it is absolutely essential that the operator observe the B-mode display as it is being developed in order to modify or correct the scanning sequence. Some skill is required before uniform B-mode images are possible using the contact scanning method.

A scanning arm, shown schematically in Fig. 2-27, is designed for contact scanning. The transducer that rests on the skin is attached through a series of arm links L_1, L_2, and L_3 to a base support attached to the wall or to a movable base on the floor near the patient. As the transducer is moved, the angles theta (Θ), phi (ϕ), and alpha (α) will change as the arm is positioned. At each joint, coupled through a series of pulleys and cables, are potentiometer resistance type transducers that measure these angles. A set of trigonometric formulas are solved using the values of the angles to determine the x, y position and direction of the sound beam emanating from the transducer face. This information is converted into x and y deflection signals for the cathode ray tube display.

Fig. 2-27 shows a simple abdominal scan through the region of the liver. The transducer is shown in a typical position, the arrows indicate a pi sector scan. At the same instant, a trace is developed on the cathode ray tube that corresponds, in a one-to-one relationship, to the direction of the sound beam position. The trace is not visible on the screen because only the echoes shown in the A-scan display (center of the illustration) are used to intensity-modulate the cathode ray tube. As the transducer is scanned about, the intensity-modulated echoes will write and store an image on the cathode ray tube face. Eventually, as the scan progresses, a complete image will be built up.

The quality of the resulting image will depend on the scanning rate and settings of the receiving amplifiers in the electronic package. All of the controls previously discussed will have an influence on this image. For example, time-compensated gain can influence the uniformity of the writing rate of the stored image.

Fig. 2-28 shows the effect of the time-compensated gain on these images. In Fig. 2-28, *A*, the time-compensated gain is turned off, the far echoes are not amplified adequately, and their intensity-modulated output on the cathode ray tube will show echoes fading away in long range. When the time-compensated gain is turned on and adjusted properly, distant echoes will write essentially at the same brightness or intensity as near echoes. The object here is for the operator to adjust the time-compensated gain to achieve the proper uniformity in the echoes. The effects of the various instrument settings apply equally well to both contact scanning and immersion water-bath scanning.

The B-mode scanner can be used to develop a series of sections of the abdomen, in order to build up a three-dimensional representation of various organs. The scanning plane can be shifted or oriented by adjusting the angle of the mounting on the support mechanisms. B-mode images are best suited for stationary structures since any movement will cause blurring of the image. In order to image moving structures, it may be necessary to time-gate the display. For example, if we wished to image a section through the left

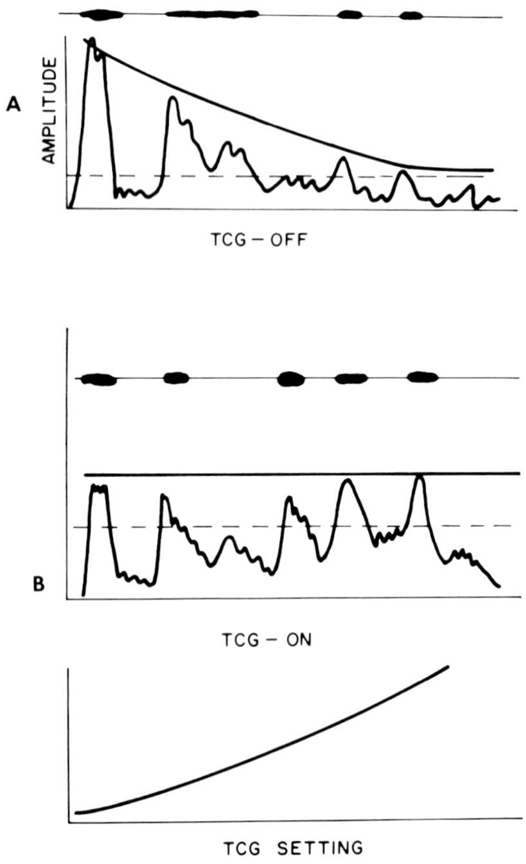

Fig. 2-28. Careful adjustment of the time-compensated gain function is necessary to produce uniform density B-mode scans.

ventricle, it would be necessary to synchronize and gate the display system with the electrocardiogram. This technique permits displaying data only at a particular instant in the cardiac cycle. If the motion is regular and periodic, then ideally the same interface should return to the same location at the same instant in the cardiac cycle. The time gate blocks out all echo movements except those that occur at the moment of the gating.

The resolution of the B-mode scan is dependent on the pulse length and the beam width just as in A mode. Therefore, to do imaging of detail structure, it would be necessary to go to higher frequencies to develop very short duration bursts to give adequate depth resolution. Beam width can be reduced to some extent by the use of focusing. However, the depth of the field may be limited.

Basic Doppler techniques

Doppler devices, in contrast to pulse echo instruments, operate on the scattered ultrasound from moving blood. The scattering phenomenon as it occurs in the bloodstream can be utilized to measure velocity of blood flow. It is conceivable that the scattering mechanism can also be used to measure velocity of valves directly. The simplest form of Doppler device is the continuous wave Doppler.

The block diagram in Fig. 2-29 shows the essential components of the system. The transducer is placed directly on the skin and contains two crystal elements, a transmitting element and a receiving element. A continuous wave sound beam is projected into the tissue in the direction of the blood vessel. At the point where the sound field intercepts the vessel, scattering caused by the red cells will occur. A certain amount of this energy will be backscattered toward the receiving element. The frequency of the backscattered signal will be determined by the Doppler shift equation:

$$\Delta f = \frac{2\,fv}{c} \cos \Theta$$

The transmitting element of the transducer is usually excited by a low-power oscillator operating in the range of 3 to 8 MHz. The excitation level is such as to produce sound field intensities under 50 mw/cm^2. Mix-

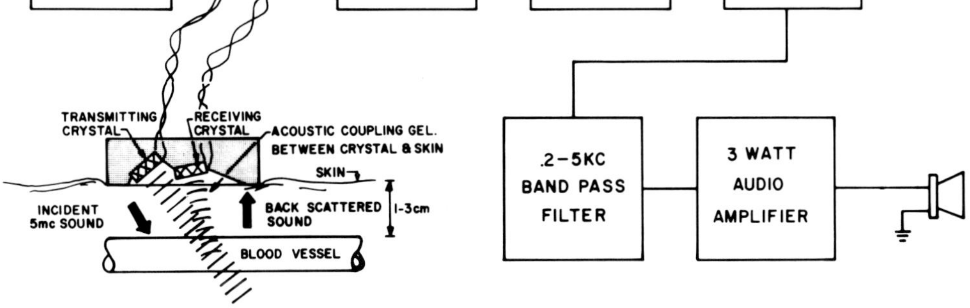

Fig. 2-29. A simple continuous-wave Doppler instrument is less complicated than a small transistor radio.

ing of the transmitted and received signals occurs acoustically at the transducer and electrically in the receiving amplifier. The effect of this is to cause an amplitude modulated (AM) wave to appear at the input of the differential 5-MHz receiver amplifier. This AM wave is essentially like a radiowave where, in this case, the frequency of the AM modulation is the Doppler difference frequency. The amplitude of the modulation will be proportional to the amplitude of the backscattered signal. A very simple radio frequency amplifier and detector can be used to separate the Doppler difference frequency. For flow velocities up to 100 cm/sec, the Doppler shift for a typical 5 MHz unit can go up to 5 to 8 kHz, depending on the velocity and the angle between the sound beam and the flow vector. This makes it possible to listen to the Doppler signal spectrum from almost all physiologic flows. With some experience a great deal of information about the blood flow can be determined. Regions of narrowing in vessels, which produce a high-velocity venturi type jet, produce high-frequency Doppler signals. These jet signals are clearly different from those either distal or proximal to it. In addition to blood flow, motion from such interfaces as the fetal heart can easily be detected as early as 8 to 10 weeks after conception. Several thousands of these units are in clinical use throughout the world and a large body of literature has been developed.[5]

Future applications of Doppler techniques probably will depend on the development of the pulse Doppler.[3] This new device incorporates features of both the continuous wave Doppler and pulse echo devices. It is capable of echo ranging to determine the depth or location of an interface as well as the velocity. Its detailed characteristics are somewhat different than the pulse echo devices.

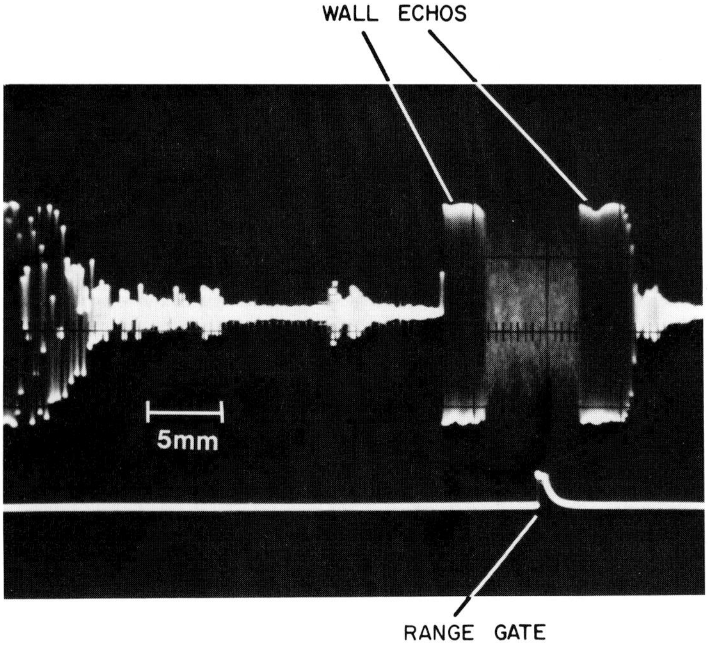

Fig. 2-30. A pulse Doppler combines the features of continuous-wave operation with pulse echo. The flow signal is apparent in the space between the wall echoes. Range gating permits selective measurement of velocity.

Fig. 2-30 shows an undetected radio frequency A-scan display from a pulse Doppler where the transducer is aimed at a plastic tube containing moving fluid. The echoes resulting from the near and the far wall are obvious. The fuzzy area between the walls is the Doppler shift signal resulting from the motion of particles within the fluid. In the pulse Doppler a short burst of ultrasound in the 3- to 8-MHz range is transmitted into the tissue. This burst is actually a series of sine waves from 2 to 10 cycles in duration. This burst is derived from a master timing oscillator and is transmitted at a relatively high pulse repetition rate compared to the pulse echo device. Each transmitted burst is in step or phase with the master oscillator, thus giving it the name "phase coherent pulse Doppler." The echoes from the tissue along the beam are compared to the master oscillator in order to determine the instantaneous phase difference. When this is done over a series of pulse repetition periods, the Doppler difference frequency can be derived. The receiver is range gated so that it is possible to dial the depth at which the operator wishes to detect the velocity.

In Fig. 2-30 the lower trace shows the position of the range gate. This gate can be scanned across the vessel, through a valve, or through any moving interface in order to selectively measure the velocity at the site of the gate. An example of the application of pulse Doppler techniques is in the measurement of velocity profiles in straight tubes used as a model of a vessel.

Fig. 2-31 shows a series of laminar profiles for a range of flow rates taken with a pulse Doppler. The vessel diameter is on the order of 6.8 mm. The shape of the profiles is very close to that which one would expect from previous knowledge of laminar flow in a straight tube. The artifacts near the far wall are caused by wall reflections and resolution factors related to the sample volume size of the pulse Doppler. While these devices are not yet available commercially, their applications

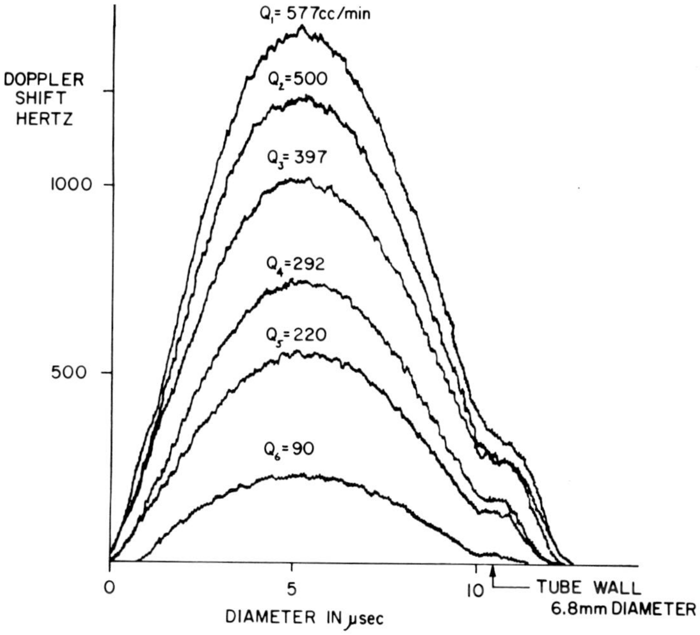

Fig. 2-31. Pulse Doppler velocity profiles of steady laminar flow in a straight tube.

are being pursued in a number of laboratories.

Doppler signal analysis

One of the difficulties of Doppler techniques is that most of the information is in the form of an audio signal spectrum that can be interpreted by the experienced operator but that is difficult to record. It is even more difficult to transmit the essence of the information from one individual to another in verbal terms. A tape recording can store the signals, but they cannot be readily duplicated or easily added to the patient record.

Two different techniques are currently being used to analyze the Doppler spectrum and to provide a graphic record; the most comprehensive procedure is to do a time domain type of spectral analysis.[6] The output from such an analyzer is shown in Fig. 2-32. The solid line superimposed on the spectral plot corresponds approximately to the true weighted average of the spectrum as a function of time. The method used to develop the average will be discussed separately in a more detailed description of the zero crossing frequency meter.

The detected Doppler difference frequency has the form of a complicated time-varying spectrum. A little study will reveal why. From Fig. 2-31 it is known that any fluid flow through a tube will produce some type of velocity profile. This profile will have a value of zero velocity at the walls and may be parabolic or blunted, depending on the circumstances.

Since there is always a range of velocities across the lumen diameter of a vessel, there will always be a corresponding spread of Doppler shifts. If the pulsatile nature of the flow is included, then the velocity profile and the signal spectrum will vary in time with the pulsations. This is apparent in the spectrum from the

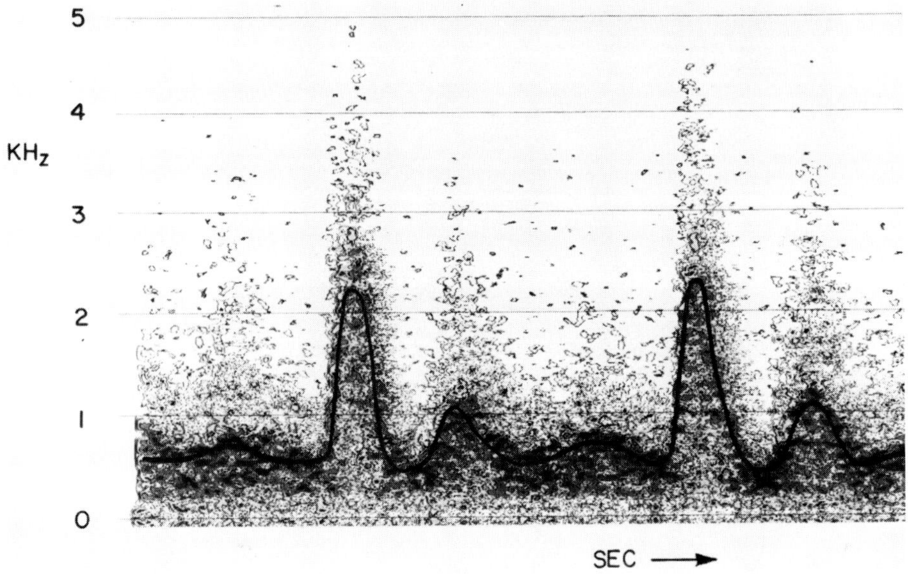

Fig. 2-32. Spectral plot of brachial flow from continuous-wave Doppler. Superimposed zero crossing output indicates average value of velocity.

brachial artery shown in Fig. 2-32. The Doppler signal spectrum is modified still further by a finite beam width of the transducer. This effect and that of the profile are summarized in Fig. 2-33. The spectral broadening is a result of the varying angle between any one scatterer and the sound beam axis as it progresses through the sound field on its way by. The example shows this effect for steady flow. If pulsatile flow is added to the model, the spectrum obviously becomes more complicated.

The shading in the spectral plot in Fig. 2-32 corresponds to the intensity of the backscattered signal. If one were to assume that the vessel were in the far field of the transducer, then the backscattered Doppler signal intensity would be proportional to the number of scatterers moving at each respective velocity. In the example in Fig. 2-32, the scatterers (red cells) have a wide range of velocities during systole owing to the broad spectrum of that instant. At the end of systole the scatterers have a narrow range of velocities as determined from the narrow spectrum. The fact that most of the scatterers are moving in this narrow span of velocities is further indicated by the higher backscattered intensity.

These spectral plots were made by first recording the signal on magnetic tape and then later processing them on a Kay* spectrum analyzer. The Kay unit can store and analyze a 2.5-second sample whose frequency span is in the range of 70 to 8,000 Hz.

Many of the continuous-wave Doppler devices available for clinical applications have an analog voltage output for writing on strip-chart type paper recorders. This type of analyzer is called a zero crossing frequency meter. It counts each time the

*Kay Electronics Corp., Pine Brook, N. J.

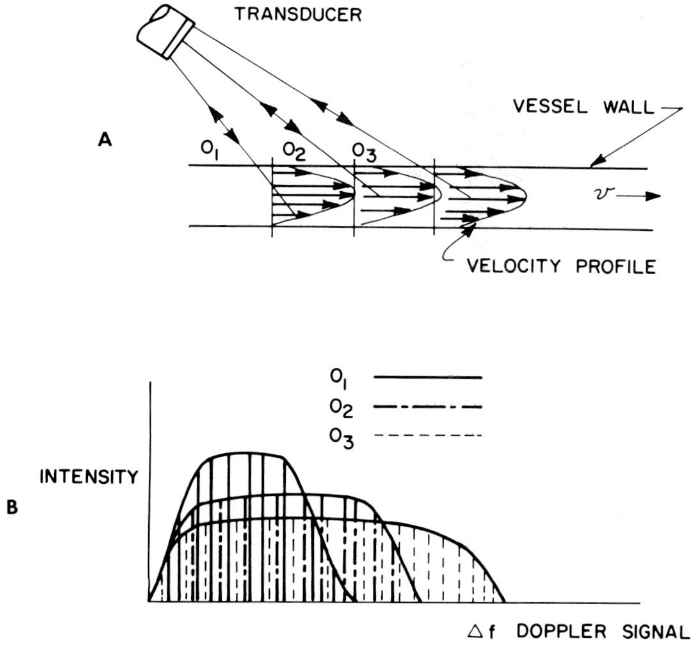

Fig. 2-33. A, Spectral broadening depends on sound beam width and velocity profile. **B,** Final spectrum is a summation of inputs from scattering region within beam.

analog form of the Doppler spectrum passes through the zero voltage level. For example, if the signal were a simple single Doppler shift of 1,000 Hz, there would be a zero crossing every millisecond corresponding to the period of the signal. The interval between zero crossings shifts rapidly as the signal becomes more complex; that is, it contains many frequencies, as in a spectrum. When the number of zero crossings per second is averaged and smoothed by an electric filter, the result is the wave superimposed on Fig. 2-32.

While the zero crossing circuitry is simple, the results depend on two important factors. These are the quality of the signal, referred to as the signal-to-noise ratio (s/n) and the zero crosser trigger threshold. There is no rigorous way to set the zero crosser circuit threshold for precise operation. The signal-to-noise ratio is usually not influenced by the operator, consequently errors can easily influence the results. These difficulties have not been resolved to anyone's satisfaction to the present time.

Special spectral analysis techniques using the fast Fourier transform algorithm on a digital computer show promise in helping to devise better signal processing methods and devices. Fig. 2-34 shows a spectral plot of ascending aorta blood flow as detected by a pulse Doppler. This method has the advantage of indicating the direction of blood flow velocity as well as the Doppler spread and the backscat-

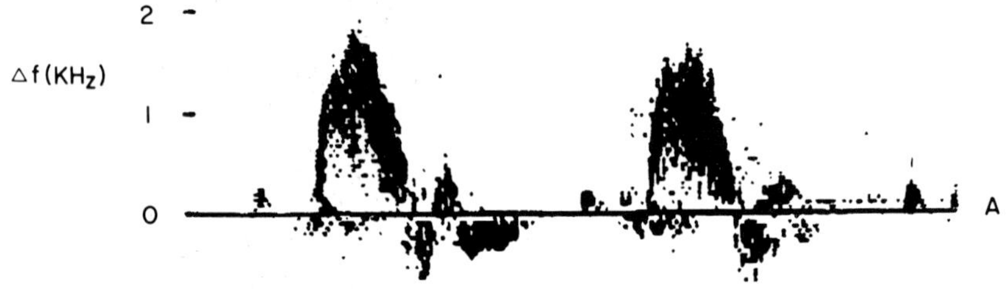

Fig. 2-34. Fast Fourier transform of ascending aortic flow taken with pulse Doppler and processed by digital computer.

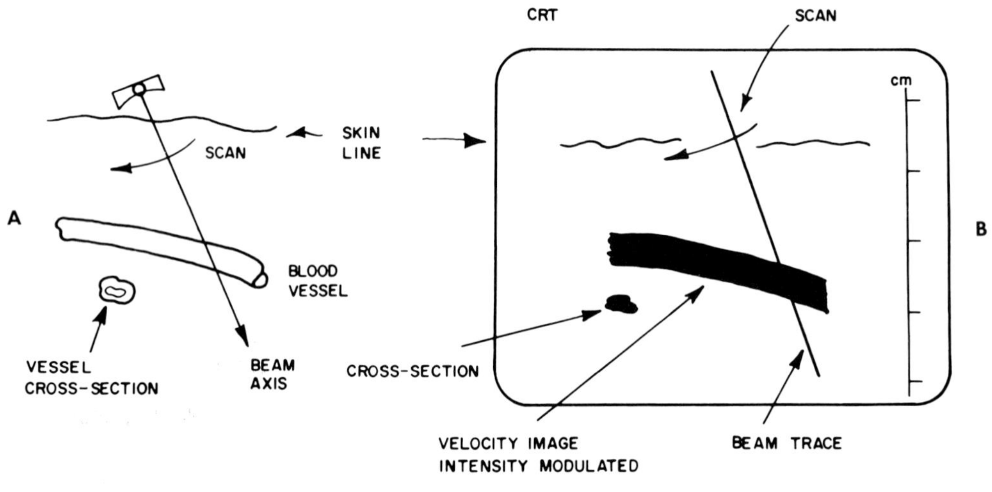

Fig. 2-35. Doppler imaging is similar to B-mode scanning except only moving blood is displayed.

tered signal intensity. These experimental methods cannot in their present form be added to an inexpensive Doppler device. They will no doubt help to develop devices that can be reproduced easily.

Both pulsed and continuous wave Dopplers are being developed for the purpose of imaging blood flow within vessels. The technique is similar to the B-mode scanning methods used with pulse echo devices. The difference in a Doppler imager is that only blood flow above a preset threshold velocity is displayed on the cathode ray tube. The transducer is affixed to a scanning arm somewhat like a B-mode scanner.[7] As the transducer is scanned, as in Fig. 2-35, *A*, Doppler signals will be detected according to the beam direction and the range gate setting. The sound beam position is mapped onto the cathode ray tube face, as shown in Fig. 2-35, *B*.

When flow signals above a certain velocity are detected, a spot will be stored on the cathode ray tube at the distance of the range gate. The cathode ray tube face (Fig. 2-35, *B*) shows a simulation of a longitudinal and cross-sectional scan. An actual image from a femoral-profunda bifurcation is shown in Fig. 2-36, *A*. The position of the beam for one instant in time is shown in Fig. 2-36, *B*. The particular pulse Doppler unit used had five range gates—three were within the vessel and two were outside.

Currently, imaging techniques are being combined with the new spectral analysis procedures to explore quantitation of transcutaneous flow signals.

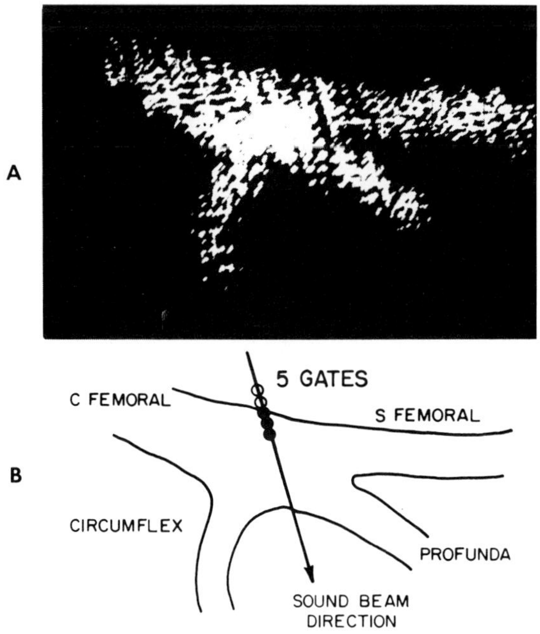

Fig. 2-36. Doppler image of femoral-profunda bifurcation using a five-gate pulse Doppler.

REFERENCES

1. Grossman, C. C., and others, editors: Diagnostic ultrasound, New York, 1966, Plenum Press, Inc.
2. Wells, P. N. T.: Physical principles of ultrasonic diagnosis, New York, 1969, Academic Press, Inc.
3. Baker, D. W.: Pulsed ultrasonic Doppler blood flow sensing, IEEE Transactions on Sonics and Ultrasonics SU-17, No. 3, July, 1970.
4. Hueter, T. F., and Bolt, R. H.: Sonics, New York, 1955, John Wiley & Sons, Inc.
5. Strandness, D. E., Jr.: Techniques in the evaluation of vascular disease, 1971, Surg. Annu. **3:**181-197, 1971.
6. Strandness, D. E., Jr., and others: Ultrasonic flow detection: a useful technique in the evaluation of peripheral vascular disease, Am. J. Surg. **113:** 311-320, 1967.
7. Mozersky, D., and others: Ultrasonics arteriography, Arch. Surg. **103:**663-667, 1971.

3 Echoencephalography

WILLIAM M. McKINNEY, M.D.

The introduction of midline echoencephalography is credited to Leksell in 1955.[1,2] Following his initial description of the technique, he stressed the role of the pineal body as a source of the midline echo.[3] De Vlieger and Ridder[4] reported results on a small series of cases in 1959. In 1960 Lithander described the use of the transmission signal as a control method.[5,6] In 1961 the monographs of Jeppson[7] and Lithander[8] each reported a large series of cases, as well as comprehensive discussions of the subject. Further data were reported by Taylor and associates[9] in 1961, Jefferson[10] in 1962, Ford and Ambrose[11] in 1963, and Brinker, King, and Taveras[12] in 1965. More recently, comprehensive reviews and textbooks on echoencephalography by Kazner,[13] Grossman,[14] and White[15] have appeared. These studies indicate a definite clinical use for echoencephalography in the detection of space-occupying lesions of the brain. The introduction of ventricular size measurements aided the clinician in rapid determination of ventricular size as a screening method.[16] A wide acceptance of midline echoencephalography and ventricular measurements has followed. Recently, dynamic studies of pulsations in selected areas of the brain have added a new dimension to an understanding of the brain.

The following discussion is designed to systematically present practical clinical echoencephalography.

INSTRUMENTATION

Echoencephalography depends on reflection of pulsed ultrasound from internal structures of the brain. Echoes arise from structures that are perpendicular to the direction of the sonic beam. Standard echoencephalographic instruments now available are designed to transmit small pulses of ultrasound into the brain at a low power level and high repetition rate. Reflections, or echoes, are displayed on an oscilloscope as vertical deflections along a calibrated horizontal baseline and are generally photographed by a Polaroid camera (Fig. 3-1).

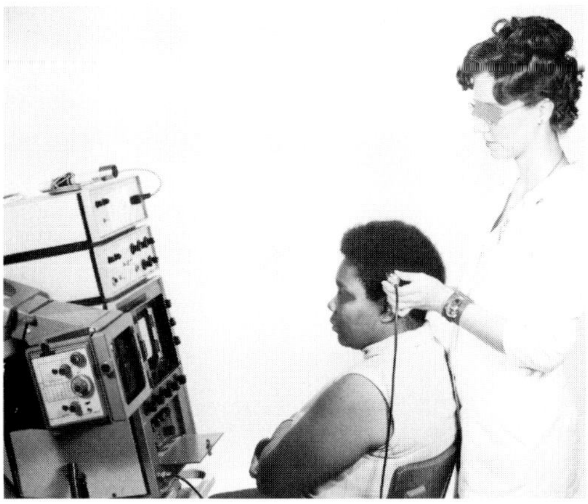

Fig. 3-1. A standard echoencephalographic instrument with the transducer placed at the temporoparietal area.

Proper instrument settings are very important for the particular instrument being used. Power levels in many instruments may be varied to use minimum power required for identification of internal landmarks of the brain. Children require a lower power setting than adults because of the thinness of the skull and the presence of less calcification. Gain controls are very important in the determination of internal landmarks varying from person to person. The time-varying gain must be set appropriately to demonstrate internal structures in the far field.

Transducers vary in size and shape and may be focused or nonfocused. Standard commercial transducers are primarily in the 1- to 5-MHz range. A 2- to 2.5-MHz transducer is used as a good compromise in most cases. A 1-MHz transducer will transmit through a thick skull and should be used in more difficult cases. A 5-MHz transducer may be used in children with higher resolution made possible by the higher frequency. The display is usually in A mode although B mode may be used. Through transmission from one transducer to the other to determine the acoustic midline of the brain has received some attention. The through transmission yields a theoretic midline for comparison with the midline determined by echo reflection. This requires placing a transducer at both sides of the head. The distance between the two transducers is measured acoustically and displayed on the oscilloscope. Although this may appear to be a useful method, errors may result from interpreter bias and misidentification of the internal landmarks. It is an additional step and not in current daily use in many laboratories. New instrumentation has been developed for a "computer midline," or automated determination. Although this instrument has been developed to make the definition of a maximum echo possible, it has a marked disadvantage in that the signals are not seen and internal landmarks are difficult to identify. As a screening device, using untrained personnel, this may have some value. However, it is a limited examination using a very simple device. The "computer midline" may be compared to a one-lead electrocardiogram or electroencephalogram.

TECHNIQUE

Various methods for echoencephalography have been reported; however, a simple, useful "ABC" approach is presented here. The patient may be examined in the sitting or recumbent position. Artifact and error caused by contraction of the temporal muscle may be avoided by asking the patient to open his mouth. In order to have reproducible studies, the head is measured in three standard positions, A, B and C. A coordinate system has been developed for daily clinical use (Fig. 3-2). The head is measured from the nasion to the inion and a grease pencil mark is placed halfway between the two. A measurement is then taken from the superior external auditory canals through the mark. Point A is placed one tenth of this distance superior to the external auditory canal. Point B is marked same distance superior to point A. On a perpendicular to point B,

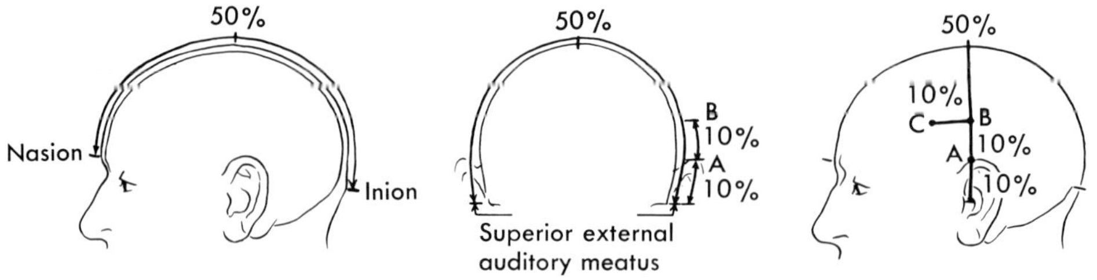

Fig. 3-2. ABC coordinate system for standard positions.

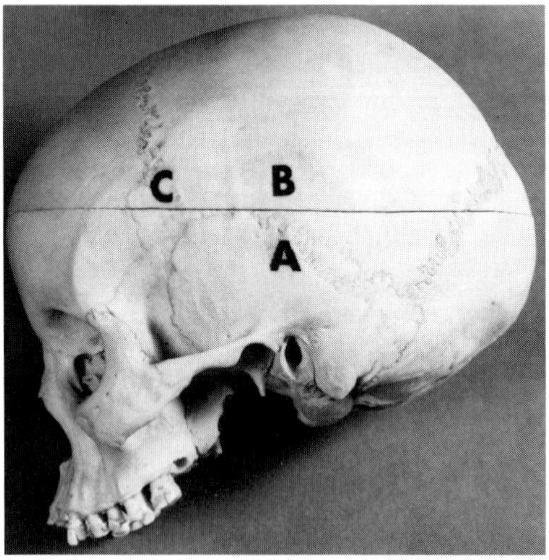

Fig. 3-3. Standard positions in relation to skull surface.

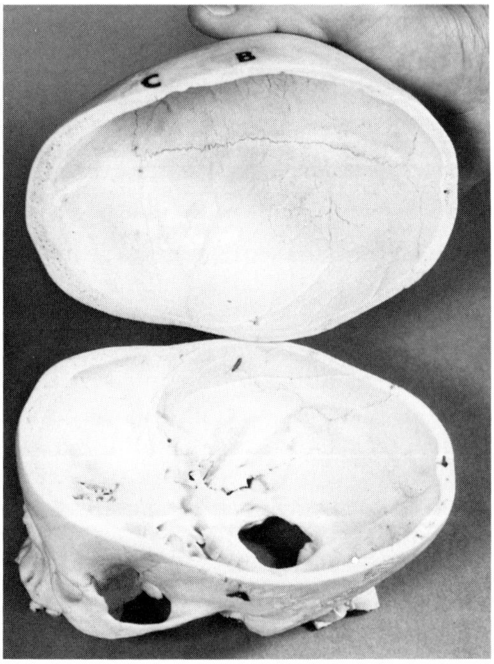

Fig. 3-4. The skull surface is irregular, with the thinnest area in the temporoparietal area.

the same one tenth measurement is used to locate point C. This provides a reference for all clinical studies and aids in reporting of these studies.

The anatomic basis of echoencephalography consists of the identification of echoes arising from major structures that present an interface perpendicular to the sound beam. These include the walls of the third ventricle, cisterna ambiens, pineal body, temporal horn, septum pellucidum, walls of the lateral ventricles, sylvian area, skull, skin, vessels, and abnormal structures. It has been of interest that gray and white matter interfaces may be detected at high gain settings based on the difference in vascular supply of these areas. Gray matter has approximately two to four times the vasculature of white matter. Abnormalities of these standard internal landmarks result in abnormal studies indicating the presence of pathology. Calcification, edema, infarction, unusual pulsations, and other density changes produce abnormal echoes.

The landmarks on the skull represent three specific areas in relation to the skull surface (Fig. 3-3). The skull is irregular and standard echoencephalography is primarily in the temporoparietal area. The skull thickness is less in this area and, al-

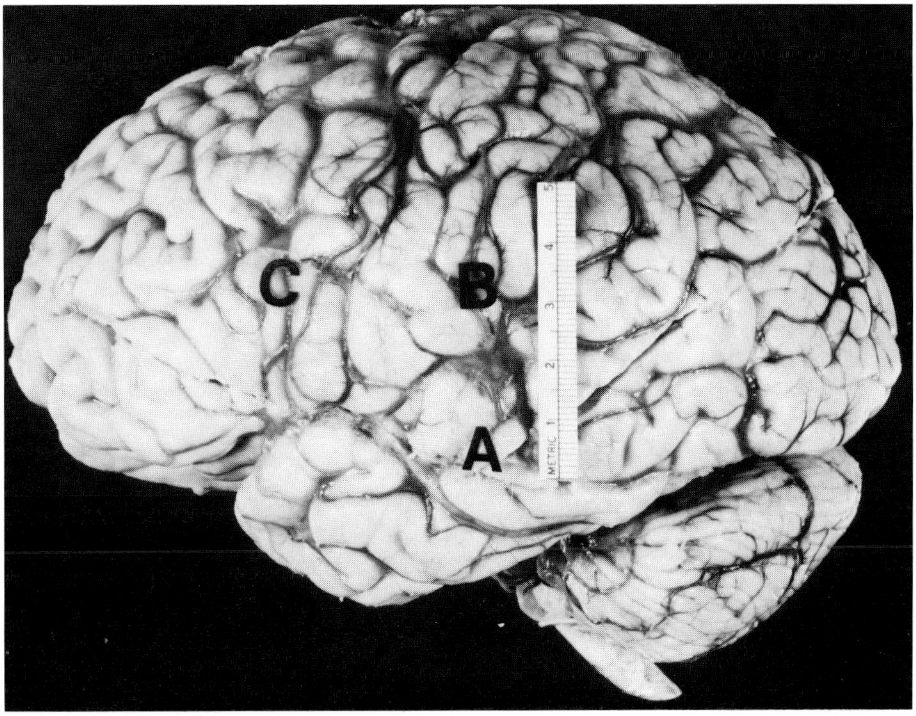

Fig. 3-5. Pathologic correlation of standard positions on the surface of the brain.

though irregular, allows the sonic beam to penetrate (Fig. 3-4). Pathologic correlation with the coordinate system on the surface of the brain has resulted in a better understanding of internal structures (Fig. 3-5). When the brain is sectioned, the average sonic beam may be thought of as being perpendicular to internal structures, with position A passing through the walls of the third ventricle and position B superior to this (Fig. 3-6). By slight rocking of the transducer, the sonic beam is varied slightly in order to penetrate the irregular surface of the skull. Position C is a frontal position and is a more difficult position to obtain because of irregularities of skull thickness and angulation with curvature of the skull (Fig. 3-7).

Standard echoencephalography is performed by placing the transducer on the right side of the head with the A-scan representation deflected upward on a Polaroid film. By changing the electronic setting, a double exposure is made with the A scan downward to represent the transducer on the left side of the head (Fig. 3-8). By comparison of the echoencephalogram with the transducer on the right and left side of the head, midline echoencephalography may be performed.

A series of illustrations represents the steps in performing standard echoencephalography with the ABC coordinate system. The transducer will have reverberations with higher gain settings and produce multiple echoes that appear as an artifact called a transducer ring (Fig. 3-9). Since a part of the sonic energy is returned from each interface, a smaller amount of energy is then transmitted through the next interface. This requires an internal electronic setting (compensated gain) so that the echoes will appear to be similar in amplitude although the amount of returned sonic

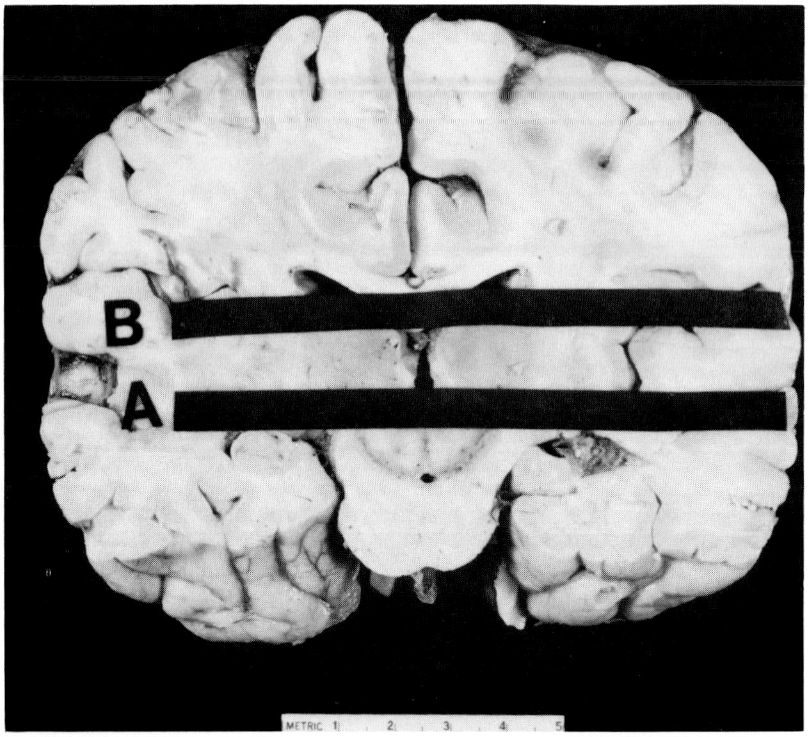

Fig. 3-6. The average sonic beam is illustrated in positions *A* and *B*.

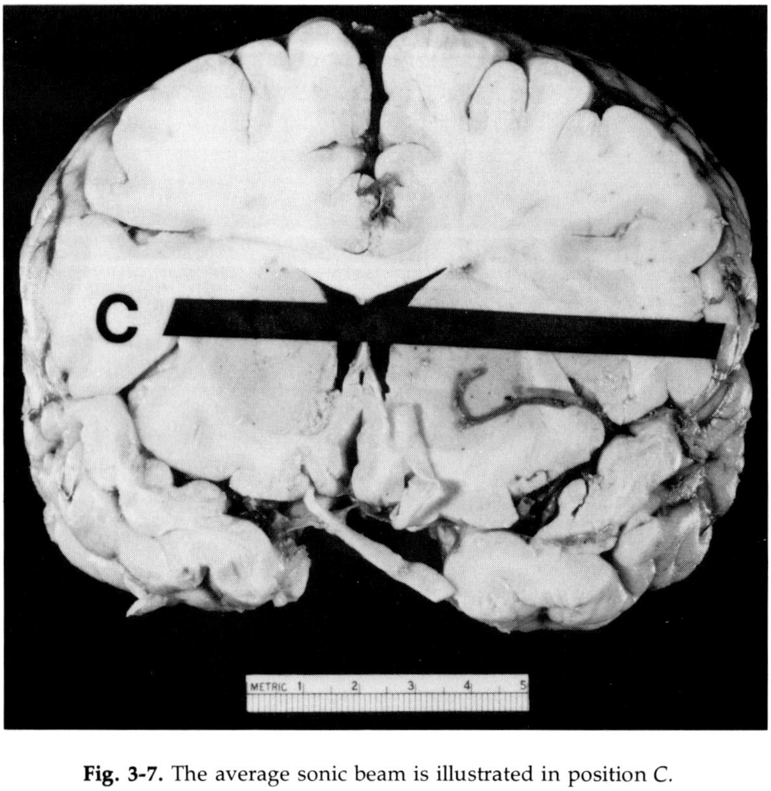

Fig. 3-7. The average sonic beam is illustrated in position *C*.

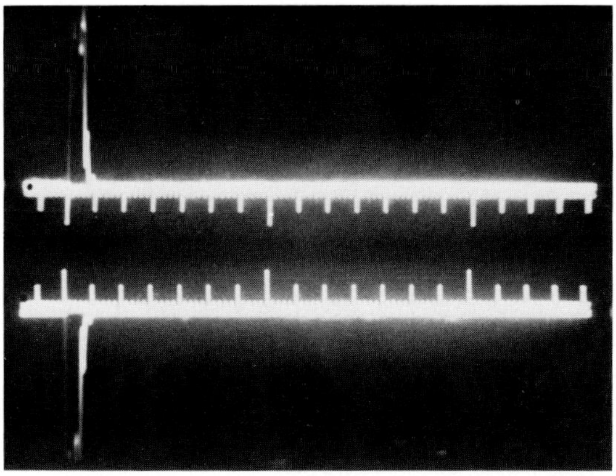

Fig. 3-8. Echoencephalograms are recorded by double exposure on Polaroid film. The top trace represents the transducer at the right side of the head. The lower trace is inverted and represents the transducer at the left side of the head.

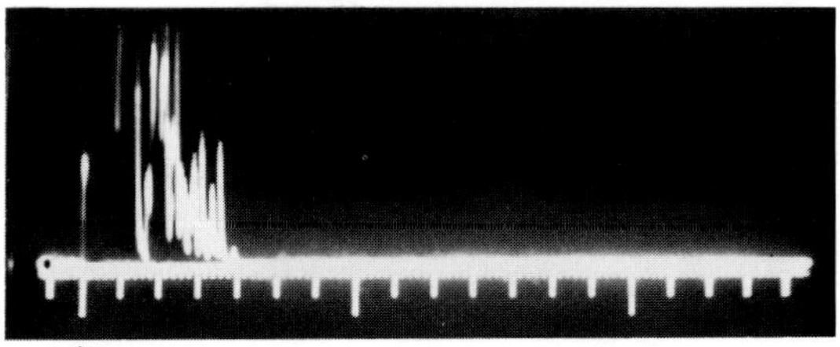

Fig. 3-9. The gain has been increased to demonstrate the transducer ring with multiple echoes from the transducer.

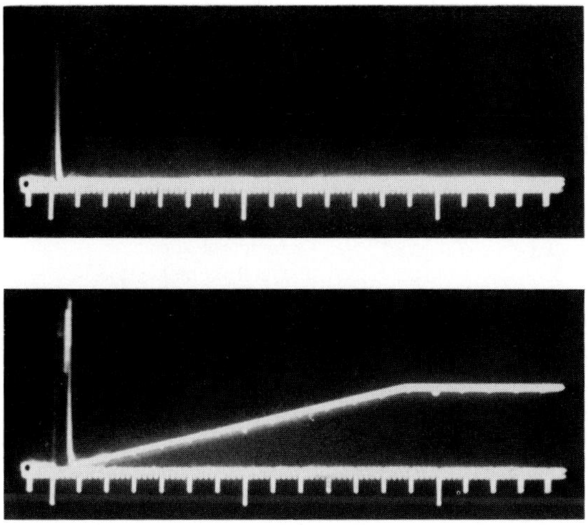

Fig. 3-10. The setting is now with the transducer at the right side of the head. The compensated gain is illustrated with gradual increase and gain setting with depth and tissue.

energy is less. This appears as a sloping line that represents the increase in decibels at various distances (Fig. 3-10). When coupling media are applied, artifacts are produced with multiple reverberations of the sound beam at the coupling gel surface (Fig. 3-11).

It is essential to identify internal echoencephalographic landmarks in a systematic method. The primary landmarks are illustrated (Fig. 3-12). In normal patients, these internal landmarks may be readily identified. However, when a pathologic condition exists, it will become more difficult, and in some cases impossible, to identify any of the internal landmarks. The following description and illustrations of positions A, B, and C are given in a step-

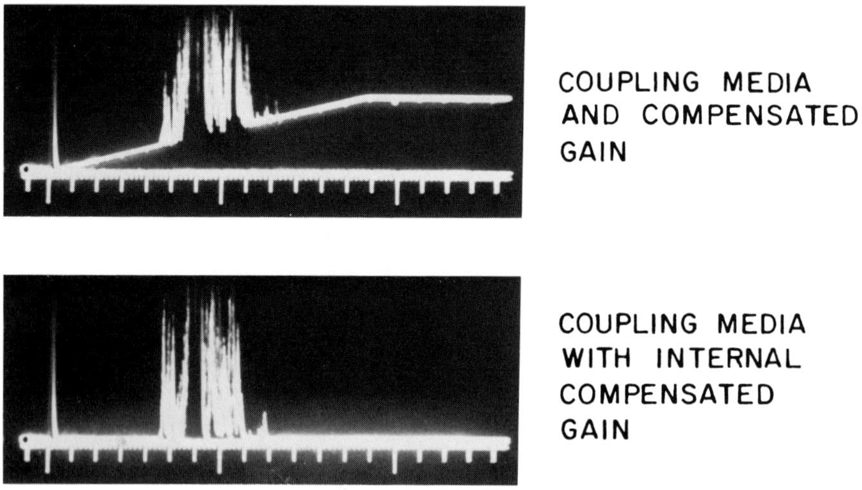

Fig. 3-11. Coupling gel is applied to the transducer with compensated gain illustrated. The compensated gain is still being used to process the signal; however, it is not identified on the trace because of an internal electronic control.

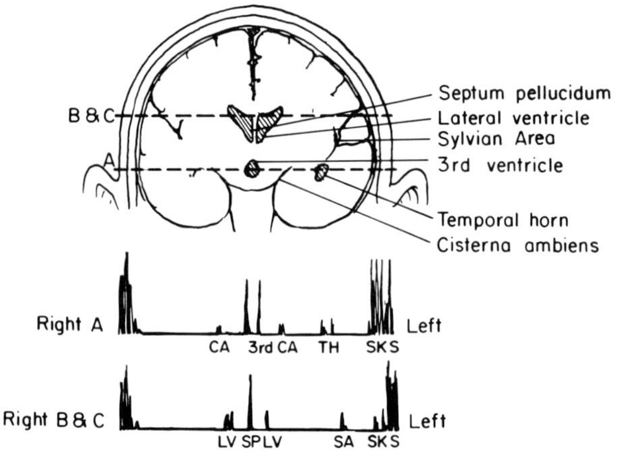

Fig. 3-12. Primary internal landmarks. *SP,* Septum pellucidum; *LV,* lateral ventricle; *SA,* sylvian area; *3rd,* third ventricle; *TH,* temporal horn; *CA,* cisterna ambiens; *SK,* skull inner and outer table; *s,* skin.

wise presentation as a method for examination and viewing of the oscilloscope.

Position A. The transducer is placed at the right side of the head with coupling gel in position A. By regulation of gain controls, various internal landmarks may be identified (Fig. 3-13). By increasing the gain, the transducer ring and echoes from reverberations of the hair, air, and subcutaneous tissues may be obtained in the first 3 to 4 cm on the oscilloscope. With low gain controls, the inner and outer tables of the skull as well as the skin surface may be identified. The skin surface may be easily identified by simple tapping on the opposite side of the skull to determine the exact location of this area. The skull thickness as well as the distance from the outer table of the skull to the skin surface may be measured. By increasing the gain control, both walls of the third ventricle may be identified. These are shown, in Fig. 3-13 at 7.2 and 7.6 cm. The skull and skin echoes have been increased with increasing gain. By a steady increase in the gain and by a slight rocking of the transducer, the cisterna ambiens and temporal horn echoes may be identified. It should be recognized that at high gain these echoes may be seen as a composite; however, their specific identity and direct measurement may be more difficult without alteration of the gain controls. With experience, the examiner may readily identify these internal landmarks in the normal case. In general, the cisterna ambiens will lie 12 to 16 mm lateral to the anatomic midline of the third ventricle and the temporal horn echoes at approximately 2 cm from the inner table of the skull.

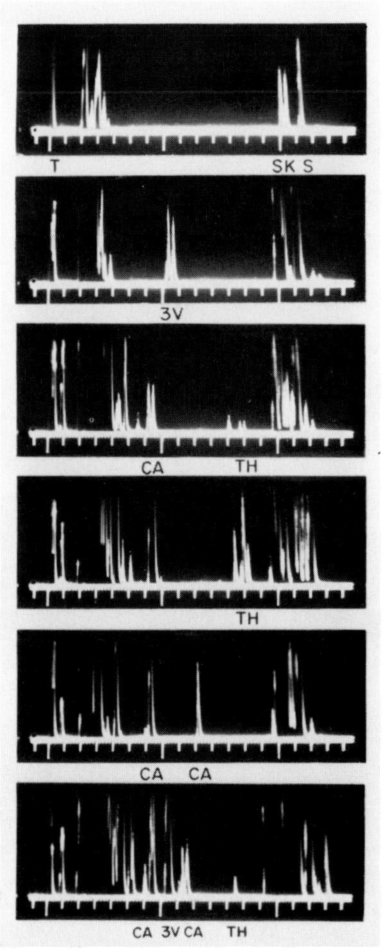

Fig. 3-13. Identification of internal landmarks in the A position. *T*, Transducer; *SK*, skull; *S*, skin; *3V*, third ventricle; *CA*, cisterna ambiens; *TH*, temporal horn.

Position B. The transducer is placed in position B with changes in gain control as in position A. The skull, inner and outer tables, and skin echoes are identified. By increasing the gain, the septum pellucidum may be identified. Since the septum pellucidum is a rather large structure, identification is more easily accomplished by anterior-posterior rocking of the transducer and cephalad and caudad rocking. The septum presents the most perpendicular surface with this technique and can be separated from ventricular echoes. By increasing the gain, small lateral ventricular echoes may be obtained (Fig. 3-14). However, in normal patients the angulation of the ventricles may be such that identification of lateral ventricular echoes will be difficult. As the ventricles enlarge, these echoes are more easily obtained. The sylvian area is identified by angulation of the transducer toward the opposite ear. Echoes will be obtained approximately 2 cm inside the inner table, and with careful examination pulsations may be seen from the middle cerebral artery and surrounding sylvian area.

Position C. This position is more frontal and the curvature of the skull as well as thickness of the skull make it more difficult to obtain. The skull surface distal to the transducer is more irregular and lining up the far wall of the skull is more difficult. The position can be obtained, however, in a high percentage of patients. It is particularly important for detection of frontal lobe lesions when there is no shift in A and B positions. With experience the number of studies obtained in this area will markedly increase. The internal landmarks are again obtained by rocking the transducer and by variations of the gain control (Fig. 3 15). In this position, the sylvian area is usually more easily obtained. These echoes will have pulsation and are seen approximately 2 to 2.5 cm from the inner table of the skull.

It has been found with experience that if one position is difficult to obtain, the movement of the transducer to an intermediate position between A and B or between B and C may help to identify internal structures. With variations in skull symmetry and certain abnormalities, the falx cerebri may be obtained in the B and C positions. When this occurs along with a shift, the

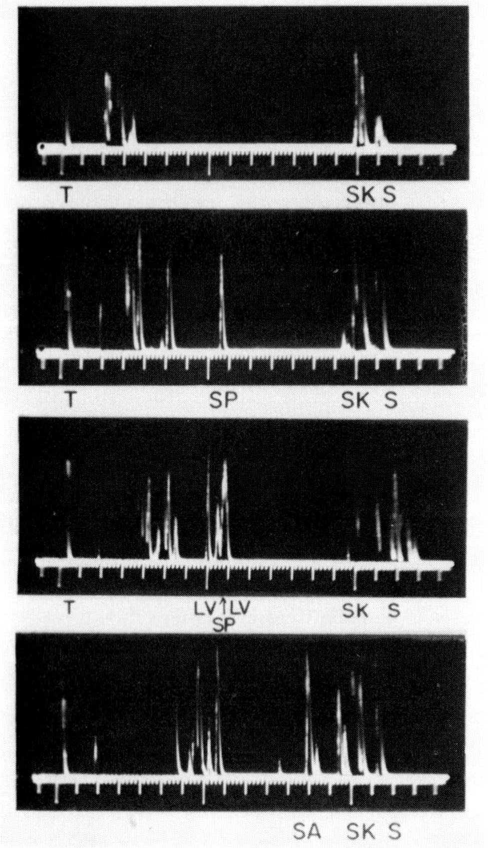

Fig. 3-14. Identification of internal landmarks in the B position. *T,* Transducer; *SK,* skull; *S,* skin; *SP,* septum pellucidum; *LV,* lateral ventricle; *SA,* sylvian area.

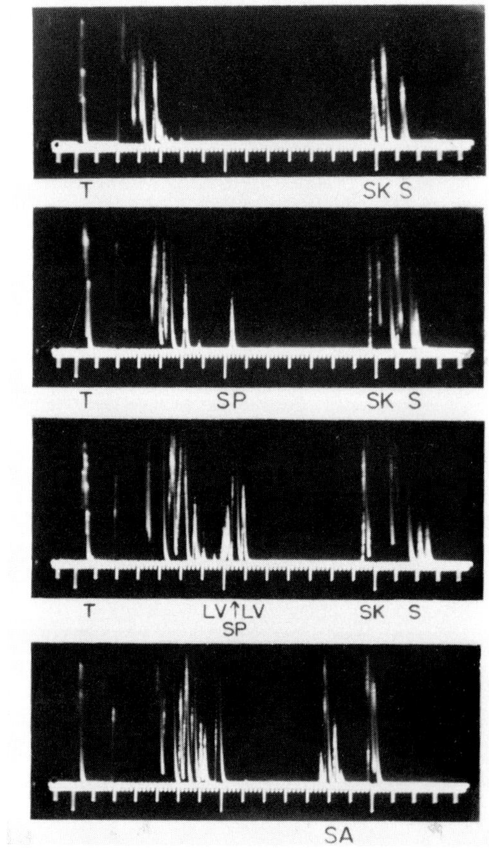

Fig. 3-15. Identification of internal landmarks in the C position. *T,* Transducer; *SK,* skull; *S,* skin; *SP,* septum pellucidum; *LV,* lateral ventricle; and *SA,* sylvian area.

falx may be used as an internal landmark while the shift beneath the falx indicates the presence of pathology.

The method presented for obtaining echoencephalograms at standard positions and for identifying internal landmarks provides an easy framework for standardization and interpretation of the procedure.

INTERPRETATIONS OF ECHOENCEPHALOGRAMS

The permanent Polaroid record obtained in all three positions is inspected. More than one photograph may be necessary in any position to readily identify internal landmarks. These are numbered A1, A2, and so on. This allows the interpreter to understand the order in which the photographs were taken to assist him to identify landmarks. A rapid inspection of these positions will give the interpreter an overall view of internal structure for further analysis. Echoes in the far field (from midline to far wall inner table) provide an indication of gain settings and alignment of the far wall inner table echoes of the skull. The far wall echoes should be aligned within 5 mm, the upper limit of normal. It is preferable to have these aligned within 1 to 2 mm from the right and left sides in a final picture. The position of all internal landmarks should be noted during the initial inspection. Unusual echoes that may occur should also be noted. Fig. 3-16 shows anatomic structures or features and technical problems that should be noted for each examination.

Echoencephalographic measurements of these internal landmarks are of great value in clinical diagnosis. The measurements are made along the baseline in range, or depth. Standard echoencephalographic equipment is calibrated in centimeters and millimeters. The measurements should be made at the initial break from the baseline and not from the peak of the echo signal. By measuring the peak of the echo, an error of several millimeters may be introduced. The initial point of measurement is extremely important since small errors may be significant and lead to a false interpretation. If two echoes are superimposed, extrapolation of the echo should be done in order to determine the position of the break from the baseline. Measurement to the closest millimeter should be accomplished, and if there is any doubt, the smaller measurement should be used. For example, 7.55 mm should be read as 7.5 mm in order to have a standard error.

The internal landmarks are then measured. The third ventricle is measured from its near wall to its far wall. The anatomic midline will be half the distance between the two walls of the ventricle. It must be stressed that echoes from both walls of the third ventricle must be present on the film. The mantle index may be measured from the ventricular wall to the surface of the skull in a comparison to the total distance from midline. In general, the measurement is made from the transducer to all internal landmarks. However, with extracranial swelling, internal measurement may be made from the closest measurement of the inner table of the far wall of the skull. This measurement has been suggested by other authors as a standard way of measurement; however, there are inherent errors caused by the irregularity of the skull that may lead to difficult interpretation. It must be remembered that skull shape and size vary considerably. External landmarks on the skin do not always correlate with internal brain structure. For this reason the transducer may have to be moved to a slightly different position from that externally marked in order to obtain internal landmarks. When this is done, the examiner must note the position in reference to standard positions so that the interpreter may make a proper reading.

Although various authors differ in normal values, the following has been useful in day-to-day interpretation of echoencephalograms with a high reliability. In adults, the third ventricle should not measure greater than 10 mm, with 8 to 10 mm a borderline range. In children, the upper limit of normal for the third ventricle is 6 mm. The lateral ventricular echo should not be greater than 20 mm from the septum pellucidum, with 18 to 20 cm in a suspected category.

Patient____________________

Date______________ Time_______

Location___________ Tech._______

MIDLINE

Position	Right	Left	Shift
A			
B			
C			

INTERNAL FEATURES NOTED:	Check Here	
Enlarged third ventricle		
Cisterna ambiens		
Sylvian area		
Lateral ventricular wall		
Epidural echo		
Flutter of septum pellucidum		
Pulsation		
Lateral movement		
Unusual echoes (i.e., tumor)		

TECHNICAL DIFFICULTIES NOTED:	Check Here	
Uncooperative patient		
Skull thickness		
Numerous echoes at midline		
Unable to transmit through one side		
Equipment		
Insufficient cranial asymmetry		

REMARKS:

Fig. 3-16. Form showing anatomic structures or features and technical problems that should be noted for each examination.

APPLICATIONS

Indications for echoencephalography

There are a number of indications for echoencephalography, as follows:

Fetal head size
Newborn
Rapid head size growth
Mental retardation
Head injury
Psychiatric disorder
Seizure disorder
Cerebrovascular disease
Suspected tumor
Brain death
Space-occupying lesion
Follow-up examinations

The determination of fetal head size has proved to be of great value in determining the fetal age. In the newborn, the detection of brain injury with hemorrhage is a rapid and easily performed procedure. In children, the rapid growth of head size may be frequently associated with dilation of the ventricles. An atraumatic method for following this ventricular enlargement is quite valuable. Mental retardation is a major problem affecting approximately 3% of the population. The detection of midline shift and ventricular enlargement may lead to prompt and proper therapy in these cases. The evaluation of epidural and subdural hematoma as well as swelling with edema in head injury is of utmost importance. It is well known that neurologic disorder may result in a psychiatric disturbance.

Rapid screening of psychiatric patients is available by echoencephalography for the recognition of neurologic problems. The incidence in mental populations of dementia caused by normal pressure hydrocephalus is as yet unknown. The detection of enlarged ventricles in dementia may lead to a satisfactory diagnosis and treatment. In seizure disorders, the use of echoencephalography may be well correlated with an electroencephalogram. The expanding lesions may be found in follow-up examinations.

A major use of echoencephalography is in the diagnosis and treatment of cerebrovascular disease. Rapid discovery of expanding lesions or edema may lead to proper treatment. Follow-up examinations may be used to document the effects of treatment. The development of hydrocephalus following subarachnoid hemorrhage is an indication for use of echoencephalography. Although other studies may be used for suspected tumors, echoencephalography may detect a space-occupying lesion that would not be known without contrast procedures.

Space-occupying lesions

Intracranial space-occupying lesions may result from tumor, edema, intracerebral hematoma, cysts, arteriovenous malformation, and subdural or epidural hematoma (Fig. 3-17). Space-occupying lesions will shift the midline in one, two, or all three positions, depending on the area and size of the lesion. By a comparison of the A, B, and C position shifts, the location of the lesion may be determined (Fig. 3-18). The upper limit of normal for midline echo displacement is 3 mm. A very high correlation with pathologic conditions is obtained in the presence of a shift greater than this.

Posterior fossa lesions, bilateral equal size subdural hematoma in the frontal

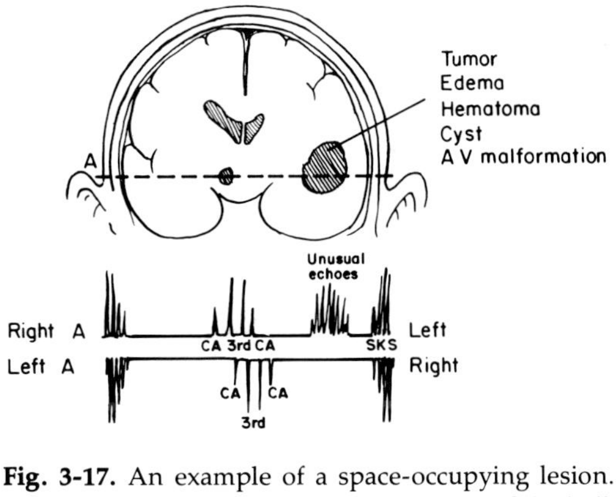

Fig. 3-17. An example of a space-occupying lesion. *CA,* Cisterna ambiens; *3rd,* third ventricle; *SK,* skull; *S,* skin.

area, and some temporal and occipital lesions may exist without shift of the midline and represent limitations to this technique as a screening measure. Because of the change in density of abnormal tissue, unusual echoes may be obtained if tumors are in the path of the sonic beam. These unusual echoes are seen in the far field from midline to inner table. They should not be confused with markedly enlarged ventricles, temporal horn echoes, or echoes from the sylvian area. The echoes are much more prominent with calcification of certain types of tumors. In arteriovenous malformations they may have a markedly pulsatile character.

It is not possible to identify the type of pathologic condition on the basis of unusual echoes using simple A-scan techniques. Deep brain hemorrhages may give rise to unusual echoes at or near midline, making identification of midline structures quite difficult (Fig. 3-19). In some cases, however, the unusual echoes will be helpful in a diagnosis.

Since changes of density cause a reflection of sound, gain settings must be increased in these areas in order to obtain echoes from structures more distant to the transducer. There may be a shielding or shadow effect of these echoes, making landmarks distal to the transducer from the abnormal echoes difficult to obtain.

Although initial reports stated that subdural echoes were easy to obtain, this is not the case. The subdural hematoma interface must be in the path of the sonic beam and perpendicular to it for return of the echo. In acute subdural hematoma, the interface may not be in the proper posi-

A

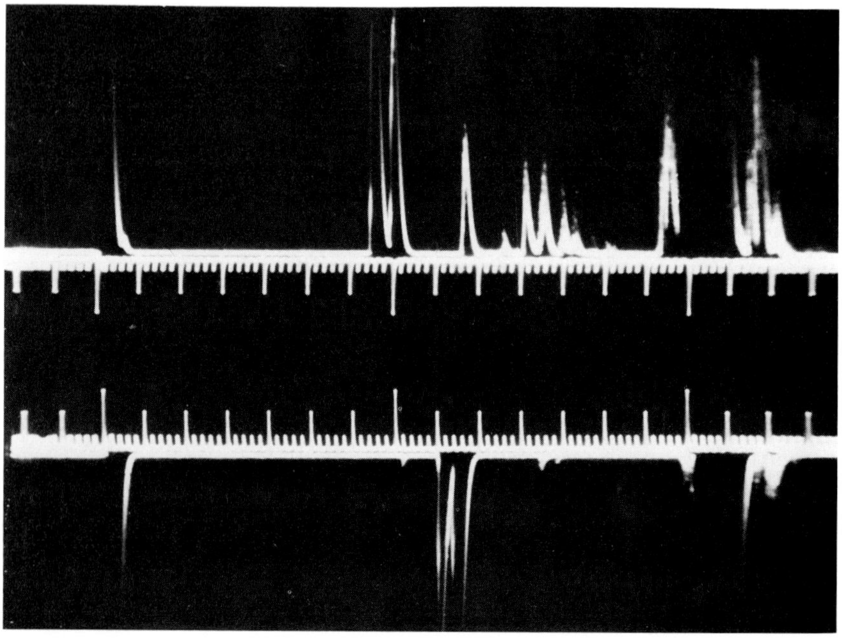

Fig. 3-18. A, In the A position, the third ventricle is identified easily 6.7 cm from the right and 8.2 cm from the left with a shift of 7.5 mm from left to right. Unusual echoes are noted in the left hemisphere. **B,** The septum pellucidum in the B position measures 6.4 cm from the right and 7.5 cm from the left with a shift of 5.5 mm from left to right. **C,** The septum pellucidum in the C position measures 6.4 cm and 7.2 cm with a shift of 4 mm from left to right. Unusual echoes are noted in the left hemisphere.

tion to obtain this echo (Fig. 3-20). In chronic subdural hematoma, however, a more definite interface may be obtained because of the formation of the membrane. The subdural hematoma may also act as an unusual echo and shield the echo from the far wall of the skull, making increased gain necessary. The primary criteria for diagno-

B

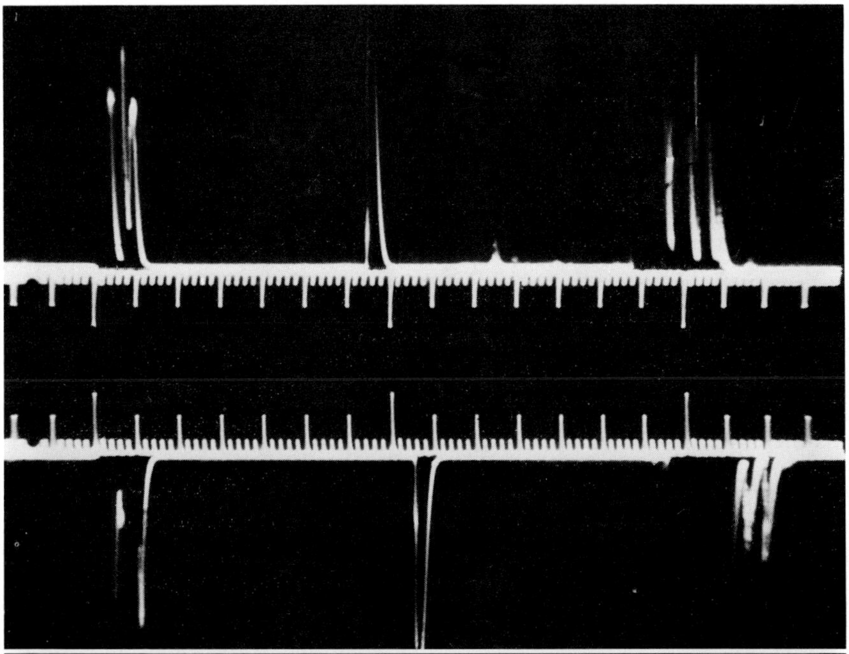

C

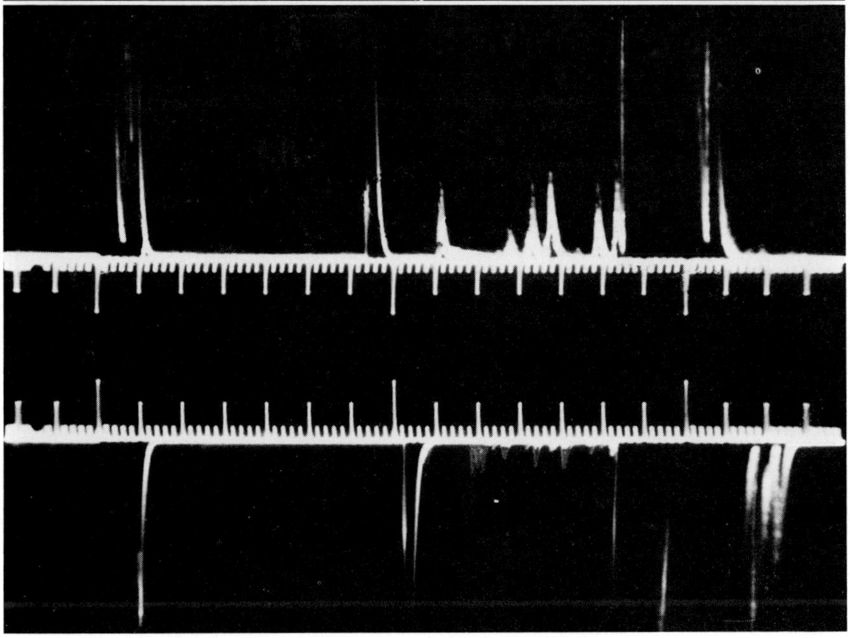

Fig. 3-18, cont'd. For legend see opposite page.

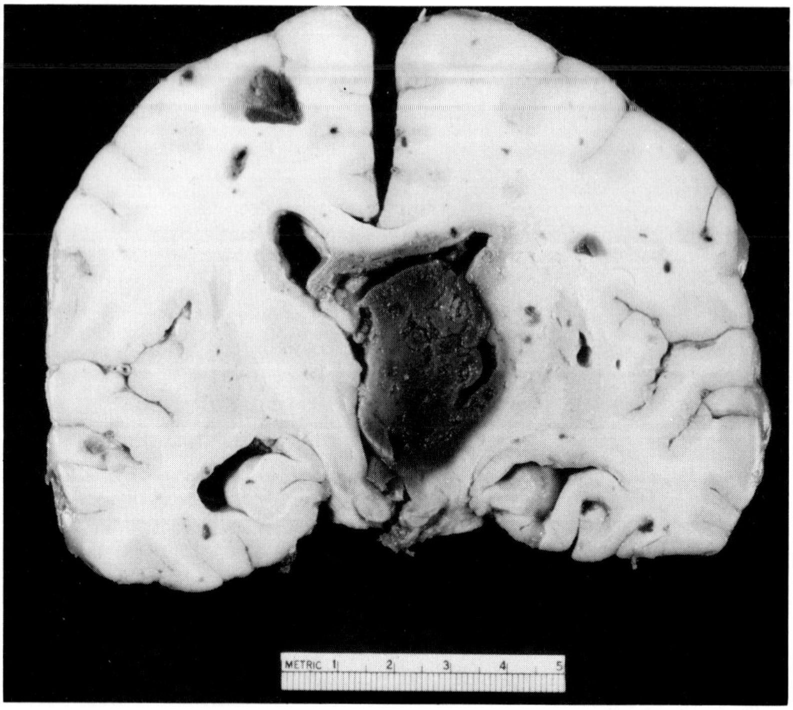

Fig. 3-19. An example of a deep space-occupying lesion.

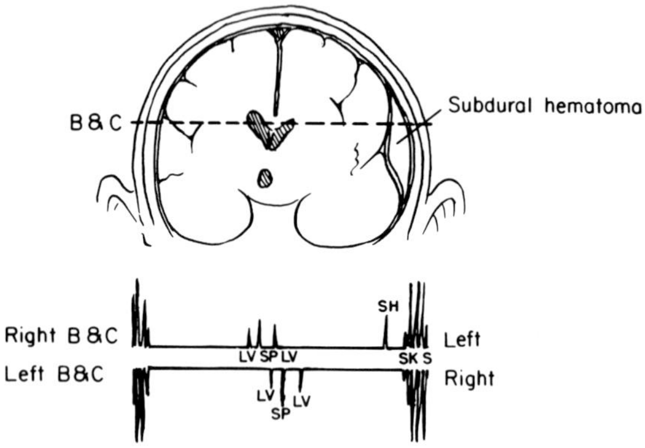

Fig. 3-20. A subdural hematoma with the criteria of subdural echo and shifted midline.

sis of a subdural hematoma include a shift of the midline, the subdural echo, and increased gain needed through the area of the subdural hematoma for identification of internal landmarks. Epidural hematomas are quite similar in their criteria.

Following removal of a subdural hematoma, the brain may or may not reexpand. The reexpansion may be followed by repeated studies with echoencephalography. When head injury occurs, the transducer may be used to scan the inner table of the skull to look for unusual echoes that may represent subdural hematomas. It must be emphasized that confusion with normal landmarks from the sylvian area and temporal horn may result.

Ventricular measurements

Measurement of the third and lateral ventricular size by echoencephalography has developed into a screening technique for hydrocephalus in children and, more recently, in the adult for the detection of normal pressure hydrocephalus and atrophy. Measurements can also be made on patients before and after shunt procedures. Detection of ventricular size becomes easier

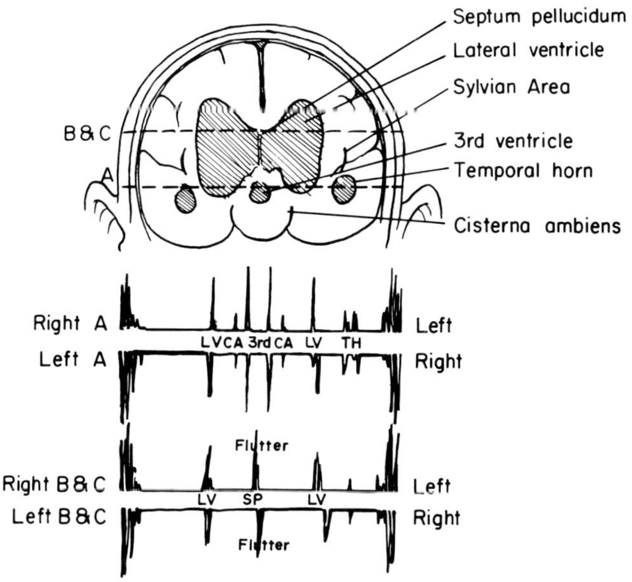

Fig. 3-21. The ventricles are enlarged, presenting a more perpendicular surface.

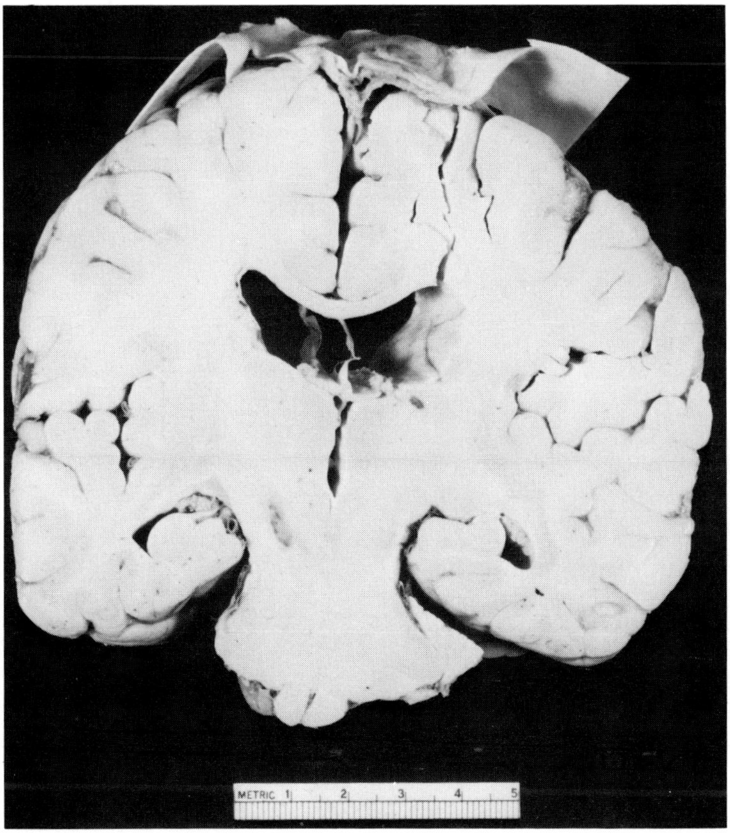

Fig. 3-22. A flutter type echo may be seen with a tear in the septum pellucidum.

as the ventricles dilate, presenting a more perpendicular surface to the sonic beam. In the A position, large ventricles may be seen because of their increased size (Fig. 3-21). Internal landmarks must also be identified in this case in order to avoid confusion of the sylvian area and temporal horn with enlarged ventricular echoes. Careful examination of the septum pellucidum by moving the transducer in a direction from B to C position may reveal a most unusual echo that has a characteristic fluttering. This is thought to be caused by a tear in the septum pellucidum as a result of stretching of the ventricular walls (Fig. 3-22). On occasion, a flutter may be seen at the lateral walls of the lateral ventricles. This may result from the forces on the wall from blood pulsation. The flutter is generally three to five movements per cardiac cycle. If measured carefully, all structures within the brain have movement with the cardiac cycle. When the ventricles are enlarged, a brief inspection of the echoencephalograms from all three positions will provide an unmistakable indication of this (Fig. 3-23).

RELIABILITY

The reliability of echoencephalography depends upon inherent limitations of the technique, the skill of the examiner, and adequacy of interpretation. There is definitely a skill requirement that is based on the motor skill of the examiner. Slight changes in transducer angulation may produce major changes in the reflected echo patterns. Although many attempts have been made to standardize equipment for the examination, this motor skill continues to be the best method for identification of internal landmarks.

There are many investigations of the reliability of echoencephalography reporting

A

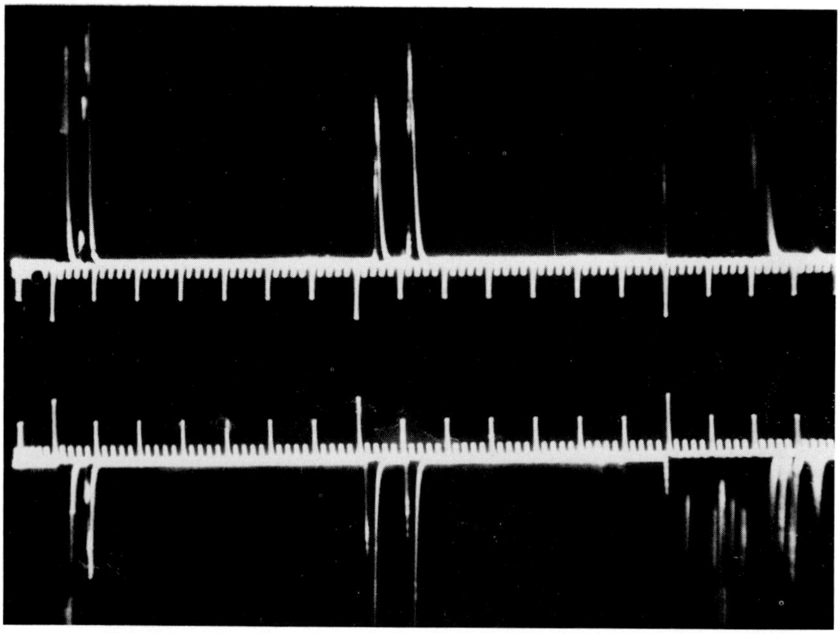

Fig. 3-23. A, The third ventricle is easily identified. **B,** The lateral ventricles are easily identified. **C,** The lateral ventricle measures 24 mm from the septum pellucidum. The C position far walls do not line up, making the midline appear shifted. A flutter was observed between the B and C position.

good correlation with radiographic procedures. Inherent problems exist in knowing exactly the area of measurement for correlation. In addition, many studies that report correlation have only studied one area of the brain without a standardized technique. It is generally accepted that the procedure is approximately 95% accurate. When used in conjunction with other studies, the echoencephalogram is a valuable

B

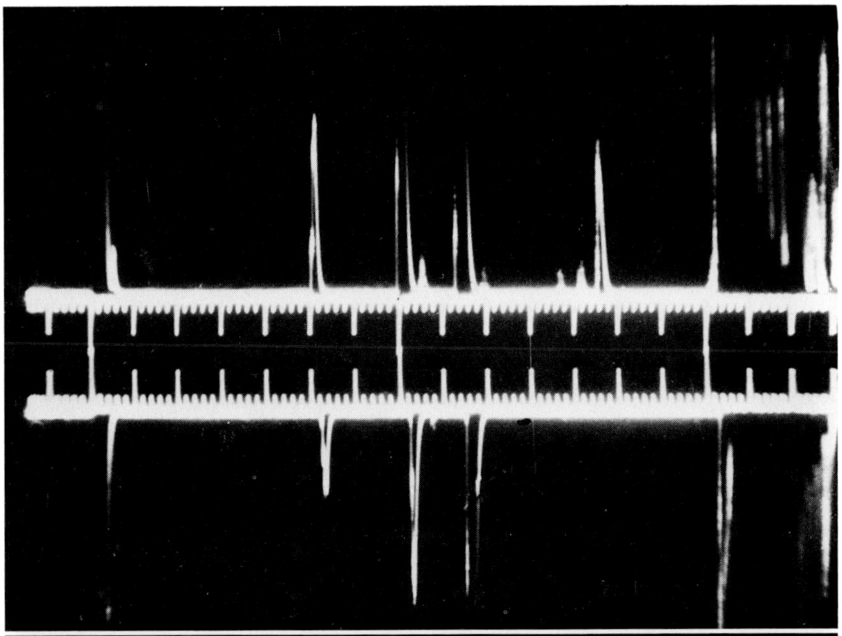

C

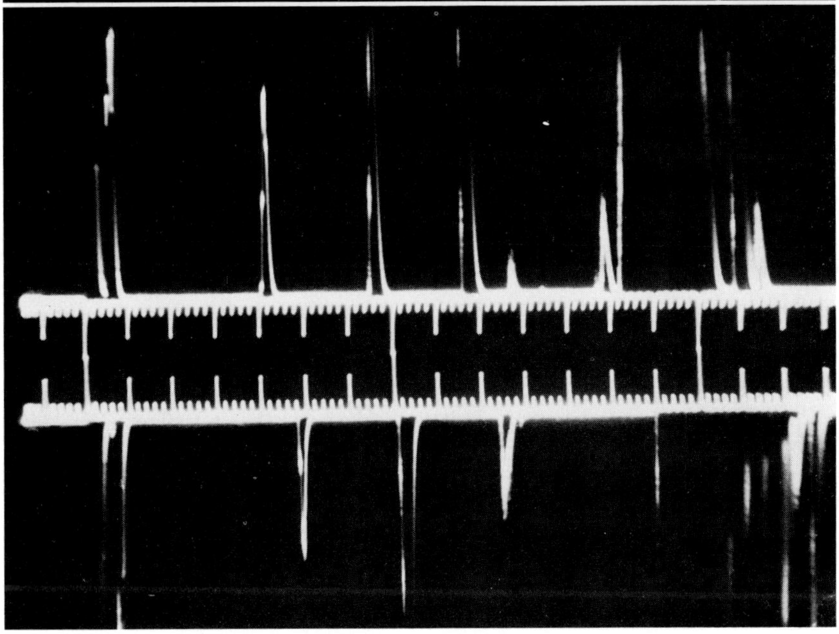

Fig. 3-23, cont'd. For legend see opposite page.

aid for the detection of space-occupying lesions and ventricular dilation. It has particular value since demonstration of atrophy on one side of the brain, when correlated with an electroencephalogram, will avoid a contrast study. A midline shift from the direction of a space-occupying lesion with a lateralized electroencephalogram may be considered an indication for contrast studies. Reliability of echoencephalography in acute trauma cases is more difficult to measure since the patient's condition may be changing rapidly after the time of the examination and extracranial lesions may make the examination difficult. Follow-up examinations are extremely important in cases of head trauma and suspected expanding lesions.

SUMMARY

This chapter presents a standardized method of performing echoencephalography. The reader is referred to selected references for additional study. Echoencephalography has become a valuable and useful technique in the detection and management of brain disease and promises to expand man's knowledge in the future.

Acknowledgments

My sincere appreciation is expressed to the large number of students, residents, physicians, and investigators who have contributed to this work. Specific appreciation to Mrs. Vera Biddix who typed the manuscript, Mrs. Patricia Nuss, Chief Sonographer, Mr. George Lynch of Audiovisual, and to members of the Sonic Laboratory staff.

REFERENCES

1. Leksell, L.: Kirurgisk behandling av akuta skallskador, Nord. Med. **54:**1444, 1955.
2. Leksell, L.: Echoencephalography; detection of intracranial complications following head injury, Acta Chir. Scand. **110:**301-315, 1956.
3. Leksell, L.: Echoencephalography. II. Midline echo from pineal body as an index of pineal displacement, Acta Chir. Scand. **115:**255-259, 1958.
4. de Vlieger, M., and Ridder, H. J.: Use of echoencephalography, Neurology **1:**216-259, 1959.
5. Lithander, B.: Control method for echoencephalography, Acta Psychiatr. Neurol. Scan. **35:**235-240, 1960.
6. Lithander, B.: Clinical use of echoencephalography, Acta Psychiatr. Scand. **35:**241-244, 1960.
7. Jeppson, S.: Echoencephalography. IV. The midline echo; an evaluation of its usefulness for diagnosing intracranial expansivities and an investigation into its source, Acta Chir. Scand., Suppl. 272, pp. 1-151, 1961.
8. Lithander, B.: Clinical and experimental studies in echo-encephalography, Acta Psychiatr. Scand., Suppl. 159, pp. 1-53, 1961.
9. Taylor, J. C., Newell, J. A., and Karvounis, P.: Ultrasonics in diagnosis of intracranial space-occupying lesions, Lancet **1:**1197-1199, 1961.
10. Jefferson, A.: Clinical experiences with echoencephalography, Acta Neurochir. **10:**392-409, 1962.
11. Ford, R., and Ambrose, J.: Echoencephalography; measurement of position of midline structures in skull with high frequency pulsed ultrasound, Brain **86:**189-196, 1963.
12. Brinker, R. A., King, D. L., and Taveras, J. M.: Echoencephalography, Am. J. Roentgenol. **93:**781-790, 1965.
13. Kazner, E., Schiefer, W., and Zulch, K. S.: Proceedings in echoencephalography, New York, 1968, Springer-Verlag.
14. Grossman, C. C.: The use of diagnostic ultrasound in brain disorders, Springfield, Ill., 1966, Charles C Thomas, Publisher.
15. White, D. N.: Ultrasonic encephalography, Basel, 1971, Schwabe & Co.
16. Ford, R., and MacRae, D. L.: Echoencephalography—standardized technique for the measurement of the width of the third and lateral ventricles. In Grossman, C. C., and others, editors: Diagnostic ultrasound, New York, 1966, Plenum Press, pp. 117-129.

ADDITIONAL READINGS

Avant, W. S., Jr.: Pulsatile echoencephalography, Neurology **16:**1033-1040, 1966.

Barrows, H. S., Dyck, P., and Kurse, T.: The diagnostic application of ultrasound in neurologic disease: the intracerebral midline, Neurology **15:**361-365, 1965.

Brownhill, D.: The clinical value of echoencephalography, Aust. N. Z. J. Surg. **48:**74-78, 1970.

Campbell, J. K., and others: Ultrasonic studies of brain movements, Neurology **20:**418, 1970.

Campbell, J. K., and others: Pulsatile echoencephalography, Acta Neurol. Scand. **45**(Suppl.):1-57, 1970.

Clarke, L. G.: Brain midline structure position in mentally handicapped subjects measured by ultrasonic echoencephalography, Am. J. Ment. Defic. **74:**594-598, 1970.

Cristian, C., Constantinovici, A., and Arseni, C.: Echoencephalography (echo), and EEG in craniocerebral injuries, E.E.G. Clin. Neurophysiol. **30:**359-360, 1971.

de Vlieger, M.: Evolution of echoencephalography in neurology—a review, Ultrasonics **5:**91-97, 1967.

de Vlieger, M., ter Braak, J. W. G., and Scandia, W. A. M.: Echoencephalography as an aid in the diagnosis of subdural and extradural hematomas. In Biemond, A., editor: Recent neurological research, New York, 1959, American Elsevier Publishing Co., pp. 37-45.

de Vlieger, M., and others: Movements of cerebral structures, E.E.G. Clin. Neurophysiol. **29:**319-320, 1970.

de Vlieger, M., and others: Cerebral echopulsations in cardiac arrhythmia, Psychiatr. Neurol. Neurochir. **74:**279-289, 1971.

de Vlieger, M., and Parys, J. A.: EEG paroxysms and echoencephalography, Epilepsia **13:**813-817, 1972.

Fernandez, H., McKinney, W. M., and Spudis, E. V.: Pulsatile echoencephalography: correlations with k-complexes and epileptic discharges, Neurology **21:**225-231, 1971.

Galicich, J. H., and Williams, J. B.: A computerized echoencephalograph, J. Neurosurg. **35:**453-460, 1971.

Gordon, D.: Echoencephalography; ultrasonic rays in diagnostic radiology, Br. Med. J. **1:**1500-1504, 1959.

Hagberg, B., and Naglo, A. S.: The conservative management of infantile hydrocephalus, Paediatr. Scand. **61:**165-177, 1972.

Heimburger, R. F., Eggleton, R. C., and Fry, F. J.: Ultrasonic visualization in determination of tumor growth rate, J.A.M.A. **224:**497-581, 1973.

Jeppson, S.: Echoencephalography. V. A method for recording the intracranial pressure with the aid of the echoencephalographic technique; a preliminary report, Acta Chir. Scand. **128:**218-224, 1964.

Kazner, E.: Echoencephalography with simultaneous A and B mode display, J. Neurol. Neurosurg. Psychiatr. **33:**718, 1970.

Kienast, H. W., and Boshes, L. D.: The values, limitations and future of echoencephalography, Behau Neuropsychiatr. **3:**2-4, 1971.

Kossoff, G., and Garrett, W. J.: Intracranial detail in fetal echograms, Invest. Radiol. **7:**159-163, 1972.

Kurze, T., Small, R. B., and Rumbaugh, C. L.: Diagnostic concepts of cerebral injuries, Clin. Neurosurg. **19:**220-239, 1972.

Lapayowker, M. S., and Christen, G. E.: Echoencephalography in general hospital practice, Am. J. Roentgenol. **93:**803-810, 1965.

Lindsay, K. W.: Echoencephalography—an evaluation in general medical wards, Scot. Med. J. **17:**130-139, 1972.

McKinney, W. M.: The value of B-mode determination of midline in echoencephalography, Neurology **14:**259, 1964.

McKinney, W. M.: Echoencephalography. In Toole, J. F., editor: Special techniques for neurologic diagnosis, Philadelphia, 1969, F. A. Davis Co.

McKinney, W. M., and others: Evaluation of five hundred psychiatric in-patients by midline echoencephalography, Acta Radiol. **5:**865-870, 1966.

Mostafawy, A.: Pediatric sonoencephalography, New York, 1971, Springer-Verlag.

Pia, H. W., and Geletneky, C. L.: Echoenzephalgraphic, Stuttgart, 1968, Georg Thieme Verlag.

Pin, C., and Fournet, A.: Study of ultrasound displacement in cases of recent cranial trauma: comparisons with the EEG data, E.E.G. Clin. Neurophysiol. **29:**529, 1970.

Reese, C. L.: Two dimensional echoencephalography: a clinical study, Neurology **20:**417-418, 1970.

Reiwer, J., Karnes, W. E., and Sandok, B. A.: Intracranial midline echo shift and width, Mayo Clin. Proc. **46:**593-596, 1971.

Sandok, B. A.: A-mode echoencephalography in the evaluation of cerebrovascular disease, Stroke **2:**452-455, 1971.

Sandok, B. A., Henson, T. E., and Skaggs, H., Jr.: Analysis of echoencephalograms: an evaluation of interpreter consistency, Neurology **20:**933-938, 1970.

Schiefer, W., Kazner, E., and Kunze, S.: Clinical echo-encephalography, New York, 1968, Springer-Verlag.

Schlagenhauff, R. E., and Mazurowski, J.: Ultrasonic measurement of cerebral ventricular system: a critical and comparative study of echoencephalographic and pneumoencephalographic determinations in 100 patients, Neurology **21:**1134-1139, 1971.

Sjogren, I.: Echo-ventriculography in infantile hydrocephalus: preliminary report, Acta Neurol. Scand. **41**(Suppl.):13:13-18, 1965.

Sugar, O., and Uematsu, S.: The use of ultrasound in the diagnosis of intracranial lesions, Surg. Clin. North. Am. **44:**55-64, 1964.

Tanaka, K.: Diagnosis of brain disease by ultrasound, Tokyo, 1968, Shindan-To-Chiryo, Sha Co., Ltd.

Uematsu, S., and Walker, A. E.: A manual of echoencephalography, Baltimore, 1971, The Williams & Wilkins Co.

Wealthall, S. R., and Todd, J. H.: Ultrasonic B-scans in the diagnosis and assessment of hydrocephalus in infants, Br. J. Radiol. **46:**566, 1973.

White, D. N.: Ultrasonic encephalography, Neurology **20:**419, 1970.

White, D. N., and Clar, J. M.: Amplitude averaged A-scan echoencephalography of a mental hospital population, Can. Psychiatr. Assoc. J. **15:**453-460, 1970.

4 Echocardiography: contrast techniques and cardiac anatomy

RAYMOND GRAMIAK, M.D.

Inspection of an echocardiogram can be a confusing experience to an uninitiated observer because the ultrasonic record bears no resemblance to the heart itself and contains no familiar landmarks. These very difficulties led Edler[1] to compare excised and transected specimens of the heart to the distribution of echoes obtained from the specimens in order to provide an anatomic basis for structure recognition. He also used the technique of passing needles into cadavers in duplication of the ultrasonic beam path and thereby identified the mitral valve as the source of the familiar echo pattern seen in living patients. Joyner pioneered the use of intracardiac injections of saline in studies of the mitral valve but never published his technique or findings.[2]

It was the fortuitous examination of a patient in the cardiac catheterization laboratory during cardiac output studies with indocyanine green that initiated our interest in the use of intracardiac contrast agents for ultrasonography and eventually resulted in publications utilizing this technique for the identification of structures. The first of these was published in 1968, when we used contrast injections to identify the aortic root and valve cusps and to separate this portion of the heart from the left ventricular outflow tract.[3] Subsequently, a systematic study was done to validate ultrasonic cardiac chamber anatomy and to demonstrate various functional changes, including the abnormal mitral valve movement pattern seen in hypertrophic obstructive cardiomyopathy, intracardiac shunts, and aortic regurgitation.[4]

The source of the signal from the indocyanine green injection was identified by Kremkau,[5] who proved that it was the gas content of the indocyanine green solution that produced the echoes. He was also able to show that rapid catheter injections of any material produced signals, presumably bubbles arising in the blood as a result of cavitation. Since these original publications, other investigators have also used intracardiac injections of indocyanine green to verify anatomy. Feigenbaum[6] identified the components of the left ventricular wall to provide anatomic support for his studies of cardiac output. Goldberg[7] examined the heart and great vessels from a suprasternal transducer position and used the indocyanine green injection technique to validate the anatomy. By this method the innominate vein, the aortic arch, the right pulmonary artery, and the left atrium were identified lying in that order in the beam.

Hipona[8] timed the arrival of radiographic contrast material in peripheral vessels by using a rapid injection technique in the abdominal aorta and noting an ultrasonic signal when the agent arrived in the peripheral vessels. This permitted accurate timing of radiographic exposures. More recently, this useful method has been applied in our laboratory to the validation of the echocardiographic anatomy of the pulmonary valve.[9]

ULTRASONIC CONTRAST AGENTS

Intracardiac contrast echoes have been produced by two basic methods. The first requires the injection of minute amounts of gas to form microbubbles while the other forms microbubbles from the gas content of the blood as a result of cavitation stemming from rapid injection rates.

Indocyanine green has been the most effective and widely accepted agent for the delivery of minute gas volumes into the heart. Its safety has been established by extensive use for cardiac output determination. Preparation requires vigorous shaking of the dry agent and the fluid medium for solution. Sufficient gas enters solution and produces microbubbles when injected into the heart. The volume of this injected gas was estimated by allowing a typical syringe of indocyanine green to separate out its gas content by standing at atmospheric pressure. In 2 ml of dye solution (5 mg indocyanine green) the gas content was approximately 0.02 ml.[4]

The other technique that has produced successful intracardiac contrast signals involves a very rapid injection of any liquid through a catheter at rates commonly used in angiocardiography. We have injected physiologic saline, 5% dextrose in water, and the patient's own blood to produce intracardiac echoes. The source of the signal is believed to be microbubbles that have formed as a result of cavitation related to the high flow rate at the catheter tip.

In the laboratory animal hydrogen peroxide has produced an intense intracardiac signal after peripheral vein injection of 5 ml of peroxide diluted 1:10. These injections produce no recognizable deleterious effect on the animal's electrocardiogram and intracardiac pressure in a very small series of studies. Small amounts of ether have been similarly used by Ziskin,[10] who detected intense intracardiac echoes in animals following injection of small volumes. The echo source is probably related to rapid vaporization and bubble formation of the ether.

The bubbles that form in the circulation as a result of cavitation or those injected in minute amounts do not last long in the circulation. They do not recirculate following left heart injection nor can they cross the pulmonary capillary bed after intravenous injection. Left atrial contrast injection may be difficult to recognize in the aortic arch. No harmful effects have been noted in any of the patients we have studied as a result of the microbubbles that have been injected into the left heart. Other work carried out in our laboratory may indicate that similar bubbles can be generated in the heart as a result of circulatory dynamics.[11]

STUDIES OF CARDIAC ANATOMY

The introduction of intracardiac contrast agents during cardiac catheterization with simultaneous recording of the echocardiogram has proved to be an excellent technique for the validation of ultrasonic anatomy and the development of recognizable patterns that correlate with the anatomy of the heart. The fluoroscopic position of the catheter and the observation of pressure patterns has allowed definitive identification of cardiac structures. By means of this technique we have identified the mitral valve, the aortic valve, the tricuspid valve, the pulmonic valve, the cardiac chambers and septa, as well as the coronary sinus. Intracardiac shunts have been identified and valvular regurgitation studied.

Mitral valve. The mitral valve represents a landmark in the heart that has been well identified by other methods as well as by contrast injections. It is usually located by a left parasternal transducer position with the beam directed posteriorly or slightly medially. Its deep position in the

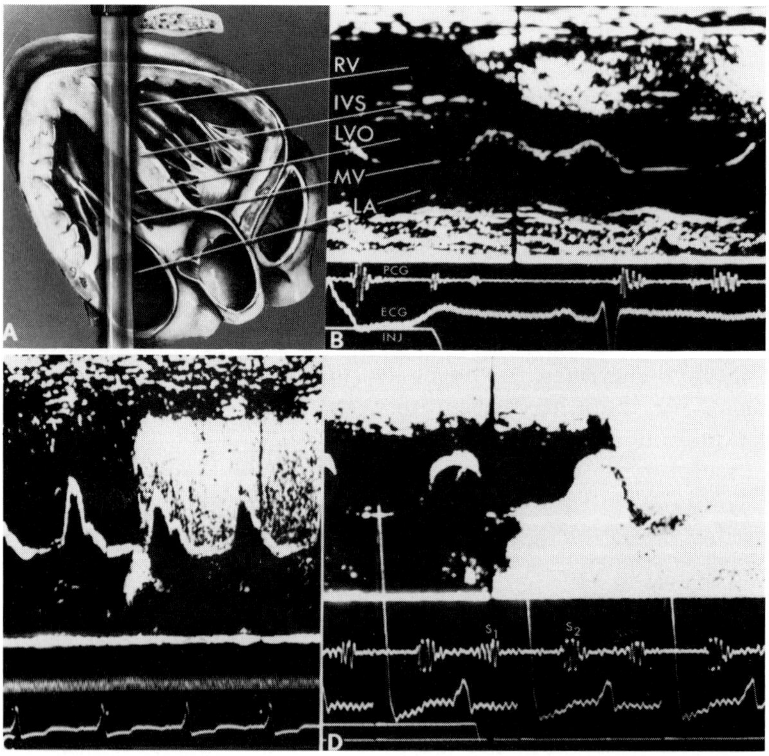

Fig. 4-1. Contrast identification of the mitral valve. Beam direction and structures encountered are shown in **A.** Right ventricular *(RV)* contrast injection fills the space before the interventricular septum *(IVS)* in **B.** Left ventricular injection **(C)** identifies the left ventricular outflow space in front of the mitral valve echo. In **D** the contrast was injected into the left atrium and held there during systole. In diastole the contrast agent appears in the left ventricular outflow tract. *LVO,* Left ventricular outflow tract; *RV,* right ventricle; *MV,* mitral valve; *LA,* left atrium; *PCG,* phonocardiogram; *ECG,* electrocardiogram; *INJ,* injection signal. (From Gramiak, R., Shah, P. M., and Kramer, D. H.: Radiology **92:**939-948, 1969.)

heart and its rapid motion pattern are characteristic. Representative echocardiograms obtained during contrast injection into different heart chambers are shown in Fig. 4-1. Right ventricular injection filled an anterior space and identified the interventricular septum as the posterior margin of the right ventricular cavity. The space in front of the mitral leaflet always filled during left ventricular injection, delineating the left ventricular outflow tract and the left side of the ventricular septum, which represents the structure recorded anterior to the mitral leaflet. When injection took place in the left atrium, on the other hand, dense echoes were recorded first behind the mitral valve and the left ventricular outflow tract filled later during diastole. When the left ventricular cavity was enlarged, the space behind the mitral valve was often identified as left ventricle also. Observation of posterior heart wall motion can be used without contrast injection to recognize left ventricular exit of the ultrasonic beam by noting that the posterior (left ventricular) wall moves anteriorly in systole and posteriorly in diastole, as compared to the left atrial wall, which usually moves anteriorly in diastole.

Aortic valve. Echoes from the aortic root

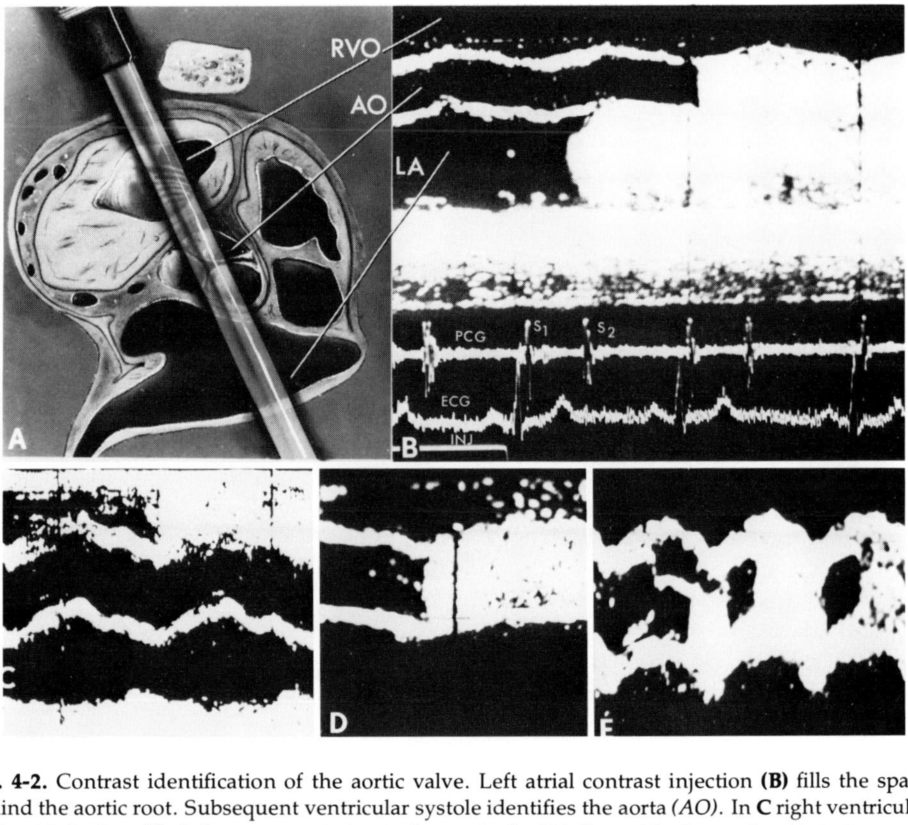

Fig. 4-2. Contrast identification of the aortic valve. Left atrial contrast injection **(B)** fills the space behind the aortic root. Subsequent ventricular systole identifies the aorta *(AO)*. In **C** right ventricular contrast injection filled the space anterior to the aorta. In **D** left ventricular contrast injection produced systolic filling of the aorta. In **E** a supravalvular contrast injection identifies the valve leaflets as a result of the delivery of noncontrast blood in systole. *RVO,* Right ventricular outflow tract; *LA,* left atrium; *PCG,* phonocardiogram; *ECG,* electrocardiogram; *INJ,* injection signal. (From Gramiak, R., Shah, P. M., and Kramer, D. H.: Radiology **92:**939-948, 1969.)

and valve leaflets represent another stable ultrasonic configuration that can be used as a landmark of intracardiac anatomy. When the ultrasonic beam is directed medially and cephalad from the usual mitral valve recording position, it passes through the aortic root (Fig. 4-2). Two parallel signals 3 to 5 cm apart represent the margins of the aortic walls, and these are flanked by echo-free spaces posteriorly and anteriorly. The injection of contrast agents into the left atrial cavity fills the space behind the aortic root, and there is subsequent systolic appearance of contrast material within the aorta. The right ventricular outflow tract is identified as the echo-free space that lies in front of the aortic root. When contrast is injected into the left ventricle, only the space between the aortic margins fills, since the left ventricle lies at a plane outside that of the recording beam. Supravalvular injection of contrast into the aorta fills only the space between the margins of the aortic root. This is a good technique to show the identity of the aortic valve cusps, which occupy a midaortic position in diastole, and to demonstrate rapid movements toward the periphery in systole. The ejection of noncontrast blood from the left ventricle is limited by these leaflet echoes in systole, which identifies their valvular origin and establishes their relationship to the aortic orifice.

If the transducer is angulated slowly from the mitral to the aortic recording position, continuity between the interventricular septum and the anterior aortic margin can be demonstrated. Similarly, there is continuity between the posterior aortic margin and the anterior mitral leaflet that lies at the same depth as the aorta in systole. Beam angulation techniques of this type have proved useful in development of orientation of intracardiac anatomy, especially in patients with congenital heart disease, where the relationships may be altered.

Tricuspid valve. The tricuspid valve is

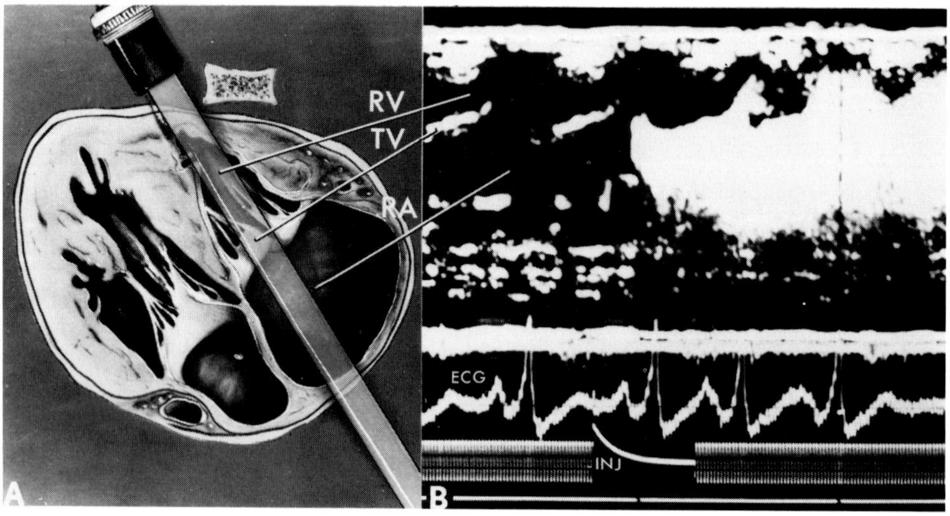

Fig. 4-3. Contrast identification of the tricuspid valve. The beam is angled medially and inferiorly from the mitral valve recording position **(A).** Contrast injection into the right atrial cavity fills the space behind the fragmentary echoes arising from the tricuspid valve *(TV).* There is subsequent filling of the right ventricular cavity *(RV)* lying anterior to the tricuspid valve. *ECG,* Electrocardiogram; *INJ,* injection signal. (From Gramiak, R., Shah, P. M., and Kramer, D. H.: Radiology **92:**939-948, 1969.)

somewhat more difficult to detect than the mitral and aortic valves, and its clinical usefulness is somewhat limited as compared to the left heart structures. The tricuspid leaflets can be detected by directing the ultrasonic beam medially, usually at a rather steep angle from the mitral valve recording position, and directing the beam under the sternum (Fig. 4-3). Tricuspid leaflet echoes are usually situated in an anterior position, approximately at the depth of the anterior margin of the aortic root. Most often the position in systole is recorded with a rapid anterior opening movement in diastole. If an entire cardiac cycle can be recorded, the configuration is very similar to that of the mitral valve. Contrast injections into the right atrium fill the space behind the tricuspid valve and move anteriorly into the right ventricular cavity in diastole.

Pulmonic valve. Recording pulmonic valve motion is a new ultrasonic technique that has already shown some usefulness in the evaluation of congenital heart disease and that may be of value in the assessment of pulmonary hypertension. We have used two different techniques for the detection of the pulmonic valve. The most commonly employed technique begins with identification of the aortic valve. The displacement of the transducer one interspace toward the head passes the beam through the supravalvular portion of the aorta. Slow gradual angulation of the beam toward the left shoulder replaces the well-

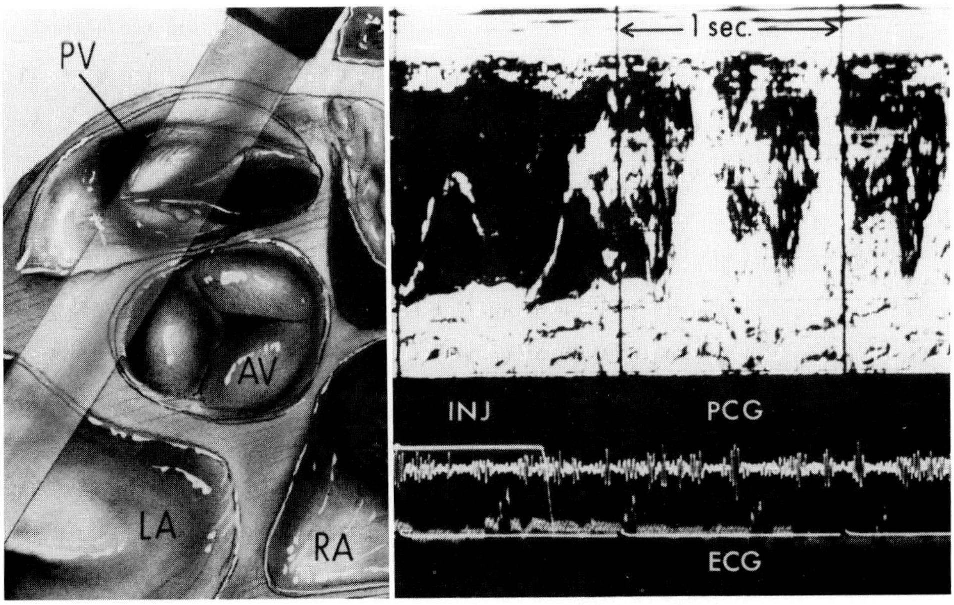

Fig. 4-4. Contrast identification of the pulmonic valve. The beam has been angled toward the patient's left shoulder from a position one interspace above the aortic valve. It passes through a portion of the right ventricular outflow tract and detects the left pulmonic cusp. Pulmonary artery contrast injection fills the cusp with dense echoes. Fragmentary echoes in front of the cusp are probably caused by catheter-induced pulmonic regurgitation, while the dense narrow bands represent diastolic filling of a cusp that is normally out of the ultrasonic beam. *PV*, Pulmonic valve; *AV*, aortic valve; *RA*, right atrium; *LA*, left atrium; *INJ*, injection signal; *PCG*, phonocardiogram; *ECG*, electrocardiogram. (From Gramiak, R., Nanda, N., and Shah, P. M.: Radiology **102:**153-157, 1972.)

known configuration of the aortic root with an echo-free space lying anterior to the aorta (Fig. 4-4). This space is bounded posteriorly by characteristically thick echoes, while the anterior margin moves relative to the stationary echoes of the chest wall. Minute changes in the position and angulation of the transducer result in detection of pulmonic valve cusps. These are recognized as rapidly moving reflectors, synchronous with the heart cycle and usually located posteriorly in this space. An alternative method that we have used begins with identification of the mitral valve. Movement of the transducer one interspace cephalad has often resulted in recording of the pulmonic valve leaflet.

Solinger[12] has used another technique in the pediatric patient. He has utilized a transducer position near the second interspace, further toward the head than those we have reported. With the transducer directed somewhat downward, he passes the beam across the pulmonic ring and records two valve cusps that move in counter directions in systole and show some resemblance to aortic valve cusp movement.

Utilizing the transducer positions with which we are familiar, injection of contrast material into the pulmonary artery has filled the space behind the moving cusp echo and identified it as the left pulmonary cusp. Since the beam is placed rather low and angled upward, the space in front of the cusp very likely represents the right ventricular outflow tract. Other contrast-filled pulmonic valve cusps, lying at a plane above the ultrasonic beam, may appear in diastole and produce bar-like echoes. Scattered echoes seen in the outflow tract and shown in Fig. 4-4 probably result from catheter-induced pulmonic regurgitation. We have also identified the left atrial cavity lying behind the pulmonic valve, and the thick echo complex between these cavities probably represents the atriopulmonic sulcus. This may develop into a significant echocardiographic structure at some future date, since it contains the proximal part of the left coronary artery.

Interatrial septum. Placement of the transducer to the right of the sternum can be used to study intracardiac structures when there is some cardiac enlargement or when the lung is excluded from this area because of the patient's chest configuration. Placement of the transducer 1 cm caudad from the ideal mitral valve recording position and direction of the beam medially and cephalad will pass it through the interatrial septum, as shown in Fig. 4-5. The usual depth of the atrial septum is 4 to 6 cm in an adult and can be recognized by its oscillating motion. The amplitude may be as much as 2 cm, and the direction of movement is usually toward the transducer in systole. The echo-free space in front of the septum has been identified as the right atrium by means of contrast injections. Similarly, the left atrium has been identified behind the septum.

Coronary sinus. Unusual echo patterns that do not conform clearly to the left ventricular or left atrial wall have been recorded in our laboratory in patients who have enlargement of the coronary sinus. In one who showed clinical and hemodynamic evidence of mitral regurgitation from chordae rupture, an unusual linear echo pattern was found behind the mitral valve, with a free space behind it and dense "heart wall" echoes still more posterior. The linear echo moved posteriorly during systole with the resultant narrowing of the space. Widening occurred in diastole as the margin moved forward. This patient was shown to have an anomalous left superior vena cava by angiography, and an injection of ultrasonic contrast identified an enlarged coronary sinus that communicated with the anomalous vessel (Fig. 4-6). In a pediatric patient an enlarged coronary sinus produced an echo deep in the atrial cavity near the atrioventricular junction. This case has not been verified by ultrasonic contrast

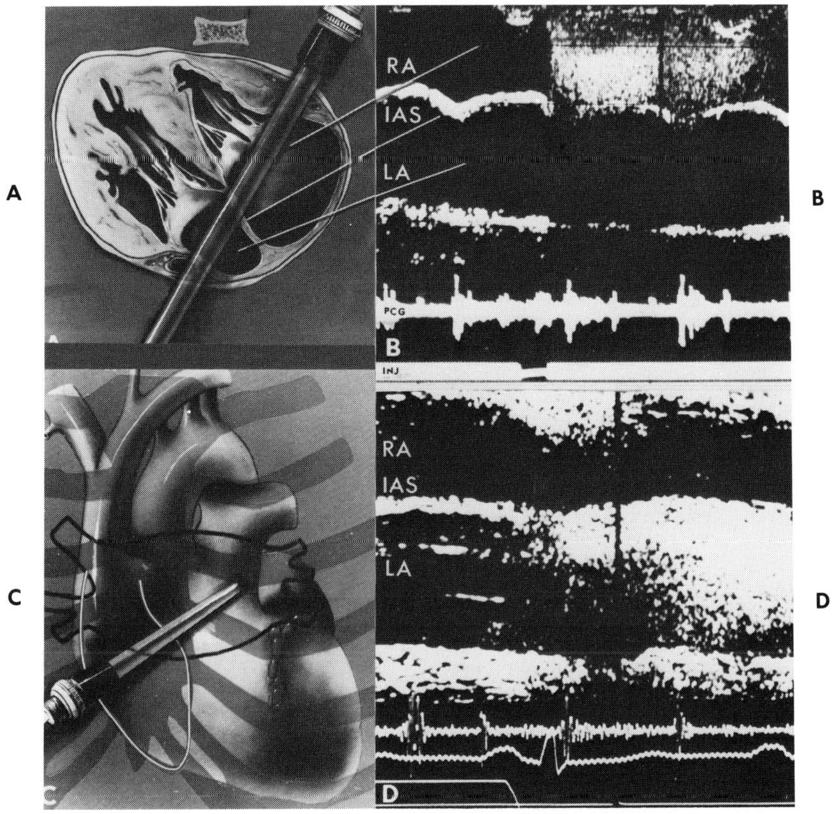

Fig. 4-5. Contrast identification of the atrial septum. The beam is positioned to the right of the sternum, one interspace lower than the mitral valve recording position and angled medially. The interatrial septum *(IAS)* is the central echo pattern that limits the contrast echoes in the right atrium (*RA* in **B**) and in the left atrium (*LA* in **D**). (From Gramiak, R., Shah, P. M., and Kramer, D. H.: Radiology **92:**939-948, 1969.)

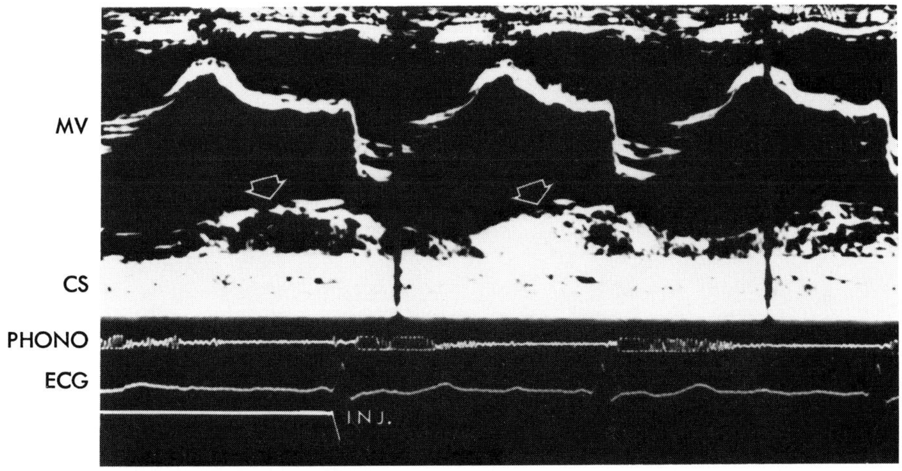

Fig. 4-6. Contrast identification of the coronary sinus. Contrast medium was injected into an anomalous left superior vena cava that drained into the coronary sinus *(CS),* identified by arrows. Note arrival of contrast agent (second arrow). *MV,* Mitral valve; *PHONO,* phonocardiogram; *ECG,* electrocardiogram; *INJ,* injection signal.

injection, though it was demonstrated angiographically and the enlarged coronary sinus was identified at surgery.

Intracardiac shunts. The detection of intracardiac shunts at the time of cardiac catheterization using ultrasonic contrast injections is relatively easy. Patterns of flow can be observed and conventional radiologic studies can be better planned with this information. Different patterns are produced by atrial septal defects as compared to ventricular septal defects when the beam is directed at the mitral valve and left heart contrast injection is employed. Left atrial contrast injection in atrial septal defects results in simultaneous filling of the right and left ventricles in diastole. On the other hand, ventricular

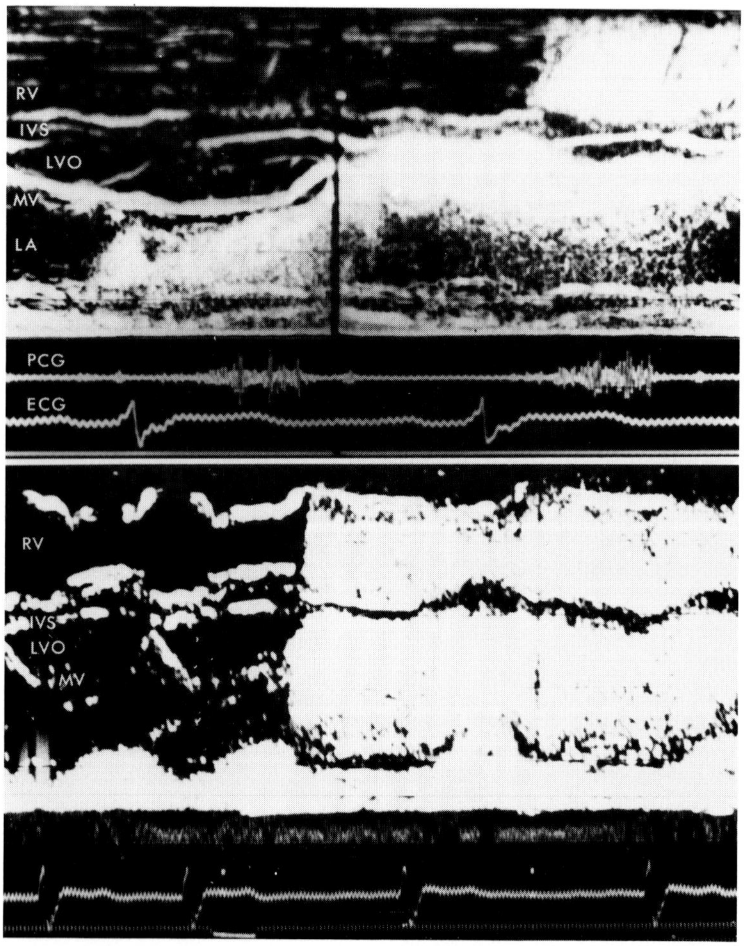

Fig. 4-7. Contrast differentiation of intracardiac shunts. In both instances the contrast injection occurred into the left atrium. In the upper panel contrast is held in the left atrium *(LA)* during systole and enters the left ventricular outflow tract *(LVO)* in diastole. On the subsequent systole, it passes through a VSD into the right ventricle *(RV)*. In the lower panel left atrial contrast injection (not in examining beam) is followed by simultaneous filling of both ventricular cavities in diastole. An ASD permitted both atria to fill simultaneously. *IVS*, Interventricular septum; *MV*, mitral valve; *PCG*, phonocardiogram; *ECG*, electrocardiogram. (From Gramiak, R., Shah, P. M., and Kramer, D. H.: Radiology **92:**939-948, 1969.)

septal defects show filling of the left ventricular outflow tract in diastole followed by filling of the right ventricle on next ventricular systole after left heart contrast injection (Fig. 4-7). We have studied a patient with a defect in the membranous portion of the ventricular septum using contrast injections and the atrial septal recording position (right of the sternum). Injection of contrast material during ventricular diastole into the left atrium filled the left atrial cavity but not the right. Contrast material appeared in the right atrium on the next ventricular systole. The presence of this shunt passing from the left ventricle to the right atrium was verified by angiocardiography.

Valvular regurgitation. The supravalvular injection of contrast material in the aortic root during recordings of the mitral valve has demonstrated aortic regurgitation by the appearance of the contrast effect in the left ventricular outflow tract during diastole. Furthermore, observation of the left atrium from the aortic root recording position has demonstrated mitral regurgitation after left ventricular injection of contrast material.

CONCLUSION

Ultrasonic contrast techniques, as described here, have been useful to validate the source of intracardiac echoes and to demonstrate some functional changes. Certain important limitations are present, however, that restrict current methods. The pulmonary capillary bed presents a substantial barrier and does not permit the passage of peripherally injected materials into the left heart. The requirement to carry out cardiac catheterization for left heart studies presents a serious deterrent. The contrast effect obtained is quite variable in intensity and makes it hazardous to attempt quantitation of shunts or valvular regurgitation.

The development of an ideal contrast agent is particularly important in the advancement of cardiac ultrasound. A suitable material could give us information about altered blood flow patterns such as those produced by valve stenosis or regurgitation as well as those resulting from intracardiac shunts. Requirements for an ideal contrast agent are that it should be harmless, well tolerated, and easily administered. Its contrast effect should be consistent and reproducible, and it should be easily administered to left heart structures either by passage through the pulmonary capillary bed or directly through an inhalation technique. The development of such an ideal agent represents one of the important goals of echocardiographic research.

REFERENCES

1. Edler, I.: The diagnostic use of ultrasound in heart disease. In Kelly, E., editor: Ultrasonic energy: biological investigations and medical applications, Urbana, 1965, University of Illinois Press.
2. Joyner, C. R.: Personal communication.
3. Gramiak, R., and Shah, P. M.: Echocardiography of the aortic root, Invest. Radiol. **3**:356, 1968.
4. Gramiak, R., Shah, P. M., and Kramer, D. H.: Ultrasound cardiography: contrast studies in anatomy and function, Radiology **92**:939, 1969.
5. Kremkau, F. W., and others: Ultrasonic detection of cavitation at catheter tips, Am. J. Roentgenol. **60**:177, 1970.
6. Feigenbaum, H., and others: Identification of ultrasound echoes from the left ventricle by use of intracardiac injections and indocyanine green, Circulation **41**:615, 1970.
7. Goldberg, B.: Suprasternal ultrasonography, J.A.M.A. **215**:245, 1971.
8. Hipona, F. A., Sear, H. S., and Boyle, R. N.: Precision arteriography with ultrasonic timing, Invest. Radiol. **6**:64, 1971.
9. Gramiak, R., Nanda, N. C., and Shah, P. M.: Echocardiographic detection of the pulmonary valve, Radiology **102**:153, 1972.
10. Ziskin, M. C., and others: Contrast agents for diagnostic ultrasound, Invest. Radiol. **7**:500-505, 1972.
11. Gramiak, R., and Shah, P. M.: Detection of intracardiac blood flow by pulsed echo-ranging ultrasound, Radiology **100**:415, 1971.
12. Solinger, R., Elbl, F., and Minhas, K.: Echocardiography in the normal neonate, Circulation **47**:108-118, 1973.

5 Echocardiography in acquired heart disease

RAYMOND GRAMIAK, M.D.

INTRODUCTION

History

The extensive development of sonar techniques for submarine detection around the time of World War II initiated activity that resulted in application of pulse echo techniques to the study of the human heart. High-speed oscilloscopes used in nondestructive testing of metal provided the link between long-range naval echoing devices and the short-range methods needed to image cardiac structures.[1] Hertz is credited with the first application of such an instrument to a patient, and his collaboration with Edler resulted in the first clinical studies of mitral valve motion.[2] Edler subsequently imaged many of the structures in the heart now under study, and his early work in the 1950's dealt primarily with the recognition and evaluation of mitral stenosis.[3-5] Effert contributed early in the same area and added the first description of a left atrial tumor.[6]

In the early 1960's John Reid built a clinical instrument and introduced ultrasound cardiography into the United States. Joyner in 1963 published the first American effort in cardiac ultrasound in a study dealing with mitral stenosis.[7] Shortly after this, Feigenbaum published data on the recognition of pericardial fluid behind the left ventricular wall[8] and later developed the concepts and techniques for measuring left ventricular volume.[9] Intracardiac contrast injections were introduced by Gramiak in 1968[10] and have been shown to be a useful method for the validation of cardiac anatomy as recorded by the ultrasonic beam as well as the delineation of certain functional abnormalities. Numerous other workers have contributed significantly in the description and evaluation of various acquired cardiac lesions.[11–15]

Basic principles

Since echocardiographic technique utilizes a single transducer that acts as both the sender and the receiver, maximal echo returns are obtained when the surface being examined lies perpendicular to the ultrasonic beam. Tilting of a moving heart valve can readily direct the returning echoes away from the receiver and produce image dropouts that detract from the clinical usefulness of the record. This problem can usually be controlled by careful selection of the transducer position and angle to ensure recording of movement throughout the entire cardiac cycle. In the mitral valve it is regularly possible to record complete cycles of anterior leaflet motion, but detection of the posterior leaflet may be more difficult. Similarly, tricuspid recording is degraded because of signal dropout. This also affects the results of aortic and pulmonic valve recording.

The examiner must be constantly aware of the fact that the ultrasonic beam has a finite width that may vary according to the physical characteristics of the transducer crystal, interposed focusing elements, and receiver sensitivity. All structures in the ultrasonic beam will be depicted on the axis of that beam despite the fact that they may be as much as 10 to 20 mm apart in lateral realtionships. This fact must be constantly borne in mind during echocardiographic interpretation to prevent erroneous conclusions.

Reverberations of ultrasound waves may produce image degrading clutter and be extremely important in the heart. These are produced by multiple reflections within solid structures and are imaged deep to the structures, depending on the delay in echo return produced by these internal reflections. Thus chest wall echoes regularly produce heavy clutter, which tends to obscure the images of the right heart, particularly the tricuspid and pulmonic valves. This same type of clutter may create difficulties in imaging the left side of the ventricular septum or a pericardial effusion space lying behind the muscular left ventricular wall. Meticulous control of instrument sensitivity may suppress these clutter patterns but usually also results in suppression of the image of important anatomic structures such as the tricuspid valve.

Occasionally, one may detect the image of a moving structure that resembles a heart valve behind the left ventricular wall, particularly in thin-chested individuals. This phenomenon probably results from the illumination of a heart valve by reflected or refracted ultrasonic energy away from the main axis of the ultrasonic probe. Since the ultrasonic path is lengthened by this off-axis illumination, echoes that return will be shown in a deep position and cannot be demonstrated in the axial pathway of the ultrasonic energy through the heart. These observations represent the major sources of confusion that we have encountered to proper echocardiographic interpretation.

Examination principles

Echocardiographic diagnosis depends on several basic observations. The first of these is the determination of the size, position, or configuration of a cardiac structure or cavity. The second is the observation of the motion pattern of cardiac elements where alterations from recognized normal patterns represent reliable indicators of disease. The third is the evaluation of the intensity of echo returns. The recognition of inappropriate echo intensities can be useful for the detection of pericardial fluid by its sonolucent appearance, left atrial myxoma by the presence of abnormal echoes in the left atrial cavity and behind the mitral valve, or calcification of cardiac valves or other structural elements.

Every patient examined by cardiac ultrasound should have studies of the four heart valves, an evaluation of the anterior and posterior heart walls for pericardial effusion, the determination of septal and left ventricular wall thickness, and the determination of ventricular and left atrial chamber size. It is also useful to demonstrate the relationship of intracardiac structures by moving the beam during recording. This develops a spatial awareness of the size, position, and configuration of various cardiac chambers as well as the relationship of heart valves. It is also useful in the evaluation of pericardial fluid.

The approach to the heart is dictated by the physical characteristics of the patient and is almost exclusively from a left parasternal position, though successful recordings have been made from the right of the sternum,[16] from a subxiphoid position,[17] and from a suprasternal transducer position.[18] The lung, by virtue of its air content and multiple reflecting surfaces, represents an insurmountable barrier to the ultrasonic beam and therefore limits the extent to which the transducer can be displaced laterally. On the other hand, the sternum is almost as formidable a barrier when ossified, so that the adult heart must be examined through the cardiac window formed by these two structures.

Costal cartilages, when noncalcified, pass the ultrasonic beam without significant attenuation but may produce a sonolucent image that could be confusing in the evaluation of pericardial fluid. On occasion, patients will be encountered with a cardiac window that is so small that transducer placement is markedly limited and the ability to examine the structures of the heart severely curtailed. The emphysematous patient may, in fact, be impossible to examine. Some data may be obtained from a subxiphoid transducer position in these emphysematous patients or they may be examined tilted 45 to 90 degrees on their left side. This maneuver appears to displace the heart toward the left and to increase the size of the cardiac window. Examination in this position should always be used before the attempt to derive important echocardiographic data is abandoned.

There are other patient factors that add difficulty to the echocardiographic examination. For instance, the obese patient with a very thick chest wall may attenuate the sonic energy to the point where the returns are indistinguishable from clutter and noise. It also appears that the displacement of the transducer from the cardiac window limits the ability to maneuver the beam to secure the desired information. Chest deformities such as pectus excavatum may hinder the echocardiographic examination, especially when medial angulation of the transducer is required to locate a structure. The sloping chest wall offers little opportunity for adequate transducer seating during angulation. Patients who have had a left radical mastectomy and radiation therapy may also be difficult to examine because of difficulties in transducer coupling with the skin. The thin soft tissue layer does not permit significant depression by the transducer.

The costal cartilages present undesirable surface features, and ultrasonic energy may be lost because of poor coupling. Liberal application of ultrasonic gel may be of some help, but in general these patients are hard to examine. A severe degree of kyphoscoliosis may rotate the heart in such a manner that meaningful data cannot be obtained.

Some patients' hearts are difficult to examine because of a high "noise" level. This appears to be related to some particular physical characteristic of the patient's tissues or blood that results in a "grassy" appearance of the echo display in A mode. This finding occurs mainly in older patients, especially those with chronic pulmonary disease. The added signals result in images that appear cluttered with nonstructural signals that may interfere with clear identification of structures. Careful adjustment of instrument sensitivity may partially alleviate this problem.

Successful echocardiographic diagnosis also depends on accurate identification of the phase of the cardiac cycle. This can only be done successfully with the simultaneous recording of physiologic signals from the patient. The electrocardiogram represents the minimal physiologic data that should be recorded with each examination. We have found it useful to record a simultaneous phonocardiogram and the movements of the chest wall related to respiration. On other occasions it has been desirable to record the carotid pulse, the jugular venous pulse, or intracardiac pressure data.

The selection of an ultrasonic instrument when equipping a laboratory may be difficult. Most beginners in ultrasound are tempted to purchase an instrument with all-around capabilities so that examinations in a variety of organ systems can be made. This is a choice dictated more by economics than by technology. Many commercial devices are available with the specific features required for successful echocardiography. They have similar capabilities and can produce satisfactory results. Choice of a specific type may relate to the accessibility and ease of controls as well as the type of service offered by the manufacturer. Thus the selection becomes personal. It is difficult to obtain unbiased information, particularly from enthusiasts who have become skilled in the use of the device of a specific manufacturer.

Transducers, on the other hand, can be specified somewhat more scientifically according to their characteristics. Most adult cardiac examinations are carried out with transducers of approximately 2-MHz frequency. This appears to offer the best compromise between range resolution and sensitivity. Higher frequencies may produce better detail but their ability to penetrate is compromised. Focusing devices will produce narrower beams at specified depths, but the beam will broaden beyond the focal point. Though broad beams tend to image more off axis structures, they also tend to suffer less from signal dropout than narrow focused beams. Pulse length can also affect image quality. Long pulses (greater than 2 μsec) tend to produce thick ultrasonic images as compared to transducers with shorter pulses. On the other hand, the highly damped crystals in the short pulsed instruments tend to be less sensitive and therefore somewhat more difficult to use.

One of the areas that influences the quality of the ultrasonic examination most is that of the recording medium for the ultrasonic image. Photographic devices have been used extensively to record the sweep of the B-mode information across the face of the oscilloscope. The number of cardiac cycles recorded was limited by the size of the oscilloscope screen, and it proved difficult to image complete cardiac cycles at sweep speeds of 50 mm/sec or above. These photographic records could be made in a nonstorage mode that produced the best detail but required a photographic exposure for evaluation of results. This added to the cost as well as the time required to carry out examinations. Storage oscilloscopes permitted a quick method to evaluate the quality of a record without the expense of a photograph but have been relatively poor in detail content. They appear to be relegated to the position of preview devices in echocardiography while permanent recordings are made by other methods.

The introduction of the analog gate circumvented some of these difficulties. This device permits the rejection of all signals to a certain range, which can be adjusted for a particular examination. The first echo encountered is then converted to an electric signal that could then be recorded by a strip chart device. Much of the early mitral valve recording was done in this fashion, and continuous records as well as high sweep speeds could be obtained. In addition, multiple channels of physiologic data could be incorporated. This device has faded from the ultrasonic recording scene because dropouts resulted in spurious signals, the interjection of another echo resulted in misleading traces, as commonly occurs with wide ultrasonic beams, and, if more than one echo source was important diagnostically, it could not be imaged. Recently, various strip-chart recorders that image the entire ultrasonic pattern and several channels of physiologic data have become available. These have influenced cardiac ultrasound recording dramatically and have extended the usefulness of the technique. Some of these are especially adapted physiologic recorders, add-on strip-chart recorders, and self-contained units that incorporate ultrasonic equipment and strip-chart recorders. The images are formed on roll paper by different techniques. Some are heat-processed or ultraviolet light–processed and produce the ultrasonic image immediately for inspection. Others require chemical processing and cannot be inspected until after the completion of the examination. The feature of immediate inspection is useful for adjusting the ultrasonic instrument for optimal technical quality.

We have utilized moving 35-mm film to obtain the same type of record. The film technique has been found desirable since the image is optically compressed and therefore easy to store and manipulate. Oscilloscope record cameras provide a wide choice of film transport speeds, processing can be readily carried out in most x-ray departments, and the image is stable and of high quality. Film cost is small compared to paper. We estimate that 1 minute of recording on 35-mm film at 100 mm/sec costs approximately $0.18, while similar use of paper would cost from $1.60 to $3.00 per minute. The strip film is viewed by projection, and paper prints of selected portions are made for future comparison as well as for investigative studies. The ultrasonic signal may also be recorded on videotape and then played back through the ultrasonic device and imaged on the oscilloscope screen. This permits long recordings and editing after the examination but still requires that a photographic or strip-chart record be made from the oscilloscope. The individual user must decide which system is best suited for his particular operation.

Selection of ultrasonic instrument settings

The success of an ultrasonic examination of the heart is directly related to the skill of the examiner in selecting the proper sensitivity parameters for the production of an ideal image. Unfortunately, the ideal image cannot be defined accurately at this time. Good images are those that show the structures one expects to encounter clearly, while poor images fail in this regard. Technique charts of the type commonly found in radiology departments do not exist, and each examiner must tailor the examination for the particular circumstance at hand. The position of control knobs is not recorded, nor are the position and angle of the transducer. All influence the signal returns and their interpretation. Some general information on instrument adjustment is available and will be described subsequently when different areas of the heart are described. These will serve as guidelines for the beginner who must modify them according to his needs.

Major deficiencies in cardiac ultrasound today

A typical, well-executed M-mode study of mitral valve motion can be a bewildering experience to anyone seeing it for the first time. Without training in echocardiography an experienced cardiologist, radiologist, or pathologist with a thorough knowledge of cardiac anatomy, function, and disease usually cannot recognize the structures shown on an echocardiogram and especially cannot evaluate a disease process. This results from the fact that the M mode presentation is nonanatomic and does not conform to the large body of information that has been generated using the classic techniques to study the heart. Thus an imaging technique that demonstrates the returning echoes in their true anatomic format should be useful in diagnosis, especially in the presence of complex malformations. Furthermore, this type of image should enhance the evaluation of left ventricular function by displaying the ventricular cavity in its true size and shape.

Current ultrasonic techniques provide only the grossest estimates of the composition of the tissue studied. Though it is currently possible to recognize clear fluid in the pericardial sac as compared to the muscular heart wall, we cannot differentiate bloody from clear effusions nor can we study the structure of the heart wall in patients in sufficient detail to recognize areas of scar formation or infarction.

Current ultrasonic methods provide good information about the solid structures of the heart, but they are not readily applicable to the analysis of the blood flow patterns. Thus important information about intracardiac shunts or valvular regurgitation is not currently obtainable.

It is encouraging, however, that techniques are available to overcome these deficiencies using B-scanning methods,[19] computer processing of signals,[20] or pulsed Doppler techniques.[21] Eventually, all will be remedied.

Directions for future development

Many concepts are under development to extend the usefulness of cardiac ultrasound. Recently, a multielement transducer has been developed that displays twenty lines of information from an 8 cm wide transducer.[22] When applied to the heart, the movement of structures can be seen in real time in a coarse, raster format. Thus a moving picture image is generated on an oscilloscopic screen. Limitations are imposed by the size of the transducer, the ability to angle its beam, and resolution of deep cardiac structures. Its eventual usefulness will be determined by clinical trial.

We are currently developing a cine ultrasonic method that uses standard commercial equipment, B-scanning arm, manual movement of the transducer, and computer reformatting of the ultrasonic data into cine frames. Though feasibility of the technique has been demonstrated,[23] this approach also is unproved clinically. Others are developing ultrasonic beams that can be scanned electronically to view cardiac structures and to produce a motion picture image.[24] These are expected to provide greater flexibility than the multielement array and are also undergoing clinical trial. Ultrasonic cameras utilizing transducer mosaics for imaging echo returns may one day provide the equivalent of a clinical fluoroscope that can be applied to the cardiac window for a real-time ultrasonic motion image of cardiac function.[25] Ultrasonic holography is also expected to have an eventual impact on the recording of cardiac images by means of ultrasound.[26]

Interest is developing among ultrasonic instrument manufacturers for the development of methods to provide automatic setting of instrument sensitivity parameters. If successful, this approach will free the examiner from the need to adjust the instrument repeatedly and should result in reproducible examinations in any one institution as well as comparable results in all institutions.

CLINICAL ECHOCARDIOGRAPHY

The ultrasonic anatomy of the heart has been explored using the techniques of intracardiac contrast injections. The reader is referred to Chapter 4 for illustrations documenting anatomic relationships of structures as detected in the common ultrasound examining positions.

Successful echocardiographic examination depends on the examiner's ability to recognize specific cardiac structures. This is accomplished by notation of the depth, motion pattern, and position relative to other structures of target areas. Position can be evaluated by moving the beam during examination and determining the medial, lateral, superficial, and deep relationships of the cardiac structures. External landmarks such as intercostal spaces are of little value in the detection of specific cardiac structures.

Mitral valve

The mitral valve is the structure that has been most thoroughly studied by ultrasound and from which the most useful clinical data have been derived. It may be detected by placing the transducer in a left parasternal position with the beam directed posteriorly or slightly medially. The third, fourth, or fifth intercostal spaces can yield successful examinations. When considerable cardiac enlargement is present, it may be necessary to slide the transducer laterally. The point of maximal impulse can be a useful landmark for mitral valve detection. The mitral valve can be recognized by its large amplitude of movement (up to 40 mm) and a deep position, which is usually 6 to 8 cm from the face of the transducer.

Echoes in this location arise from the anterior leaflet of the mitral valve. The posterior leaflet can also be demonstrated and usually requires some angulation of the beam laterally and caudally toward the tip of the anterior leaflet and further into the body of the left ventricle. When the beam is directed too far into the ventricular cavity, anterior and posterior heart walls can be seen moving toward each other in systole, and linear echoes located within the space of the cavity are noted to move in a pattern similar to that of the posterior ventricular wall. These probably arise from papillary muscles and chordae tendineae. When a beam is directed too far cephalad, the movement of the mitral leaflet is severely damped and the septal motion is upward in systole. Additional cephalad movement will direct the beam through the aortic root. Excessive medial or lateral angulation of the beam from the correct mitral valve position usually demonstrates the motion of muscular heart wall elements with no mitral leaflet echoes.

Instrument sensitivity should be adjusted to produce a complete trace of the mitral valve motion without recording nonstructural echoes in the background. We do not advise the use of time-varied gain since the posterior wall echoes are usually very strong and require no additional amplification. Also, a flat gain setting helps to preserve echoes arising from the left side of the ventricular septum. Some suppression of anterior gain is required to minimize clutter and to show the right ventricular space. Care is especially required in this operation to make certain that the ventricular septum is imaged in its true width without suppressing its right side or adding to its apparent thickness by employing a sensitivity characteristic that is excessively steep and that images clutter with a sharp anterior margin.

The ultrasonic beam first passes through the anterior (right ventricular) wall of the heart, then a portion of the right ventricular cavity, then the interventricular septum, the left ventricular outflow tract, and the anterior mitral leaflet, and it exits from the heart through the left atrial cavity. On occasion, the beam may exit through the left ventricular cavity and, in this case, the posterior wall behind the mitral valve will show anterior movement in systole whereas the atrial wall motion may be flat or move mostly in diastole.[27] Intermediate motion patterns will be recorded when the beam encounters the atrioventricular junction.

The functional significance of the deflections comprising the mitral valve tracing can be summarized as follows (Fig. 5-1). The anterior mitral leaflet makes a short anterior excursion immediately after atrial systole (upward on the ultrasonogram) reaching a peak *(a)*. This is followed by a rapid posterior movement (downward on the ultrasonogram), which terminates at point *c*, the point of closure and ordinarily the deepest point of the mitral leaflet. Occasionally, the rate of movement changes between *a* and *c* at the time of the inscription of the R wave of the electrocardiogram. This is designated point *b* and signifies the beginning of ventricular contraction. During systole, the closed mitral valve moves anteriorly in a smooth continuous manner, probably the result of emptying of the ventricular cavity and drawing of the mitral ring toward the base of the heart. When diastole begins *(d)* the mitral leaflet executes a rapid anterior excursion and reaches its fully open position *(e)*. This is followed by the phase of rapid ventricular filling when the mitral leaflet coasts toward the position of closure *(f)*. The rate at which this movement occurs represents the rate of left atrial emptying and serves as an important indicator of mitral valve disease. During diastasis, the leaflet occupies a neutral position. Movements occurring during this phase of the

TABLE 3. Normal mitral valve measurements

Left ventricular outflow width	20- 35 mm
Mitral valve amplitude (c-e)	20- 35 mm
Diastolic mitral slope (e-f)	80-150 mm/sec
Systolic closing slope (a-c)	125-250 mm/sec

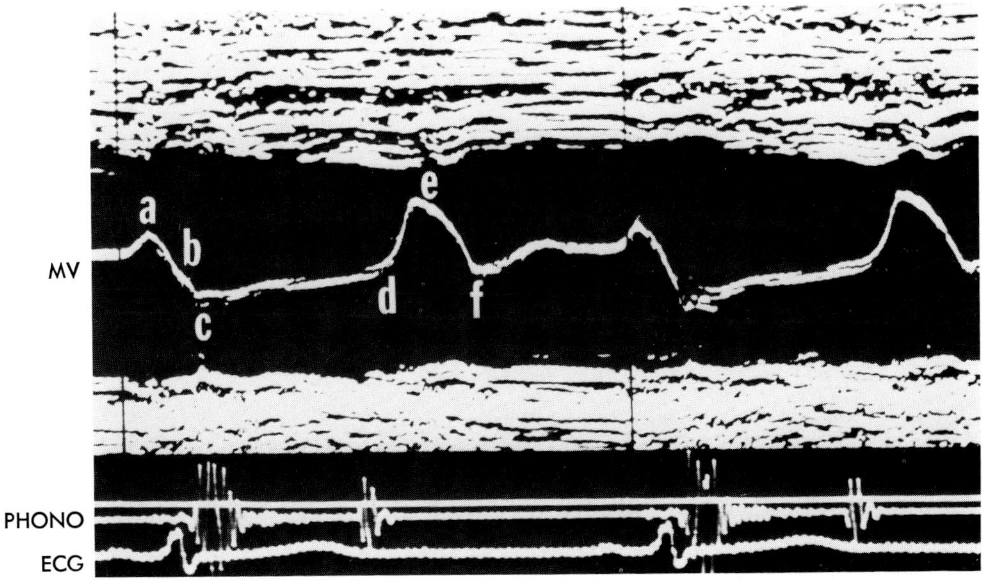

Fig. 5-1. Normal mitral valve. A normal mitral valve trace *(MV)* has been labeled to identify physiologic events. Atrial systole is followed by a peak *(a)*. Onset of ventricular systole *(b)* culminates in valve closure *(c)*. A gradual anterior motion occurs during systole. Valve opening starts at point *(d)* and the valve is fully opened at *e*. Posterior movement in diastole *(e-f)* is an indication of the rate of left atrial emptying. *PHONO,* Phonocardiogram; *ECG,* electrocardiogram.

heart cycle are poorly understood. Atrial systole reinitiates the cycle.[28]

The measurement of various parameters obtained on mitral valve echocardiograms is useful in disease evaluation. The measurement technique is illustrated in Fig. 5-2 and the important normal values obtained are listed in Table 3.

Rheumatic heart disease. Mitral stenosis has been intensely studied by early workers who showed that the slope in diastole *(e-f)* is characteristically slowed (Fig. 5-3) and that a good correlation exists between the rate of this slope and the severity of the stenosis.[29-31] Others have classified the ultrasonic findings into severe, moderate, or slight, depending on the diastolic slope.[32] Our experience has been that this slope is not a reliable predictive indicator of the usual hemodynamic correlates of severity such as mitral valve area, mitral valve gradient, or left atrial pressure. This discrepancy probably results from coexisting left ventricular disease, possibly the effects of mitral regurgitation, as well as structural changes in the valve tissue and mitral apparatus, all of which may also influence the motion of the mitral valve. The diastolic slope can be of considerable use in evaluating the effects of mitral commissurotomy and in following patients in search of indicators of restenosis.

We have found the greatest application of echocardiography in mitral stenosis in the evaluation of cusp calcification (Fig. 5-4). Patients with heavily calcified valves have regularly required mitral valve replacement. Those with lightly calcified valves need replacement approximately

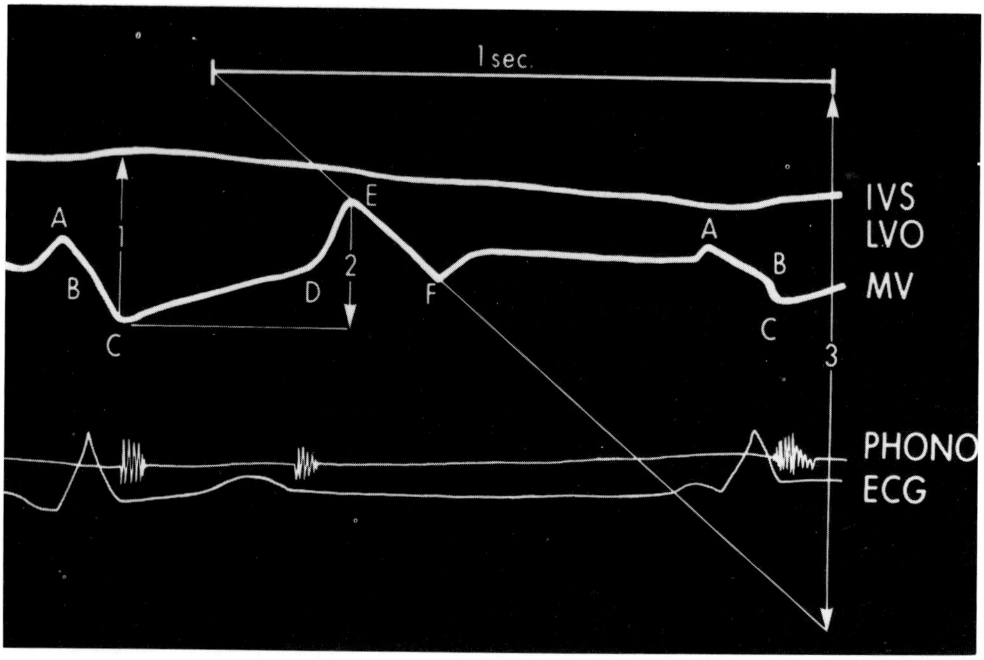

Fig. 5-2. Mitral valve measurement. The width *(1)* of the left ventricular outflow tract *(LVO)* is measured from the left side of the septum *(IVS)* to the closure point of the mitral valve *(c)*. The total excursion from closure *(c)* to the fully opened position *(e)* is shown by dimension 2. The rate of motion of a portion of the tracing may be obtained by extending it (for example, slope *e-f*) to equal 1 second of continuous motion. Then the total displacement *(3)* may be expressed as a rate in millimeters per second.

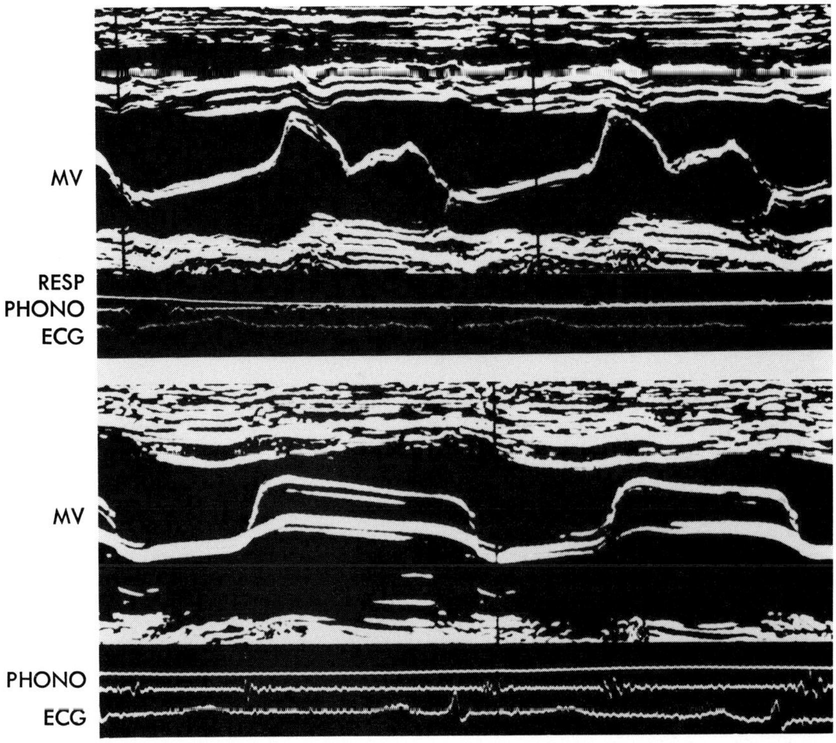

Fig. 5-3. Mitral stenosis. The upper panel is from a normal subject and shows a sharply peaked early diasolic trace, moderate sized A waves and a posterior cusp that moves in a direction opposite to the anterior cusp at the closure point. The mitral stenosis patient (lower panel) shows a flat diastolic configuration with no visible A wave and a posterior cusp that tends to follow the anterior in diastole. *MV,* Mitral valve; *RESP,* respiration; *PHONO,* phonocardiogram; *ECG,* electrocardiogram.

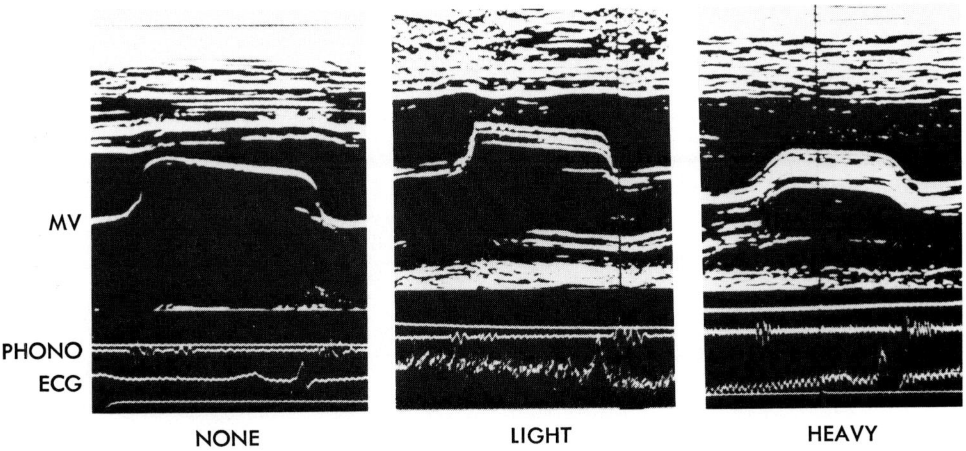

Fig. 5-4. Echocardiographic estimation of mitral valve calcification. Noncalcified valves are regularly shown as thin line traces. Lightly calcified valves will show as a multitiered collection of thin linear echoes, while heavily calcified valves are depicted as amorphous, thick conglomerate echo complexes. *MV,* Mitral valve; *PHONO,* phonocardiogram; *ECG,* electrocardiogram.

50% of the time, while those patients who clearly show evidence of thin valve leaflets without calcium almost always are candidates for commissurotomy.[33]

Another useful measurement in patients with mitral stenosis relates to the size of the left ventricular outflow tract (Fig. 5-5). This is measured from the left side of the septum to the anterior mitral leaflet at point *c*. In a series of patients studied retrospectively, it was found that those patients whose left ventricular outflow tract measured 20 mm or less did poorly when the cage-and-ball prosthesis was inserted, whereas a similar group did well with a low-profile prosthesis. Thus the routine measurement of the left ventricular outflow tract width for the preoperative selection of prosthesis type plays an important role in the preoperative management of the patient with rheumatic mitral valvular disease.[34]

The amplitude of movement of the mitral leaflet from its point of closure *(c)* to its fully opened position *(e)* is an indicator of the mobility of the valve. This amplitude of movement is reduced in patients with leaflets thickened with calcification or fibrosis or with thickening and shortening of the chordae tendineae. Patients with amplitudes of motion of 15 mm or less regularly show immobile leaflets at surgery and angiocardiography.[35] Most often these people require valve replacement.

It may be difficult on occasion to make the diagnosis of mitral stenosis on the echocardiogram. Slow slopes in diastole have been seen in other conditions where the mitral valve itself is not stenotic.[36] These usually are patients with compliance loss of the left ventricle and resultant slow emptying of the left atrium. The following observations have been useful to separate these patients from those with true mitral stenosis. The slow diastolic slope in the absence of mitral stenosis will show none of the multilayering characteristics of valve fibrosis or calcification. Furthermore, patients with mitral stenosis usually do not demonstrate A waves, whereas they can be seen when the ventricle empties poorly because of compliance loss. The rate of closure *(a-c)* in noncalcific mitral stenosis is usually rapid, in the 300 to 600 mm/sec range, while the nonstenotic valve usually closes under 300 mm/sec. In mitral steno-

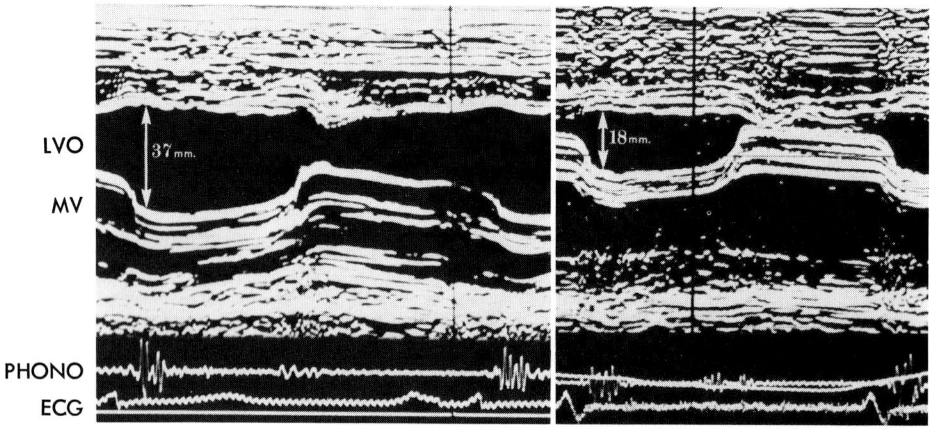

Fig. 5-5. Left ventricular outflow size in mitral stenosis. Preoperative mitral valve echograms in two patients scheduled for valve replacement are shown. On the left, the left ventricular outflow tract *(LVO)* measures a generous 37 mm and will accept a caged ball prosthesis. A narrow outflow tract is shown on the right and measures 18 mm. Outflow tracts under 20 mm require the insertion of a low profile prosthesis to avoid obstruction from a bulky prosthetic device.

sis, the closure of the valve occurs 60 to 100 msec after the inscription of the R wave, whereas the nonstenotic valve will close earlier.

An additional useful observation is the motion pattern of the posterior leaflet.[37] In the normal patient it executes a movement opposite that of the anterior leaflet, while in mitral stenosis it tends to follow the anterior leaflet and move anteriorly in diastole. The space between the anterior and posterior leaflet is probably related to the size of the mitral orifice.

When stenosis and regurgitation coexist as the result of rheumatic valvular disease, it is difficult to recognize indicators of regurgitation. A characteristic rapid early diastolic slope and a slow or late diastolic component have been found in this condition by other workers.[38] In our experience the stenotic component predominates and masks the changes that may relate to regurgitation. Regurgitation exists frequently when the valve is heavily calcified and moves poorly, but positive indicators of its presence are lacking at this time.

The value of a negative study to rule out mitral stenosis (slope over 35 mm/sec) cannot be overemphasized. This represents one of the very useful functions of echocardiography where the clinical picture may be confusing.

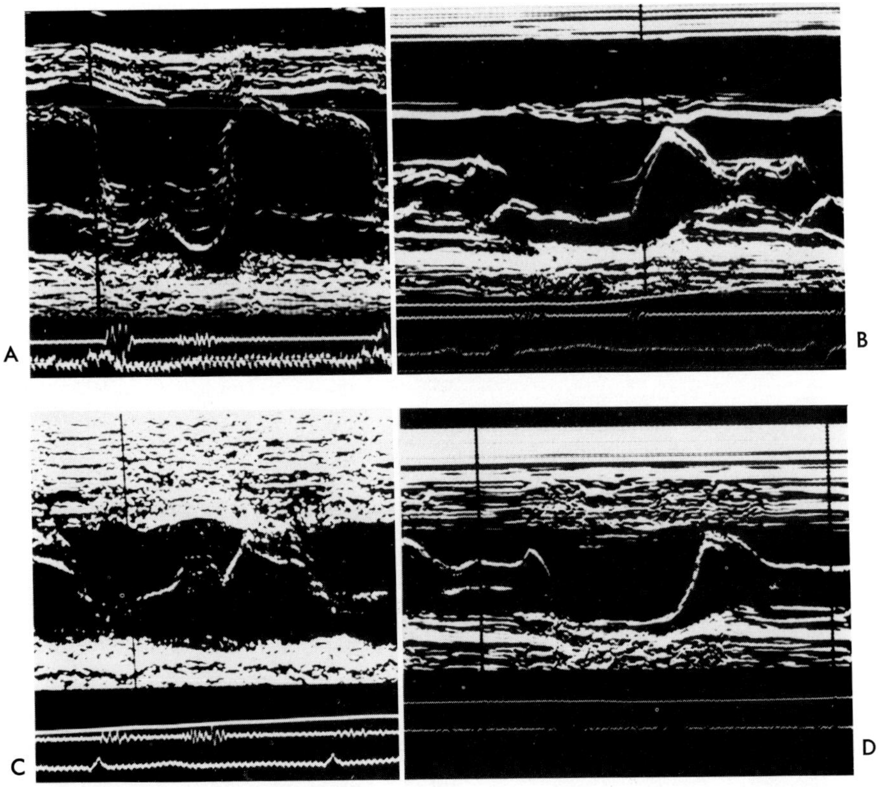

Fig. 5-6. Spectrum of systolic abnormalities in mitral valve prolapse. **A** shows a typical late systolic abrupt posterior motion and a multilayering of echoes. In **B** a generalized systolic sagging is shown. In **C** a shallow systolic hump is presented, while **D** illustrates a deep systolic position of the cusp. These illustrations are from four different patients, though it is common to find several manifestations of prolapse in most patients with this condition.

Mitral valve prolapse. Careful observation of the character of the normal systolic segment of the mitral valve has lead to the delineation of the indicators of mitral valve prolapse (Fig. 5-6). The normal gradual anterior systolic movement of the mitral leaflet is interrupted by a step-like motion of the cusp moving posteriorly.[39,40] This is usually 3 to 5 mm in magnitude, but we have seen it as large as 10 mm. The duration of this step is brief and is followed by the resumption of the normal anterior movement. This finding appears to be specific for mitral valve prolapse. We have observed other changes in mitral valve motion in the presence of prolapse. Equally reliable diagnostically is a valve that moves posteriorly in a gradual downhill fashion. The valve that sags throughout systole and forms a hammock-like configuration is also a reliable indicator of mitral valve prolapse. Early systolic plunges with rapid recovery and flattening of the systolic segment in systole have also been seen but are less reliable indicators. We have also seen low-amplitude systolic humps somewhat reminiscent to those seen in hypertrophic obstructive cardiomyopathy. However, these are not exaggerated by the Valsalva maneuver or by amyl nitrite inhalation. Septal echoes are never thickened in prolapse and outflow tracts are usually wide. Furthermore, examination of the leaflet in some other beam position usually shows one of the typical indicators of prolapse. We believe that this variation in findings probably is the result of differing movement patterns of different portions of the leaflet. The low-amplitude hump certainly appears to be related to the base of the leaflet near its attachment to the aorta, whereas the step-like prolapse pattern probably arises near the tip of the leaflet.

Identification of anterior versus posterior leaflet prolapse, in our opinion, is risky on the standard echocardiographic examination. Most often multiple lines occur, and most of them move anteriorly with the opening movement of the leaflet.

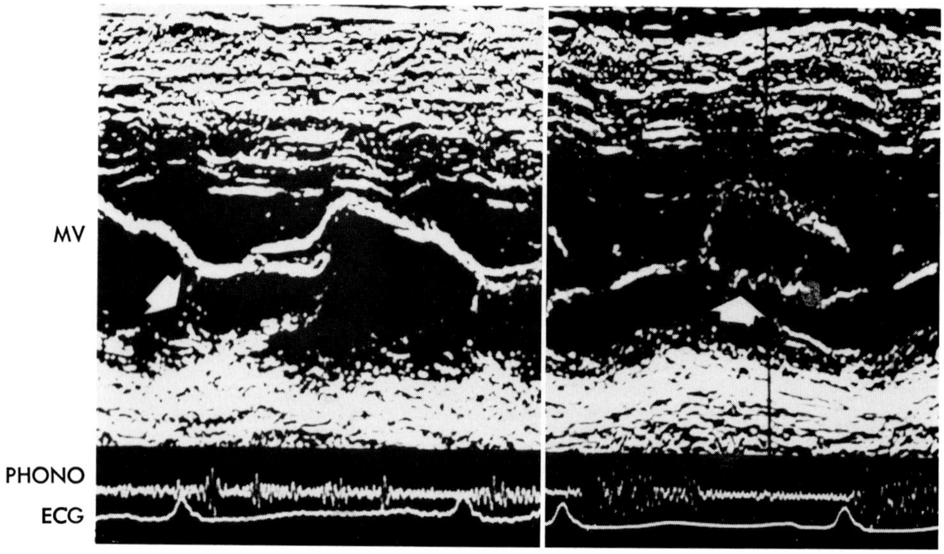

Fig. 5-7. Chordae rupture. This patient demonstrates a deep systolic plunge of the posterior mitral leaflet (left arrow) and a coarse diastolic fluttering of the posterior leaflet (right arrow). At surgery the chordae to the posterior leaflet were ruptured.

Though some of these could clearly arise from the posterior leaflet, we believe that precise identification, especially with the hope of quantitating the degree of regurgitation, is risky at this stage of development.

Chordae rupture. Rupture of the chordae tendineae results in alteration of mitral valve motion.[41] Involvement of the posterior leaflet can be recognized by an early systolic plunge of the leaflet to a very deep position, maintenance of this position throughout systole, followed by an anterior motion at the onset of diastole. A neutral position of this cusp is maintained throughout diastole. Anterior leaflet involvement results in a very coarse steplike fluttering of the leaflet in diastole. The two patterns can be noted to coexist (Fig. 5-7).

Hypertrophic obstructive cardiomyopathy. Massive asymmetric septal hypertrophy characterizes hypertrophic obstructive cardiomyopathy. Clinically and hemodynamically, there is evidence of left ventricular outflow obstruction and mitral regurgitation. The left ventricular outflow tract is regularly narrowed in these patients with diameters ranging from 10 to 20 mm. Thickening of the septal image, especially when it exceeds the thickness of the left ventricular wall, is probably characteristic. In our experience, septal images have measured up to 35 mm. When there is evidence of left ventricular outflow tract

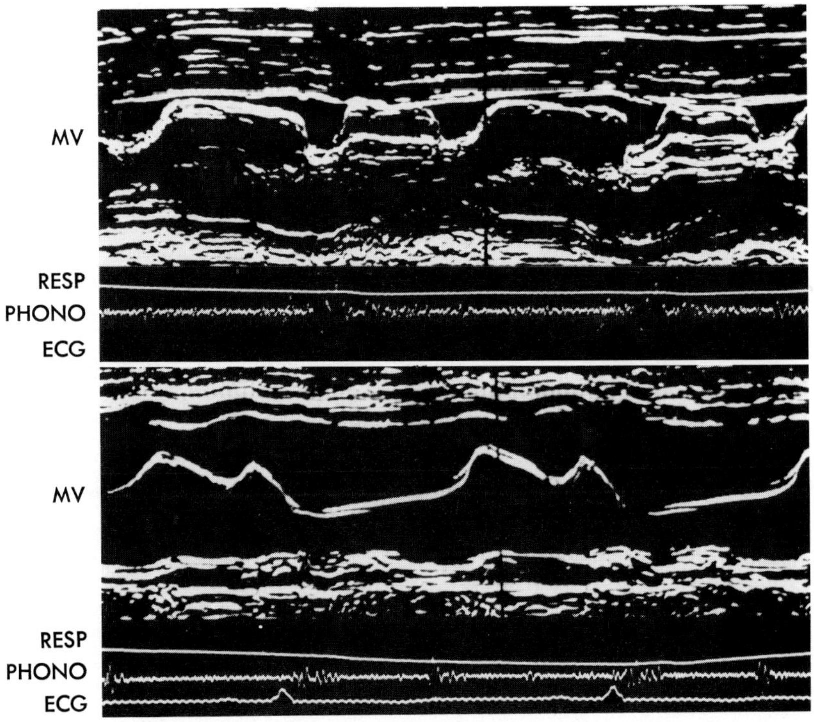

Fig. 5-8. Obstructive cardiomyopathy (IHSS, HOCM, MSS). The upper panel is from a patient with obstructive cardiomyopathy. There is an abnormal systolic anterior motion (SAM) of the mitral valve that starts soon after closure and contacts the thickened ventricular septum. The anterior leaflet returns to its closed position just before diastolic opening of the valve. Note the flat diastolic slopes of the mitral valve and the very narrow left ventricular outflow tract. A normal tracing with similar cardiac cycle length is shown below for comparison.

obstruction, a typical change in the systolic portion of the mitral valve echo pattern can be seen (Fig. 5-8). Normal closure of the anterior leaflet takes place, but this is maintained for only a brief period and is followed by a rapid anterior or reopening movement of the leaflet. This may contact the septum. The anterior leaflet usually remains in the open position for approximately 50% of the ejection time and then returns to a closed position briefly prior to diastolic reopening of the valve. Clinical and hemodynamic evidence of outflow tract obstruction and mitral regurgitation results from this systolic anterior movement (SAM).[42] When the anterior leaflet of the mitral valve reaches the septum, high gradients can be observed between the left ventricle and the aorta with every cardiac cycle. When the systolic abnormality is small, neither large enough to reach the septum nor present with every cardiac cycle, latent or labile obstruction can be demonstrated in two thirds of the patients (Fig. 5-9). Pressure gradients in the left ventricular outflow tract are usually less than in those patients where SAM reaches the septum.[43] The use of the Valsalva maneuver or amyl nitrite inhalation is a useful procedure to convert the inconstant or small systolic abnormalities to the complete form (Fig. 5-10). This will clearly identify the latent or labile variety of this disease and will rule out some of the confusing patterns that may be encountered in mitral valve prolapse or when confusion is produced by a wide beam that images the aortic root along with the mitral valve.

Echocardiography has been useful to determine the effectiveness of therapy aimed at relief of left ventricular outflow obstruction. We have compared pre- and posttreatment records of patients on long-term propranolol and have been unable to recognize any change in the systolic movement of the mitral valve. On the other

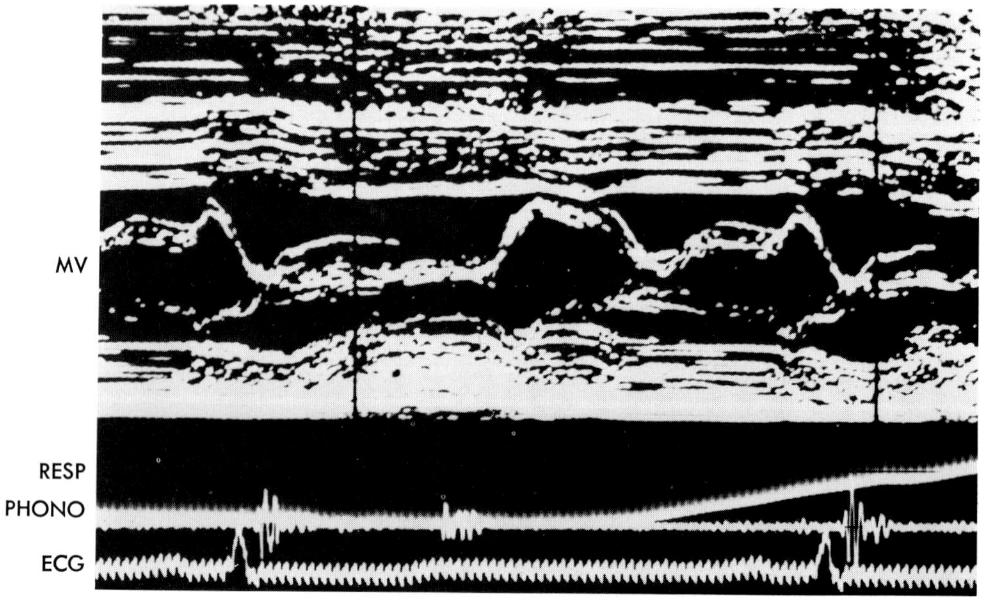

Fig. 5-9. Incomplete systolic abnormality in a patient with obstructive cardiomyopathy. The systolic abnormality is shallow and is imaged only during a portion of its excursion. These patients regularly have no gradient at rest. *MV,* Mitral valve; *RESP,* respiration; *PHONO,* phonocardiogram; *ECG,* electrocardiogram.

hand, patients who have shown good postoperative hemodynamic response to ventriculomyotomy have also shown no evidence of systolic abnormality on the echocardiogram. In one instance, a patient was studied pre- and postoperatively, and she lost the abnormal systolic anterior motion of the mitral valve as well as the gradient across the left ventricular outflow tract.[44]

It should be mentioned that the abnormal motion of the mitral leaflet usually occurs only at the tip of the cusp and should be sought by directing the sound beam toward the apex during mitral valve recording. Our best results have been obtained when the narrowest portion of the outflow tract is located, probably the apex of the asymmetrically hypertrophied septal bulge.

Echocardiography, in our experience, is an extremely sensitive detector of functional outflow tract obstruction. With the use of the provocative techniques, false positive results are extremely rare and negative examinations can be relied on to rule out hypertrophic obstructive cardiomyopathy.

Hypertrophic cardiomyopathies with out obstruction. Hypertrophic cardiomyopathy without obstruction is a less common entity than the variety associated with obstruction. The systolic segment of the mitral valve shows a persistently normal motion pattern at rest and with provocative maneuvers. Septal hypertrophy reduces the width of the outflow tract and may be shown effectively by scanning the ultrasonic beam from the mitral valve to the aorta. The transition from the thickened septum to the relatively narrow anterior wall can be demonstrated and the encroachment on the left ventricular outflow is clear.

Cardiomyopathies with chamber dilation. Cardiomyopathies with chamber dilation are clinical entities that show generally wide left ventricular outflow tracts, measuring as much as 55 mm. The amplitude of the mitral excursion is diminished, under 20 mm, but there is no evidence of thickening or calcification of the cusp.

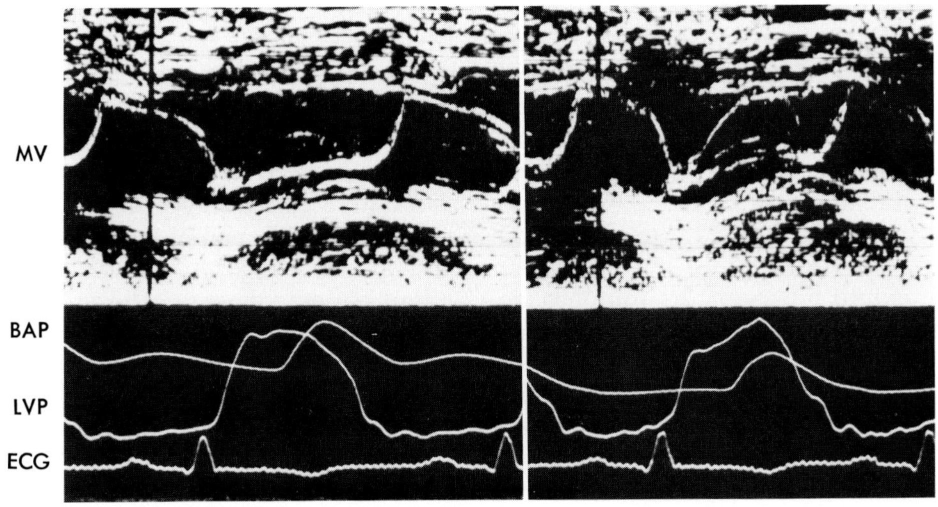

Fig. 5-10. Amyl nitrite in hypertrophic cardiomyopathy and latent or labile obstruction. The panel on the left shows a fragmentary, shallow systolic abnormality and no gradient between the brachial artery pressure *(BAP)* and left ventricular pressure *(LVP)*. After amyl nitrite inhalation (right), systolic abnormality becomes prominent and reaches the ventricular septum. A moderate gradient is demonstrated.

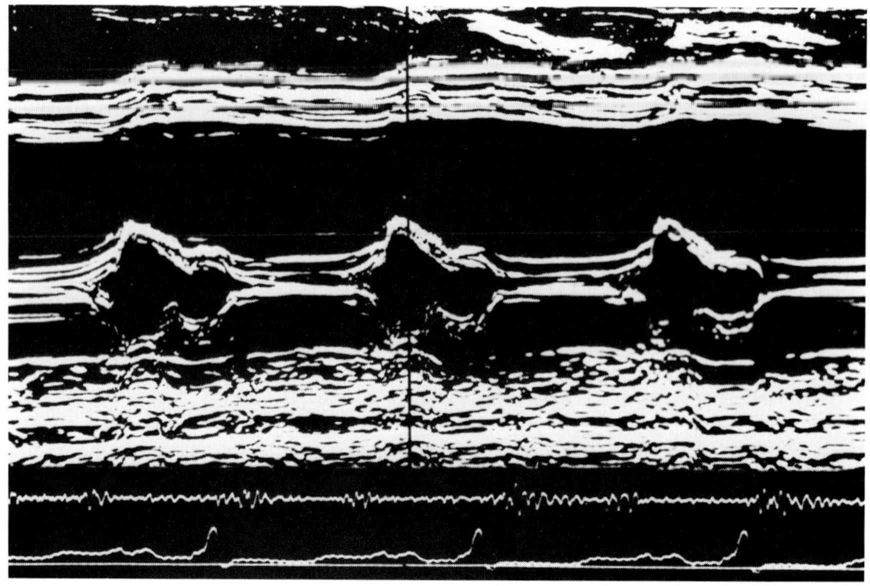

Fig. 5-11. Congestive cardiomyopathy. Mitral echoes *(MV)* are typically miniature, with frequent recording of both cusps. There is a strong tendency to record multiple linear echoes, probably arising in adjacent structures such as chordae or papillary muscles. The left ventricular outflow tract *(LVO)* is dilated. The septum is of normal width and shows poor motion. There is no systolic abnormality of mitral valve motion.

Diastolic slopes move fairly rapidly, often in the range of 100 mm/sec. Both leaflets are frequently recorded and their opposing motion clearly shown (Fig. 5-11). Additional linear echoes are often superimposed upon the mitral valve recording and are believed to arise in the aortic root, mitral annulus, or papillary muscle apparatus. Enlargement of the left ventricle probably elevates the left atrium and mitral ring and thus may bring the additional structures into line with the mitral valve during recording. The ventricular septum usually moves poorly, probably because of low cardiac output. There is no unusual thickening of the septal image. This diversified group includes those patients with congestive cardiomyopathy and severe coronary artery disease, including ventricular aneurysms and severe aortic stenosis.[45]

Prolapsing atrial tumors. The majority of left atrial tumors are atrial myxomas, though occasionally an organized thrombus may present in a similar fashion. The echocardiogram is a sensitive detector of this lesion and its image may be recognized when the tumor prolapses into the mitral orifice in diastole.[46-48] This results in obstruction to left atrial emptying and will produce a slow diastolic descent of this mitral leaflet. The mass lesion can be recognized as a complex of mixed linear and punctate echoes behind the anterior mitral leaflet in diastole. The site of attachment of the mass will result in different patterns of mobility and different echocardiographic images. The myxoma attached to the atrial septum will show free motion and will disappear into the left atrium during ventricular systole, while the immobile variety, which may be attached to the free wall of the atrium or to the leaflet itself, will stay close to the mitral valve throughout the heart cycle.[49] The mobile atrial myxoma usually arrives in the

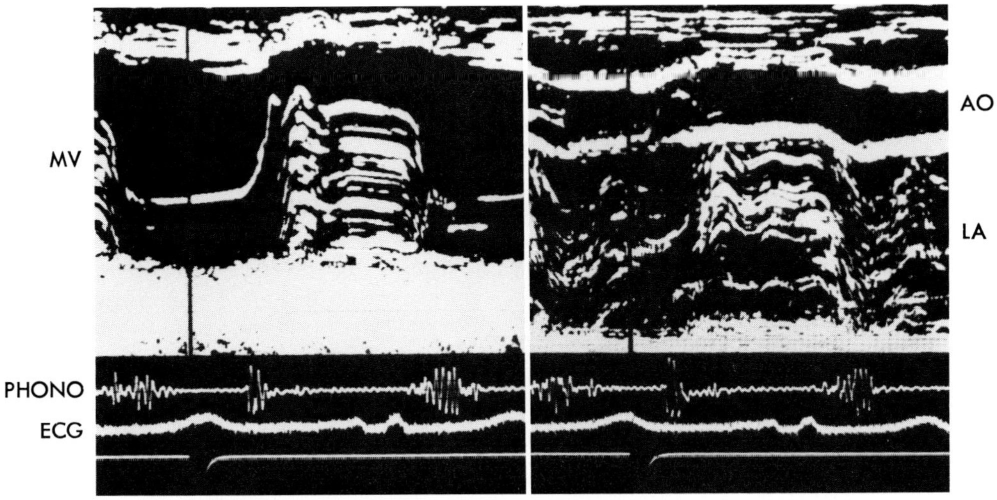

Fig. 5-12. Atrial myxoma. The recording on the left shows a characteristic grouping of linear echoes behind the mitral valve *(MV)*. Note the clear space in early diastole and the lack of a similar echoes during systole. Examination of the left atrium *(LA)* is shown on the right. Abnormal echoes are present in the left atrial cavity and their diastolic motion pattern mimics the mitral pattern. *AO,* Aortic root; *PHONO,* phonocardiogram; *ECG,* electrocardiogram.

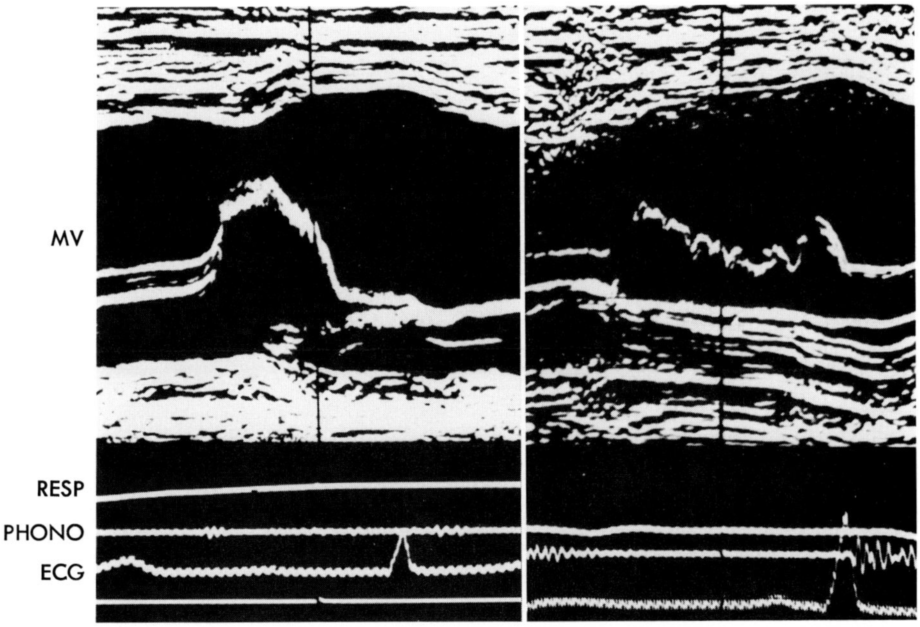

Fig. 5-13. Mitral valve flutter in aortic regurgitation. The left illustration shows a fine flutter pattern and a strong movement to closure of the valve in late diastole. On the right a coarse fluttering, restricted opening excursion, and a large A wave are seen. In both instances the left ventricular outflow tract is dilated and septal motion is vigorous. *MV,* Mitral valve; *RESP,* respiration; *PHONO,* phonocardiogram; *ECG,* electrocardiogram.

mitral orifice somewhat after opening and produces a characteristic echo free space behind the mitral valve early in diastole. This is followed by a typical multilayered tumor appearance (Fig. 5-12). Detection of atrial myxoma can be difficult and requires careful selection of instrument sensitivity. High and low gain settings should be used in these examinations to ensure that echoes arising in the mass are accurately recorded. Otherwise the abnormal mitral motion found in this condition may lead to the erroneous diagnosis of mitral stenosis.

When the mitral echogram suggests atrial myxoma, the left atrial cavity should be examined ultrasonically. Detection of linear echoes of an intensity that may be near that of the aortic wall and a motion pattern that mimics the anterior mitral leaflet will confirm the presence of a left atrial mass. An echo-free left atrium makes the diagnosis doubtful.[45]

Ultrasonic examination is probably the best technique available for the detection of left atrial tumors.

Aortic regurgitation. The motion pattern of the mitral valve is altered in the presence of chronic aortic regurgitation. A rapid diastolic flutter of 30 to 40 cps and with an amplitude usually less than 4 mm may occur and be superimposed on the opening movement or be seen only late in diastole (Fig. 5-13). This flutter is produced by the regurgitant jet as it strikes the mitral leaflet.[50] Correlation with the presence of an Austin-Flint murmur has not been good. We have also observed marked restriction of diastolic opening and very slow diastolic slopes of the anterior leaflet. The "A" wave is usually large. Delayed opening and premature closure of the mitral valve as well as rapid diastolic slopes have been reported in acute aortic regurgitation.[51] Following aortic valve replacement, the rapid flutter disappears and the mitral amplitude and diastolic slope return to normal.

The coexistence of mitral stenosis makes it difficult to document a flutter of the mitral leaflet even though it may be flexible as judged by the usual standards of mobility. The high atrial pressure probably distends the valve and dampens any tendency to flutter.

On a few occasions, we have been able to make the diagnosis of aortic regurgitation in the presence of mitral stenosis by finding fluttering of the ventricular septum in diastole. The usefulness of this observation has not been fully evaluated.

Aortic valve

The position of the aortic valve relative to the mitral valve is useful for aortic valve detection. Angulation of the beam medially and cephalad from the mitral valve recording position will pass the beam through the aortic root. It can be recognized by the parallel echoes that represent its walls, by a characteristic depth of 3 to 6 cm, and by movement synchronous with each heartbeat. The interventricular septal echo is continuous with that of the anterior aortic margin, and the posterior aortic margin can be related to the mitral valve. Valve cusp echoes can be recognized as thin linear configurations moving to the periphery in systole and occupying a midaortic position in diastole. It may on occasion be necessary to displace the transducer one interspace toward the head and to direct the beam at the aortic root from this position. When the beam is positioned too low for the detection of aortic valve cusps, the posterior margin often takes on the character of a severely dampened mitral valve movement. When the beam is directed too far medially, the anterior motion becomes exaggerated and does not parallel the posterior motion. Too much lateral angulation of the beam will pass it through the atriopulmonic sulcus (see section on pulmonary valve) and will result in a thick image that may mimic that of a diseased aortic valve. When the transducer is placed too high, the aortic wall echoes then become more anterior and the right ventricular outflow space in this supravalvular recording is lost.

The identification of aortic cusps is based on the known direction of the beam during recording as well as the position of the heart. The cusp that moves anteriorly within the aortic root represents the right coronary cusp, while that which moves away from the transducer is the noncoronary cusp. Occasionally, we see a thin linear echo between the cusps. This probably arises from the left coronary cusp moving across the ultrasonic beam. In systole, the cusps are quite steady in normal individuals. In diastole they occupy a midaortic position. The intensity of the echoes arising from the valve cusps is such that they are regularly narrower than either aortic wall and comprised of no more than three components (Fig. 5-14).

The diastolic portion of the trace is easiest to record. Since the aortic valve moves upward and laterally as it opens, slight angulation of the beam toward the patient's head may capture records with systolic movements. If only the right coronary cusp is recorded, it might be possible to locate the noncoronary cusp by minimal lateral transducer angulation. Additional movement toward the feet may also be beneficial.

Instrument sensitivity adjustment for aortic valve recording differs as compared with that used for the mitral valve. Less

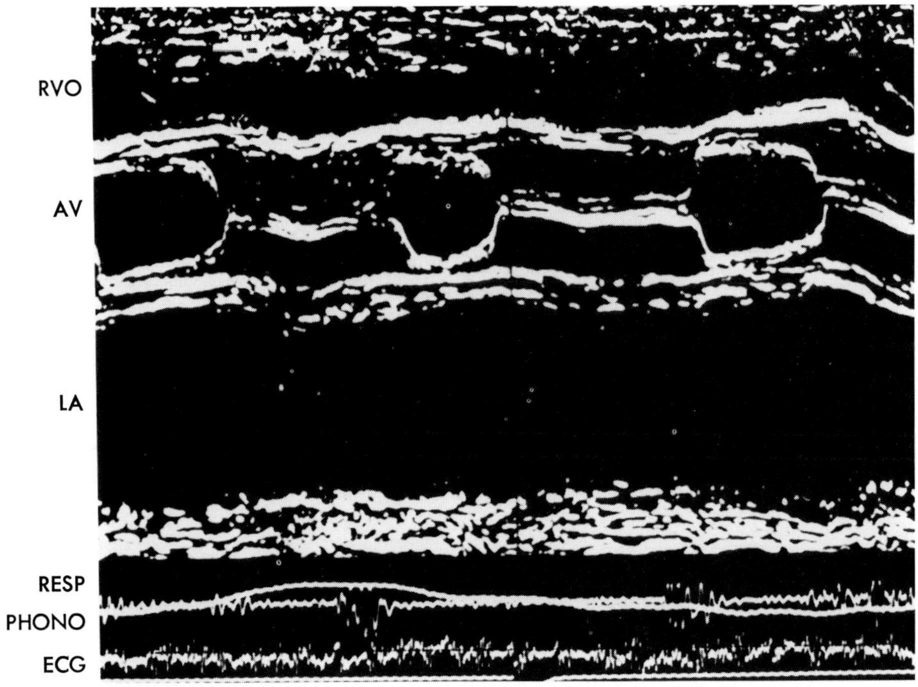

Fig. 5-14. Normal aortic cusp motion. The normal aortic valve *(AV)* is centrally placed in diastole and executes crisp opening and closing movements that form box-like configurations. During systole the leaflets are closely applied to the aortic margins and show no significant movement. The width of the diastolic echo image is regularly thinner than that of the aortic wall. *RVO,* Right ventricular outflow tract; *LA,* left atrium; *RESP,* respiration; *PHONO,* phonocardiogram; *ECG,* electrocardiogram.

overall sensitivity of the receiver is used, but the time-varied gain is employed in order to increase the amplitude of the echoes emanating from the posterior aortic wall to equal those of the anterior. This is necessary because the anterior aortic margin is an intense reflector and produces an ultrasonic shadow that results in diminished returns from the cusps and the posterior wall. With correct instrument adjustment it is possible to make accurate estimates of the intensity of the echoes arising from the aortic valve cusps. It is usually not necessary to suppress the anterior returns for clear visualization of the right ventricular outflow tract.

The physical parameters of the aortic root have been measured in the normal subject and in patients with aortic valve disease.[52] These are summarized in Table 4. Though normal has been characterized, the greatest benefits of this technique to date have stemmed from measurement of the size of the aortic root and wall thickness. Analysis of aortic valve disease based on the movements of the valve cusps has been disappointing. Some distortion of aortic valve opening and closing movements as well as limitation of cusp excursion has been seen as a manifestation of aortic valve disease. In the majority of instances, calcification of the cusps is present, masks the movements, and makes definitive measurement impossible. Calcification has been found regularly when the image of the aortic valve cusp is thicker than that of the aortic wall or when multilayered complexes (more than three) are present. In the adult patient, this has been a useful indicator of the presence of aortic valve disease.

Aortic stenosis. The echocardiographic diagnosis of aortic stenosis can be made whenever the valve echo shows evidence of thickening and normal cusp movements are obscured. It is not possible to make an accurate assessment of the severity of stenosis using available diagnostic criteria. However, gross estimates can be made using the following observations.

The degree of aortic valve calcification is related to the severity of the disease and can be evaluated echocardiographically (Fig. 5-15). Widening of the echocardiographic width of the valve complex to one third or more of the internal diameter of the aortic root is associated with severe degrees of calcification and usually high systolic pressure gradients (around 75 mm Hg). When the thickening is less than one third, then gradients are usually lower and often around 40 mm Hg. The absence of calcification on the echocardiogram is associated with no significant gradients.

The mobility of valve elements may be difficult to evaluate, but some information about the severity of stenosis can be obtained (Fig. 5-16). A thickened valve that passes through systole and diastole without change generally is accompanied by high pressure gradients, usually over 75 mm Hg. When an ill-defined change oc-

TABLE 4. Aortic valve and root measurement*

	NORMAL	AORTIC STENOSIS	AORTIC REGURGITATION
Aortic root diameter at onset systole (mm)	34	37	40
Amplitude cusp opening movement (mm)	10.3	†	9.6
Rate of cusp opening movement (mm/sec)	369	†	396
Rate of cusp closing movement (mm/sec)	293	†	406

*All figures represent mean values.
†Information obscured by disease process.

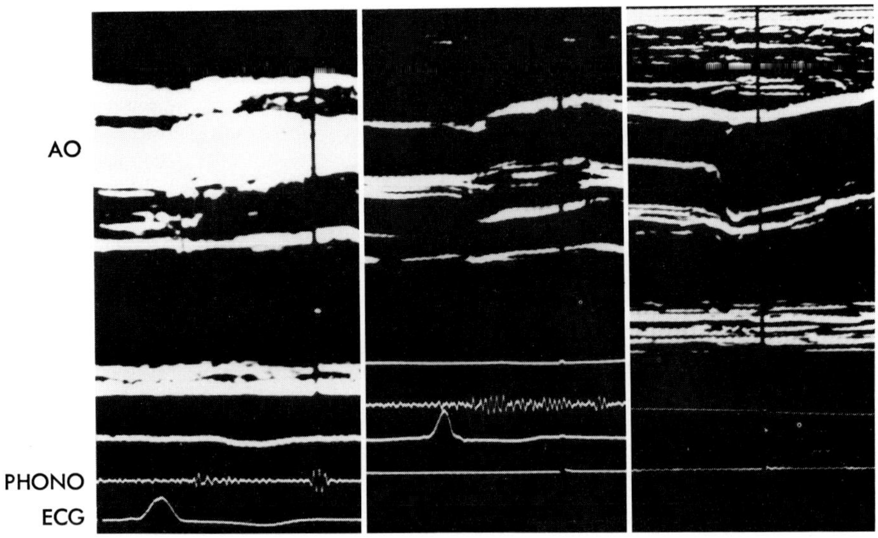

Fig. 5-15. Aortic valve calcification. A heavily calcified aortic valve *(AO)* is shown in the left panel. When valve echoes are thicker than one third of the aortic lumen, gradients are usually high. Moderate calcification of the aortic valve is seen in the central panel, where the diastolic image is somewhat thicker than the aortic walls. Patients of this type usually show moderate gradients. A normal aortic valve is shown on the right. When no calcification is demonstrated in an adult patient, there is usually no gradient present. *PHONO,* Phonocardiogram; *ECG,* electrocardiogram.

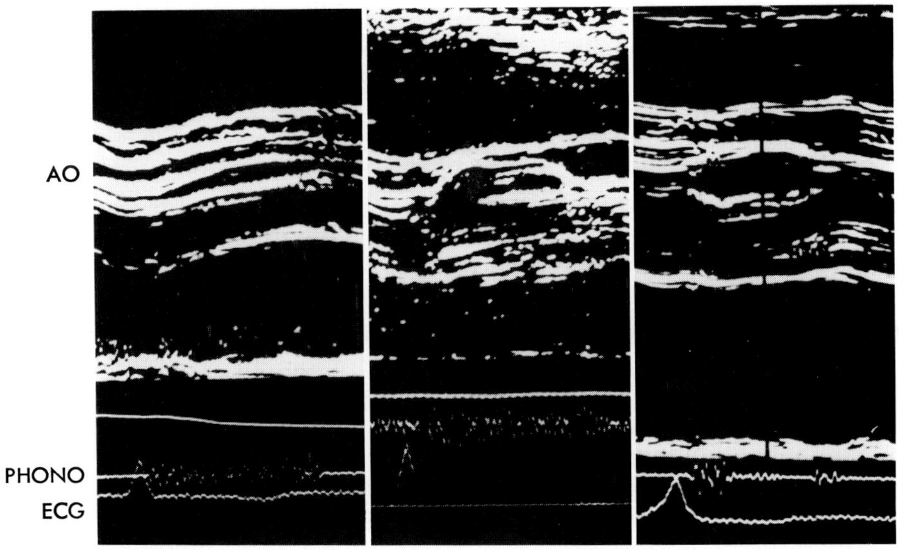

Fig. 5-16. Aortic cusp movement in aortic stenosis. In the left-hand panel thickened abnormal cusp echoes pass through systole with virtually no change. This is a finding usually associated with high gradients. In the central panel good movement of abnormal cusp echoes is present. In these patients the gradient is usually very low or nonexistent. Pure aortic regurgitation often presents with this pattern. On the right, thickened abnormal cusps show restricted systolic movement. Moderate gradients are usually found under these conditions. *AO,* Aorta; *PHONO,* phonocardiogram; *ECG,* electrocardiogram.

Table 5. Estimates of severity of aortic stenosis

GRADIENTS	CALCIFICATION	MOBILITY
High (over 75 mm Hg)	Severe—aortic valve image is wider than one third the diameter of the aortic root	Immobile—a thickened valve passes through systole and diastole without any change
Medium (50 mm Hg)	Light—aortic cusp image is thickened but less than one third the diameter of the aortic root	Altered—the pattern changes in systole but definition of the cusp movement is lacking
Low (under 50 mm Hg)	Light	One mobile cusp during systole
None*	None—normal cusp complex	Two mobile cusps during systole

*Adult patients only.

curs during systole but cusp movements are not evident, then gradients are usually lower (around 50 mm Hg). The movement of a single cusp in systole implies medium gradients, and they are usually under 50 mm Hg. When two mobile cusps are shown, then no significant gradient can be recorded in an adult patient suspected of having aortic stenosis (Table 5). It is important to emphasize that these are only gross estimates and that overlapping in these groups occurs. In very young patients, prior to the development of calcification, valve elements can be recorded as apparently moving well despite the presence of aortic stenosis.

Abnormal cusp motion in structurally normal valves. The normal aortic valve cusp maintains a steady position near the margin of the aortic root during systole. Occasionally one can see extremely fine oscillations of this cusp in normal subjects, in those with increased flow through the aortic valve, and in patients with coronary disease. Lesions producing left ventricular leaks such as mitral regurgitation and ventricular septal defects may produce a somewhat coarser flutter showing rates of 15 to 40 cps and of relatively small amplitude (approximately 2 mm). Frequently, the closing movement of the aortic valve is altered in these patients so that the cusp may show a late systolic collapse and a gradual movement toward closure rather than the sharp crisp motion seen in normal subjects (Fig. 5-17).

Patients with hypertrophic obstructive cardiomyopathy (HOCM) or idiopathic hypertrophic subaortic stenosis (IHSS) regularly show abnormal fluttering motions of the aortic valve leaflets. Occasionally one sees the normal systolic opening movement with a return to closure in midsystole followed by a late systolic reopening. The midsystolic closure is probably brought about by cessation of forward flow produced by the outflow tract obstruction and mitral regurgitation. When seen, the probability of outflow tract obstruction is quite high, though we have detected this type of movement in other causes of mitral regurgitation. Most frequently, a repetitive flutter of 5 to 50 cps is present. The amplitudes of flutter in IHSS tend to be larger (3 to 4 mm) than those encountered in other conditions.

The exact significance of these movement patterns is not always clear, but they appear to represent diagnostic clues to the presence of an abnormality. This wide

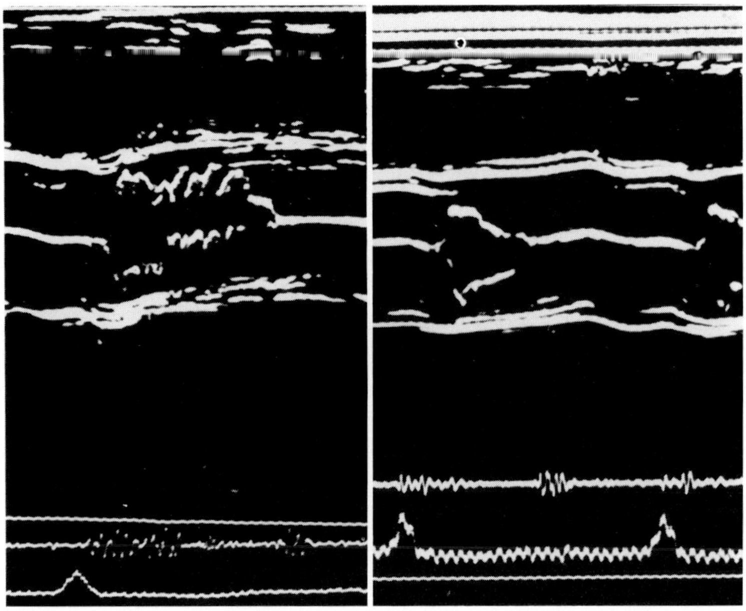

Fig. 5-17. Abnormal cusp movement in structurally normal valves. The aortic valve *(AV)* on the left shows a very coarse fluttering of the right coronary cusp and indications that the left coronary cusp moves toward a closed position in midsystole. Findings of this nature are frequently seen in patients with hypertrophic obstructive cardiomyopathy. In the right-hand panel the structurally normal aortic valve opens briskly, but the right coronary cusp rapidly collapses and does not show the abrupt closing movement characteristic of normals. This patient has a congestive cardiomyopathy with severe mitral regurgitation. Dimished systolic ejection from the mitral regurgitation probably accounts for the abnormal aortic closing pattern. *PHONO,* Phonocardiogram; *ECG,* electrocardiogram.

TABLE 6. Systolic flutter of the aortic valve in twenty-five consecutive patients

CARDIAC CATHETERIZATION DIAGNOSIS	NUMBER OF PATIENTS	COMMENTS
Coronary artery disease	9	4 left ventricular dysfunction, 1 papillary muscle dysfunction
Mitral regurgitation	5	Mixed rheumatic and nonrheumatic etiology
Hypertrophic obstructive cardiomyopathy	3	All showed associated mitral regurgitation
Ventricular septal defects	3	
Mitral stenosis	2	
Fistula from sinus of Valsalva to right atrium	1	
Atrial myxoma	1	
Pulmonary hypertension	1	

variety of conditions associated with aortic valve flutter is shown in Table 6.

Aortic root dissection. We have recently studied six patients with aortic root dissection confirmed by angiography, surgery, or autopsy (Fig. 5-18). All showed increased width of the anterior wall of the aortic root ranging from 16 to 21 mm. Similar widening of the posterior aortic wall was also found in most patients. This is in contrast with the normal mean aortic root wall thickness, which ranges from 5 to 7 mm in normal patients and in those with aortic valve disease. Recording the presence of slender aortic valve cusps in the lumen helps to identify the dissection wall. Variations in wall thickness demonstrated by transducer angulation were helpful in the identification of those dissections that were localized and did not involve the entire circumference of the aorta. The aortic root was widened in all patients (over 42 mm). Inspection of the image of the aortic wall showed that the outer margin was a strong echo complex while the inner margin of the dissection was a slender echo. The space between these margins of the dissection varies from a sonolucent one to one filled with linear and punctate echoes.

Another important feature in the identification of the dissection space is the fact that its margins retain their parallelism throughout the cardiac cycle. The combination of a widened aortic root, a widened wall with parallel margins, and a thicker outer echo as compared to the inner one is typical of aortic root dissection. Associated findings on the echocardiogram of pericardial effusion and mitral diastolic flutter help to consolidate the diagnosis.[53]

Tricuspid valve

The tricuspid valve occupies a shallow position compared to the mitral valve, seldom being more than 5 cm deep and often at the depth of the anterior margin of the aortic root or slightly deeper. It can be found by directing the ultrasonic beam

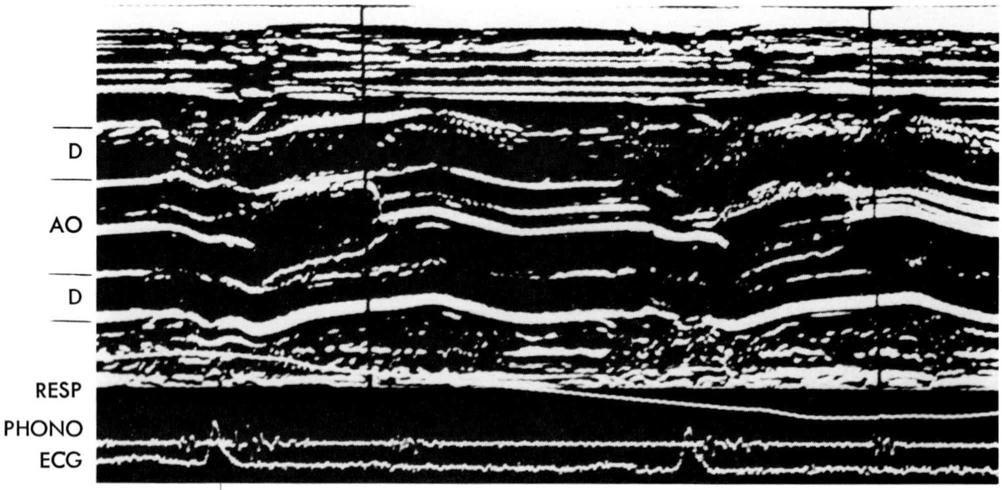

Fig. 5-18. Aortic root dissection. In this condition the aortic wall is markedly widened by the dissection space *(D)*. Characteristically the outer margin of this image is a thick echo while the inner margin is thin. Good parallelism between the outer and inner margins is maintained throughout the cardiac cycle. Aortic leaflets *(AO)* move within the true aortic lumen and their excursion is limited by the thin component of aortic wall. *RESP*, Respiration; *PHONO*, phonocardiogram; *ECG*, electrocardiogram.

medially and caudally from the aortic valve recording position. It is difficult to obtain a complete record through systole and diastole in the normal subject. Most often the segment in systole and the rapid diastolic opening movement are recorded. Inscription of a complete systolic and diastolic trace or the recording of two cusps usually indicate right ventricular enlargement, in our experience.

A steep transducer angulation required for recording the tricuspid valve results in a long sound path through chest wall tissues. Higher instrument sensitivities are therefore required than those used to record the aortic valve. Tricuspid valve recording suffers from the production of nonstructural clutter, which is imaged at approximately the plane of the tricuspid valve. We attempt to suppress the clutter by using a steep time-varied gain configuration to produce a smooth depression in the near field. Often this results in the suppression of the valve signals as well as the clutter.

The movement of the tricuspid valve is identical to that of the mitral valve (Fig. 5-19), and measurements made in normal individuals or patients with tricuspid stenosis are comparable to those obtained from the mitral valve.[54] However, we have observed a wide range of decreased diastolic slopes of the tricuspid valve in patients not affected by tricuspid stenosis. The motion of this valve is probably severely influenced by extrinsic forces such as restrictive processes involving the right ventricle or pericardium. For this reason, we advance the echocardiographic diagnosis of tricuspid stenosis with consider-

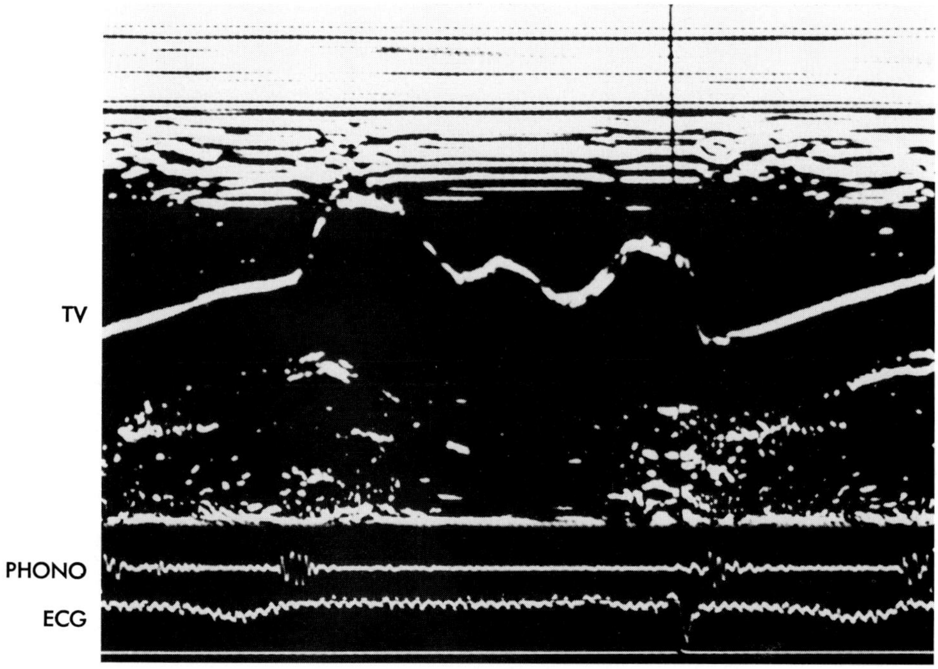

Fig. 5-19. Normal tricuspid valve. The general configuration of a normal tricuspid valve is very similar to the mitral valve. Complete traces are difficult to obtain in normal subjects and are usually found only when the right ventricular cavity is enlarged. *TV,* Tricuspid valve; *PHONO,* phonocardiogram; *ECG,* electrocardiogram.

able caution and use the method mainly to make a structural estimate of the condition of the tricuspid valve.

Diastolic flutterings of the tricuspid valve have been recorded in patients with pulmonic regurgitation. The analogy is identical to the fluttering of the mitral valve that occurs in aortic regurgitation. These are probably not specific findings for pulmonic regurgitation. We have seen them in other conditions, particularly in patients with large atrial septal defects, where flutter is believed to occur as a result of an increased flow across the valve (Fig. 5-20).

Pulmonary valve

Pulmonic valve echocardiography represents one of the newer areas in cardiac ultrasound.[55] For this reason few data are available about the movement patterns of this valve, especially about changes related to disease processes. It can be detected from a high left parasternal position by first passing the beam through the aortic root and then angling slowly toward the left shoulder of the patient. The image of the aortic walls disappears and the pulmonary artery becomes visible as a sonolucent space lying superficially near the aorta with its anterior wall within 1

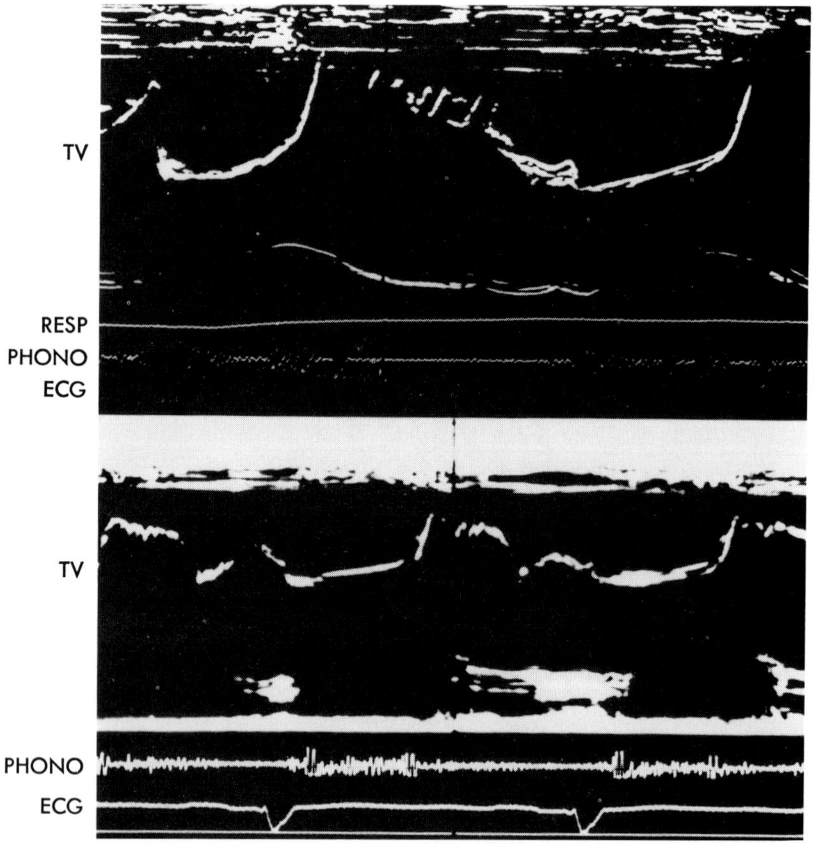

Fig. 5-20. Tricuspid valve flutter. Both patients show clinical evidence of pulmonic regurgitation. The diastolic flutter in the tricuspid valve is similar to that seen in the mitral valve with aortic regurgitation. Patients with atrial septal defects and large shunts have also shown a similar tricuspid flutter. *TV,* Tricuspid valve; *RESP,* respiration; *PHONO,* phonocardiogram; *ECG,* electrocardiogram.

to 2 cm of the inner margin of the chest. The posterior margin characteristically is a thick echo complex that usually lies 2 to 4 cm behind the anterior echo. Valve cusps appear as thin lines moving between the margins of the pulmonary artery with the heart cycle (Fig. 5-21). Another technique for the detection of the pulmonary valve depends on first localizing the mitral valve and then displacing the transducer

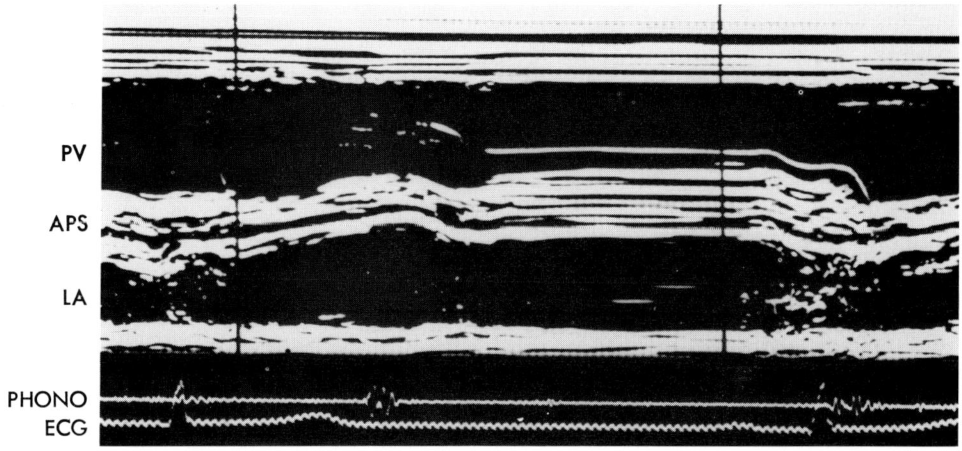

Fig. 5-21. Normal pulmonic valve. A pulmonic valve echo *(PV)* is seen in an anteriorly situated echo-free space. A prominent diastolic dip occurs following the P wave of the electrocardiogram and preceeds the normal opening pattern. The heavy echo pattern behind the valve arises in the atriopulmonic sulcus *(APS)* behind which the left atrium *(LA)* is situated. *PHONO,* Phonocardiogram; *ECG,* electrocardiogram.

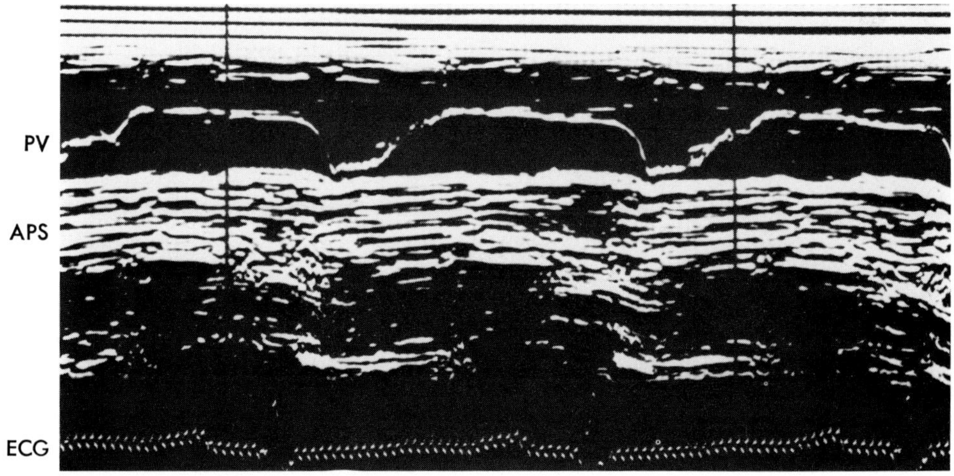

Fig. 5-22. Pulmonic valve echoes in pulmonary hypertension. The posterior dip of the pulmonic valve following atrial systole has been effaced and the valve can be seen to open more rapidly than normal. A high pulmonary artery diastolic pressure is believed to distend the pulmonic valve cusp, making it tense and less subject to displacement from low pressure events such as atrial systole.

one interspace toward the patient's head. With both techniques it is imperative to employ small movements and angulations of the transducer to find the thin valve cusp echoes.

The instrument settings for pulmonary valve detection are identical to those for the aortic valve and include relatively low overall sensitivity and considerable time-varied gain to suppress chest wall clutter.

The wide space that has been shown between the pulmonary artery and the left atrium has been designated the atriopulmonic sulcus. It contains fat, areolar tissue, the left coronary artery, and associated structures, all of which are probably the source of the thick echo complex commonly seen as the posterior margin of the pulmonary artery.

The potential usefulness of pulmonary valve studies may lie in the evaluation of pulmonary hypertension. Preliminary observations suggest that in the presence of high pulmonary artery pressure, the pulmonic valve assumes a straight diastolic configuration and rapid opening movements and resembles the aortic valve. On the other hand, with normal pulmonary artery pressure the opening movement is relatively slow, may occur slightly earlier, and also shows minor indentations related to physiologic events such as atrial systole. We presume that high pulmonary artery pressure distends the pulmonic cusp, making it difficult to displace with low pressure phenomena such as those associated with atrial emptying, while normal pulmonary artery pressure maintains a less tense pulmonic cusp that can be deflected when the atrium ejects blood into the ventricle (Fig. 5-22).[56]

Pericardial effusion

The ultrasonic detection of pericardial effusion is one of the most frequently requested clinical studies. Detection depends on the demonstration of a sonolucent space that separates a moving heart wall echo from a stationary pericardial echo (Fig. 5-23).[8] The anterior and posterior walls should be studied in all cases. Because of difficulties encountered in evaluation of echo complexes, some difference in opinion as to the reliability of the method has occurred.[12, 57-59] We recognize several of the pitfalls that have produced difficulty and can summarize them as follows.

Reliance on anterior heart wall echoes alone will produce false positives when the ultrasonic beam records the epicardial fat, which can be imaged as a sonolucent space. On the other hand, we have recorded right heart walls moving adjacent to a pericardium without an evident space in patients with large pericardial effusions. These have usually been patients with other heart disease that has enlarged the heart within the pericardial sac. The posterior wall can yield false positive examinations when the beam is passed through the left pulmonic vein, which lies behind the left ventricular wall at about the same level as the mitral valve (Fig. 5-24). False positives may also be obtained in posterior wall studies when sufficient pleural fluid accumulates and separates the heart from the lung. False negatives involving the posterior wall, on the other hand, are usually the result of poor sensitivity setting of the instrument so that nonstructural echoes or other forms of clutter obscure the pericardial effusion space.

The examination technique that we utilize involves scanning of the pericardial space by moving the transducer during recording. In this fashion, a false negative anterior space is quickly converted to a wide sonolucent space by scanning laterally toward the apex of the heart. Similarly, a false positive pulmonic vein space seen behind the mitral valve can be obliterated as the beam is scanned laterally over the free left ventricular wall. We do not ex-

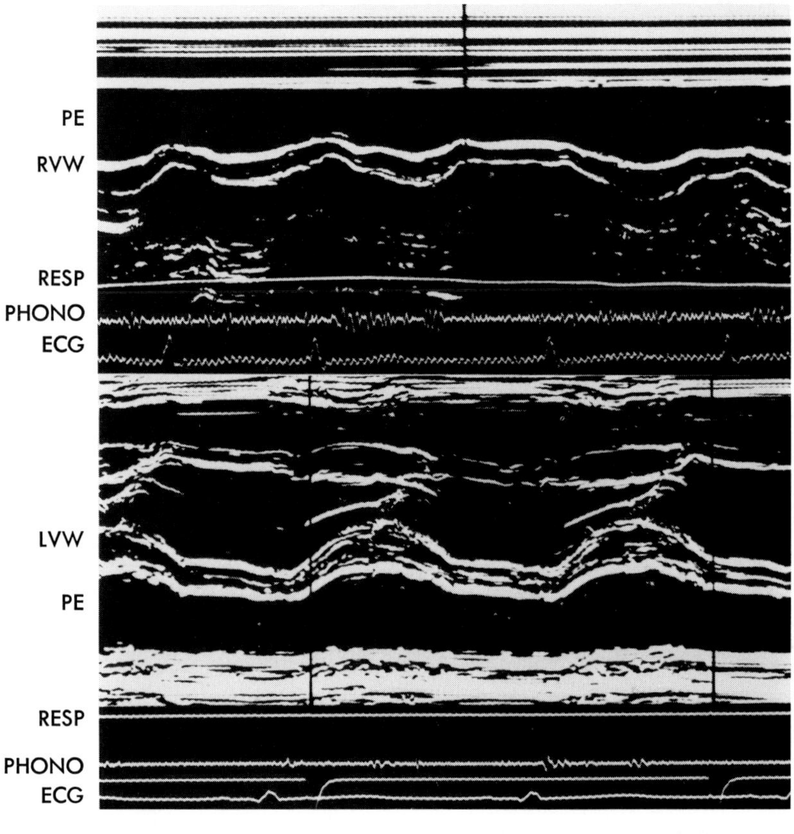

Fig. 5-23. Pericardial effusion. Individual recordings of anterior wall motion (upper panel) and posterior wall motion (lower panel) are shown. The pericardial effusion spaces *(PE)* are identified. Identification of both margins of the right ventricular wall *(RVW)* and left ventricular wall *(LVW)* helps to minimize diagnostic errors. *RESP,* Respiration; *PHONO,* phonocardiogram; *ECG,* electrocardiogram.

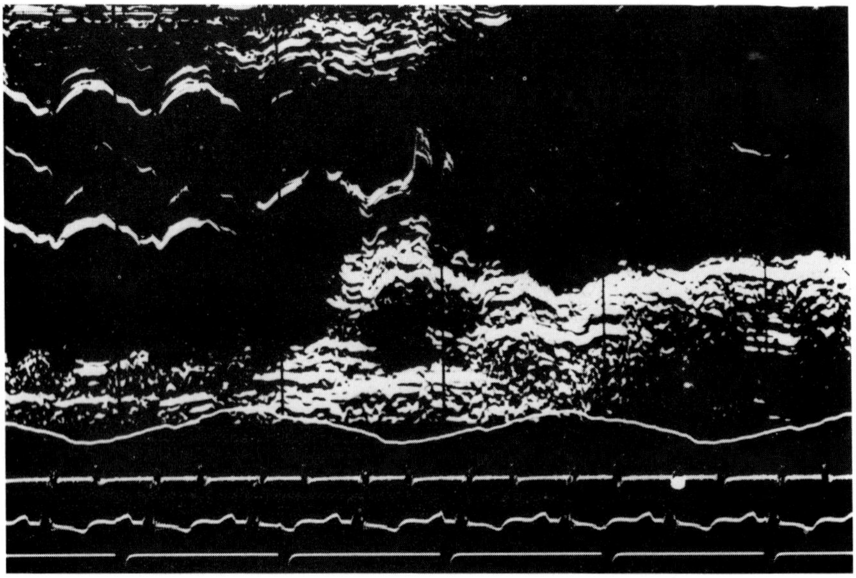

Fig. 5-24. Left pulmonic vein. In this study the examining beam was scanned from the aorta *(AO)* into the left ventricular cavity. As the beam passed the mitral valve a localized echo-free space could be identified behind it. Note that further movement of the beam into the left ventricular cavity shows a left ventricular wall *(LVW)* without a pericardial effusion space. If beam position is restricted during recording, the left pulmonic vein can produce a space behind the mitral valve which can be confused with pericardial fluid. *LA,* Left atrium; *RESP,* respiration; *PHONO,* phonocardiogram; *ECG,* electrocardiogram.

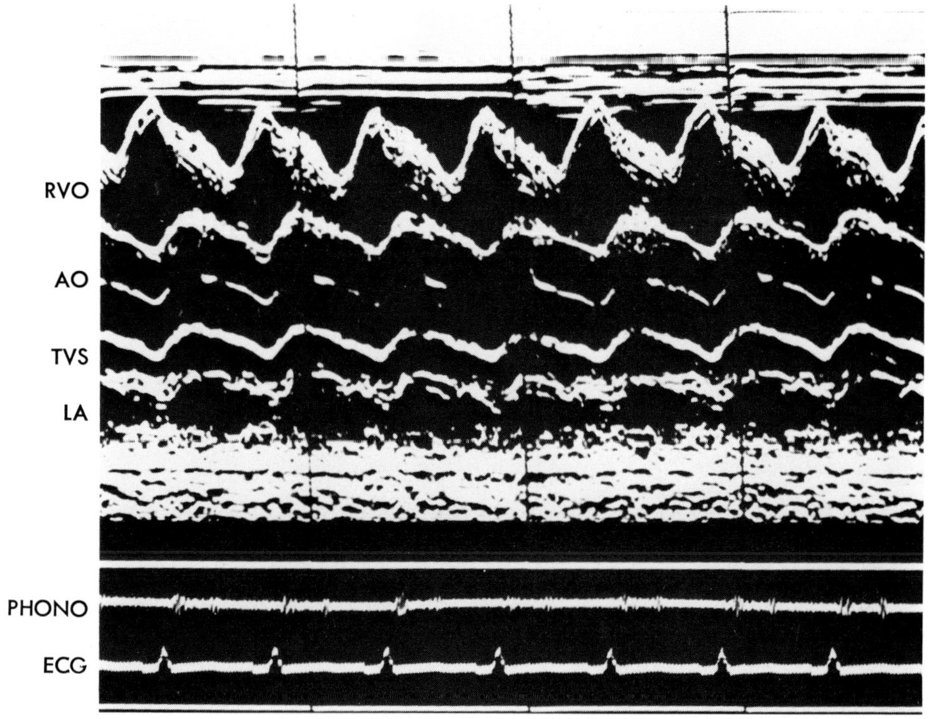

Fig. 5-25. The transverse sinus of the pericardium. This patient has a large pericardial effusion which is clearly seen in front of the right ventricular outflow tract *(RVO)*. The transverse sinus *(TVS)* is seen behind the posterior aortic wall and in front of the left atrial cavity *(LA)*. The transverse sinus characteristically shows a changing width during the cardiac cycle and has a pattern of aortic motion rather than left atrial. *AO,* Aorta; *PHONO,* phonocardiogram; *ECG,* electrocardiogram.

pect to find space behind the left atrial wall and we do not regularly look for it there.

Occasionally, one encounters an isolated posterior echo-free space that is probably caused by loculation of fluid. This is especially common in patients who have had previous cardiac surgery or malignant tumors. A solitary anterior pericardial effusion space is rare in our experience. In these difficult cases, it is of some value to study the image of the transverse sinus of the pericardium, which lies behind the aortic root in standard aortic valve echocardiograms. It may be possible to see widening of the posterior aortic image of a nonparallel nature to support the diagnosis of pericardial fluid. Similarly, the transverse sinus may be examined from a suprasternal position where it is found to lie between the image of the right pulmonary artery and the left atrium. Normally, no space is present here, though one may occur in the presence of pericardial fluid (Fig. 5-25).

We routinely examine the left pleural space in the posterior axillary line to determine the presence or absence of pleural fluid. When pleural and pericardial fluids coexist, it is possible to see a classic pericardial effusion space with a line that represents the pericardium separating it from a more deeply situated pleural effusion.

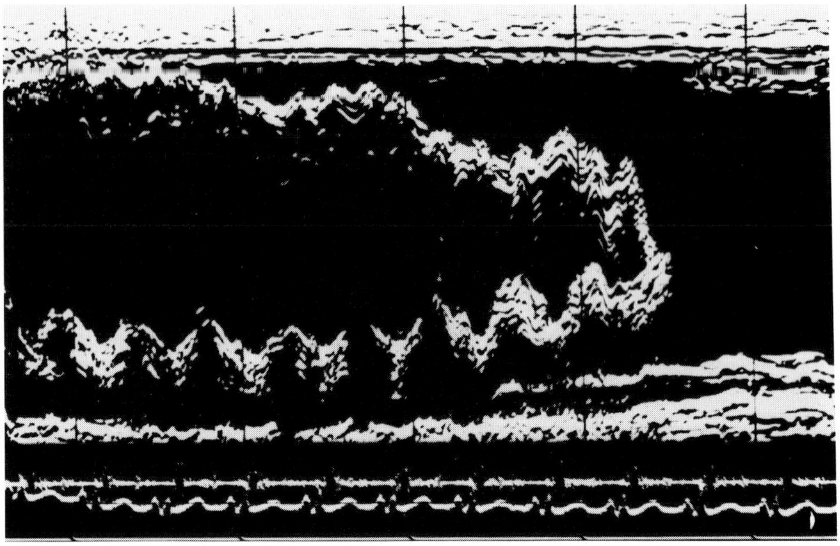

Fig. 5-26. Large pericardial effusion demonstrated by beam scanning technique. The beam is initially directed through the left ventricular cavity. No significant anterior space is present though a prominent posterior space is seen. As the beam is angled toward the apex of the heart the anterior space widens dramatically. *PHONO,* Phonocardiogram; *ECG,* electrocardiogram.

Quantitation of pericardial effusion space has been attempted by several authors, but this information should be treated with some caution.[60,61] A varying pericardial effusion width occurs frequently in our experience. The more laterally the examining beam is directed, the wider the space appears (Fig. 5-26).

The accuracy of the ultrasonic method has been compared to intracardiac carbon dioxide or radioisotope studies in animals.[62] It would appear that ultrasound is definitely superior to both of these techniques. However, accuracy in a clinical setting is less well defined. Others have shown posterior wall false positives that were found in the presence of pulmonary infiltrates.

The movement of the heart within the pericardial sac has been investigated in patients with pericardial fluid. The heart can be shown to swing in large pericardial effusions, and this is often associated with evidence of electrical alternans on the electrocardiogram.[63]

CONCLUSION

Echocardiography has developed into a reliable and useful tool for the investigation of patients with acquired heart disease. Its utility will develop as applications are increased through the medium of correlative clinical investigation. Our expectations are high that motion anatomic imaging techniques, tissue characterization studies, and intracardiac flow displays will extend the utility of this exciting new methodology and eventually displace some of the invasive investigative modalities.

REFERENCES

1. Firestone, F. A.: The supersonic reflectoscope, an instrument for inspecting the interior of solid parts by means of sound waves, J. Acoust. Soc. Am. **17:**287, 1945.
2. Edler, I., and Hertz, C. H.: Use of ultrasonic reflectoscope for the continuous recording of movements of heart walls, Kungl. Fysiog. Sallsk. Lund Forh. **24:**40, 1954.
3. Edler, I.: Diagnostic use of ultrasound in heart disease, Acta Med. Scand. **308:**32, 1955.

4. Edler, I.: Ultrasound cardiogram in mitral valve disease, Acta Chir. Scand. **111**:230, 1956.
5. Edler, I., and Gustafson, A.: Ultrasonic cardiogram in mitral stenosis, Acta Med. Scand. **159**: 85, 1957.
6. Effert, S., and Domanig, E.: The diagnosis of intra-atrial tumor and thrombi by the ultrasonic echo method, Ger. Med. Mon. **4**:1, 1959.
7. Joyner, C. R., Reid, J. M., and Bond, J. P.: Reflected ultrasound in the assessment of mitral valve disease, Circulation **27**:506, 1963.
8. Feigenbaum, H., Waldhausen, J. A., and Hyde, L. P.: Ultrasound diagnosis of pericardial effusion, J.A.M.A. **191**:107, 1965.
9. Feigenbaum, H., Zaky, A., and Nasser, W. K.: Use of ultrasound to measure left ventricular stroke volume, Circulation **35**:1092, 1967.
10. Gramiak, R., and Shah, P. M.: Echocardiography of the aortic root, Invest. Radiol. **3**:356, 1968.
11. Fortuin, N. J., and others: Determinations of left ventricular volumes by ultrasound, Circulation **44**:575, 1971.
12. Goldberg, B. B., Ostrum, B. J., and Isard, H. J.: Ultrasonic determination of pericardial effusion, J.A.M.A. **202**:103, 1967.
13. Popp, R. L., and others: Ultrasonic studies for the early detection of acute cardiac rejection, Transplantation **11**:543, 1971.
14. Segal, B. L., Likoff, W., and Kingsley, B.: Echocardiography: clinical application in mitral regurgitation, Am. J. Cardiol. **19**:50, 1967.
15. Winters, W. L., Jr., Hafer, J., Jr., and Soloff, L. A.: Abnormal mitral valve motion as demonstrated by the ultrasound technique in apparent pure mitral insufficiency, Am. Heart J. **77**:196, 1969.
16. Gramiak, R., Shah, P. M., and Kramer, D. H.: Ultrasound cardiography: contrast studies in anatomy and function, Radiology **92**:939, 1969.
17. Chang, S., and Feigenbaum, H.: Subxiphoid echocardiography, J. Clin. Ultrasound **1**(1):14-20, 1973.
18. Goldberg, B. B.: Suprasternal ultrasonography, J.A.M.A. **215**:245, 1971.
19. King, D. L., and others: Left ventricular volume determination by cross-sectional cardiac ultrasonography, Radiology **104**:201-202, 1972.
20. Waag, R. C. and others: Computer processing and display of cardiac ultrasound data (abstract), presented at the 17th Annual Meeting of the American Institute of Ultrasound in Medicine, Philadelphia, Pennsylvania, October 29-November 1, 1972.
21. Baker, D. W.: Pulsed ultrasonic doppler bloodflow sensing, I.E.E.E. Trans. Sonics Ultrasonics **SU-17**(3):170-185, 1970.
22. Bom, N., and others: Ultrasonic viewer for cross-sectional analyses of moving cardiac structures, Biomed. Engin. **6**:500-503, 1971.
23. Gramiak, R., Waag, R. C., and Simon, W.: Cine ultrasound cardiography, Radiology **107**:175-180, 1973.
24. Thurstone, F.: Personal communication.
25. Green, P.: Personal communication.
26. Korpel, A.: Acoustic imaging and holography, I.E.E.E. Spectrum **5**(10):45-52, 1968.
27. Winsberg, F., and Goldman, H. S.: Echo patterns of cardiac posterior wall, Invest. Radiol. **4**:173, 1969.
28. Edler, I.: Mitral valve function studied by ultrasound echo method. In Grossman, C. C., and others, editors: Diagnostic ultrasound, New York, 1968, Plenum Press, Inc.
29. Joyner, C. R., and others: Preoperative determination of the functional anatomy of the mitral valve, Circulation **32**(Suppl 2):120, 1965.
30. Segal, B. L., Likof, W., and Kingsley, B.: Echocardiography: clinical applications in mitral stenosis, J.A.M.A. **195**:161, 1966.
31. Winters, W. L., and others: Reflected ultrasound as a diagnostic instrument in study in mitral valve disease, Br. Heart J. **29**:788, 1967.
32. Effert, S.: Pre- and post operative evaluation of mitral stenosis by ultrasound, Am. J. Cardiol. **19**:59, 1967.
33. Nanda, N. C., and others: Ultrasound evaluation of mitral valve calcification (abstract), Circulation **46**(Suppl II):II-20, 1972.
34. Nanda, N. C., and others: Echocardiographic assessment of left ventricular outflow width in the selection of mitral valve prosthesis, Circulation **48**:1208-1214, 1973.
35. Gustafson, A.: Ultrasoundcardiography in mitral stenosis, Acta Med. Scand., Suppl. 461, p. 82, 1966.
36. Shah, P. M., and others: Determinants of atrial (S4) and ventricular (S3) gallop sound in primary myocardial disease, N. Engl. J. Med **278**:753, 1968.
37. Duchak, J. M., Chang, S., and Feigenbaum, H.: The posterior mitral valve echo and the echocardiographic diagnosis of mitral stenosis, Am. J. Cardiol. **29**:628, 1972.
38. Segal, B. L., Likof, W., and Kingsley, B.: Echocardiography; clinical application in combined mitral stenosis and mitral regurgitation, Am. J. Cardiol. **19**:42, 1967.
39. Kerber, R. E., Isaeff, D. M., and Hancock, E. W.: Echocardiographic patterns in patients with the syndrome of systolic click and late systolic murmur, N. Engl. J. Med. **284**:691, 1971.
40. Shah, P. M., and Gramiak, R.: Echocardiographic recognition of mitral valve prolapse (abstract), Circulation **42**(Suppl 3):45, 1970.

41. Sweatman, T. W., Selzer, A., and Cohn, K.: Echocardiographic diagnosis of ruptured chordae tendineae, Am. J. Cardiol. **26**:661, 1970.
42. Shah, P. M., Gramiak, R., and Kramer, D. H.: Ultrasound localization of left ventricular outflow obstruction in hypertrophic obstructive cardiomyopathy, Circulation **40**:3, 1969.
43. Shah, P. M., and others: Role of echocardiography in diagnostic and hemodynamic assessment of hypertrophic subaortic stenosis, Circulation **44**:891, 1971.
44. Shah, P. M., and others: Echocardiographic assessment of the effects of surgery and propranolol on the dynamics of outflow obstruction in hypertrophic subaortic stenosis, Circulation **45**:516-521, 1972.
45. Gramiak, R., and Shah, P. M.: Cardiac ultrasonography: a review of current applications, Radiol. Clin. North Am. **9**:469, 1971.
46. Finegan, R. E., and Harrison, D. C.: Diagnosis of left atrial myxoma by echocardiography, N. Engl. J. Med. **282**:1022, 1970.
47. Popp, R. L., and Harrison, D. C.: Ultrasound for the diagnosis of atrial tumors, Ann. Intern. Med. **7**:785, 1969.
48. Wolfe, S. B., Popp, R. L., and Feigenbaum, H.: Diagnosis of atrial tumors by ultrasound, Circulation **39**:615, 1969.
49. Johnson, M. L., and others: Echocardiographic diagnosis of a left atrial myxoma found attached to the free left atrial wall, J. Clin. Ultrasound **1**(1):75-81, 1973.
50. Winsberg, F., Gabor, G. E., and Hernberg, J. G.: Fluttering of the mitral valve in aortic insufficiency, Circulation **41**:225, 1970.
51. Pridie, R. B., Beham, R., and Oakley, C. M.: Echocardiography of the mitral valve in aortic valve disease, Br. Heart J. **33**:296, 1971.
52. Gramiak, R., and Shah, P. M.: Echocardiography of the normal and diseased aortic valve, Radiology **96**:1, 1970.
53. Nanda, N. C., Gramiak, R., and Shah, P. M.: Diagnosis of aortic root dissection by echocardiography, Circulation **48**:506-513, 1973.
54. Joyner, C. R., and others: Reflected ultrasound in the diagnosis of tricuspid stenosis, Am. J. Cardiol. **19**:66, 1967.
55. Gramiak, R., Nanda, N. C., and Shah, P. M.: Echocardiographic detection of pulmonary valve, Radiology **102**:153, 1972.
56. Nanda, N. C., and others: Echocardiographic diagnosis of pulmonary hypertension, Circulation. In press.
57. Bonte, F. J.: Referee's comments in Steinberg, J.: Angiocardiographic diagnosis of pericardial disease, Crit. Rev. Radiol. Sci. **1**:160, 1970.
58. Goldschlager, A. W., Freeman, L. M., and Davis, P. J.: Pericardial effusions and echocardiography: false results with ultrasound reflection method, N. Y. State J. Med. **67**:1854, 1967.
59. Moss, A. J., and Bruhn, B. L.: The echocardiogram: an ultrasound technique for the detection of pericardial effusion, N. Engl. J. Med. **274**:380, 1966.
60. Effert, S., Deupmann, F., and Karitsiotis, J.: Registration of movement of cardiac walls using an ultrasonic reflection procedure. In Kelly, E., editor: Ultrasonic energy, Urbana, 1965, University of Illinois Press.
61. Rothman, J., and others: Ultrasonic diagnosis of pericardial effusion, Circulation **35**:358, 1967.
62. Christensen, E. E., and Bonte, F. J.: The relative accuracy of echocardiography intravenous CO_2 studies and bloodpool scanning in detecting pericardial effusion in dogs, Radiology **9**:265, 1968.
63. Feigenbaum, H., Zaky, A., and Grabhorn, L.: Cardiac motion in patients with pericardial effusion: a study using ultrasound cardiography, Circulation **34**:611, 1966.

6

Physiologic applications of echocardiography

MORRIS N. KOTLER, M.B., BCH., M.R.C.P. (Edin.)

In recent years echocardiography has assumed greater importance in the diagnosis of various clinical disorders. Its reliability as a noninvasive technique in the evaluation of left ventricular function has been confirmed by several investigators.[1-8] Cardiac catheterization and angiography assess left ventricular function accurately but carry a risk and cannot be repeated at frequent intervals. This review will primarily emphasize cardiac function and wall motion as determined by echocardiography.

LEFT VENTRICULAR VOLUMES, STROKE VOLUME, AND EJECTION FRACTION

In Chapter 5, reference was made to the detection of pericardial effusion by recording posterior left ventricular wall movement. The calculation of left ventricular internal dimensions depends upon the simultaneous recording of left ventricular septal echoes and left ventricular endocardial echoes.

The transducer is angulated posteriorly and medially until the characteristic motion of the anterior mitral leaflet is identified. The ultrasonic beam is directed slightly laterally and inferiorly away from the mitral valve. This allows the septal echoes and left ventricular posterior wall echoes to be visualized. The distinctive septal echoes are recognized as two nearly parallel echoes 1 to 4 cm from the broad band of chest wall echoes (Fig. 6-1). By appropriate adjustments of the gain setting (or attenuator), the endocardial surface of the left ventricular posterior wall can be identified. It should be emphasized that more anterior discrete echoes ("X line" in Fig. 6-2) should not be confused with the endo-

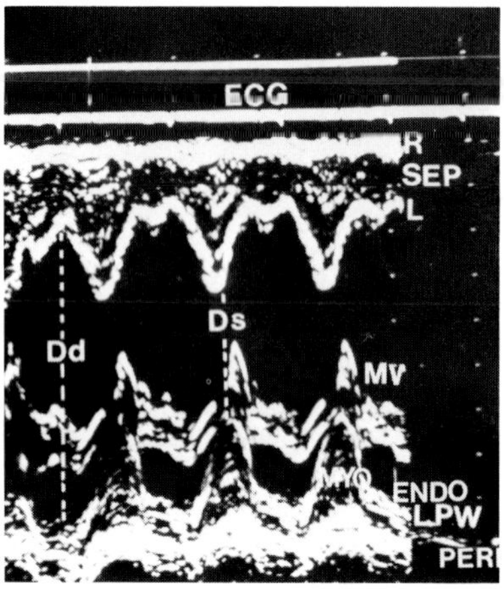

Fig. 6-1. Echocardiogram of left ventricle. The left ventricular dimension at end-diastole *(Dd)* and end-systole *(Ds)* is measured to 0.1 cm from the endocardial echo *(ENDO)* to the left side of the interventricular septal echo *(L)* during each part of the cardiac cycle. Systolic dimension *(Ds)* is defined as the smallest distance separating the endocardial surfaces of the septum and left ventricular posterior wall. Diastolic dimension *(Dd)* is usually the largest distance separating the endocardial surfaces and is measured along a vertical line drawn through the QRS complex. The left ventricular posterior wall *(LPW)* is comprised of endocardium *(ENDO)*, myocardium *(MYO)*, and pericardium *(PERI)*. *MV*, Mitral valve. Right side of the septum *(R)*, toward the top of the figure, is anterior.

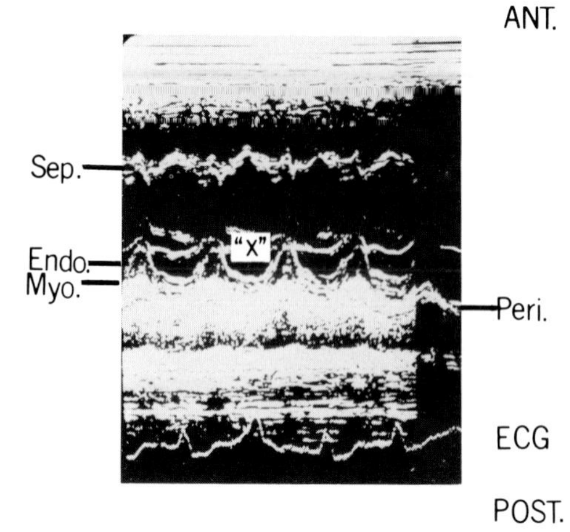

Fig. 6-2. Echocardiogram of left ventricle in a patient with volume overload of the left ventricle caused by acute aortic insufficiency. The briskly moving endocardial *(Endo)* echoes can be clearly differentiated from the sluggish anterior moving posterior chordal or "X" echoes. The myocardium and pericardium are shown; the latter is the strong posterior wall echo that is recorded when the attenuation is increased or gain setting decreased. *ANT*, Anterior; *Sep*, septum; *ECG*, electrocardiogram; *POST*, posterior.

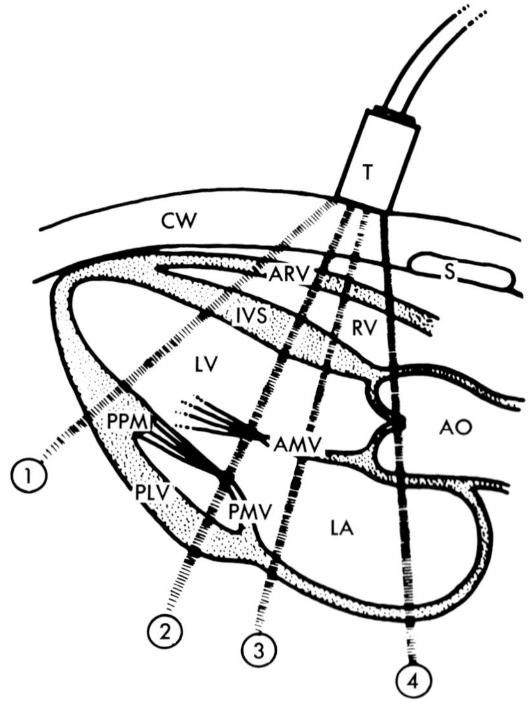

Fig. 6-3. Cross-section of heart showing structures through which ultrasonic beam passes as it is directed from apex toward base of heart. *CW*, Chest wall; *T*, transducer; *S*, sternum; *ARV*, anterior right ventricular wall; *RV*, right ventricular cavity; *IVS*, interventricular septum; *LV*, left ventricle; *PPM*, posterior papillary muscle; *PLV*, posterior left ventricular wall; *AMV*, anterior mitral valve; *PMV*, posterior mitral valve; *AO*, aorta; *LA*, left atrium. (From Feigenbaum, H.: Clinical applications of echocardiography, Progr. Cardiovasc. Dis. **14**:531, 1972. By permission of Grune and Stratton, Inc.)

cardial echoes. The "X" line is thought to represent chordal echoes or echoes from the posterior mitral valve apparatus.[9] The echoes from the posterior chordae can be distinguished from those of the posterior left ventricular endocardium by high intensity, discrete outline, and diminished amplitude of motion during systole[3] (Fig. 6-2). Epicardial echoes may also be mistaken for endocardial echoes, although motion of the endocardial echo is more rapid than the epicardial echo.

Fig. 6-3 is a diagrammatic sketch of the heart with different positions of the ultrasonic beam as the transducer is scanned from the apex of the heart to the base of the heart. Position 2 is ideal for calculation of the left internal dimension.[10] The recording of the mitral valve (predominantly the posterior leaflet and its chordae) as well as echoes from the left side of the septum and posterior left ventricular endocardium assures the examiner of a most satisfactory transducer and beam location.

If the transducer is tilted toward the apex (position 1), posterior chordal echoes merge with echoes from the papillary muscle and the true posterior endocardial echo cannot be clearly identified. It should be appreciated that if echoes from the papillary muscle are misinterpreted as arising from posterior endocardial echoes, the left ventricular cavity would be spuriously narrowed and erroneous calculation of ventricular volumes would ensue. Thus ventricular volumes derived from measurements recorded in position 1 would tend to underestimate the true ventricular volume and would be less accurate than measurements obtained from position 2.

If the transducer is tilted toward the base of the heart to positions 3 and 4, the posterior echo would represent the left atrial wall. Thus both these positions are totally unsatisfactory for recording left ventricular internal dimensions.

The left ventricular dimension at end-diastole (*Dd*) and at end-systole (*Ds*) is measured (to the nearest 0.1 cm) from the endocardial echo of the posterior wall to the left side of the interventricular septal echo (Fig. 6-1). End-diastolic dimension is usually measured at the peak of the *R* wave of the simultaneously displayed electrocardiogram and end-systolic diameter at the time of maximal anterior movement of the posterior left ventricular wall.

Based on the Dodge formula,[11] which assumes that the ventricle is similar to a prolate ellipsoid:

$$\text{Volume } (V) = (\tilde{\Pi}/6)\ D1\ D2\ L$$

where

$D1$ and $D2$ = angiographic anteroposterior and lateral minor diameters
L = longer of the major diameters from the two radiographic projections

According to Sandler and Dodge,[12] the respective minor diameters are essentially equal for the left ventricular chamber. The formula can therefore be expressed as $V = (\tilde{\Pi}/6)\ D^2L$. If the long diameter is assumed to be twice the short diameter,[11,12] the formula may be further simplified to $V = (\tilde{\Pi}/6)\ D^2\ (2D)$. The volume in both diastole and systole approximately equals the cube of the short diameter provided the formula assumes the algebraic cancellation of the factor $\tilde{\Pi}/3$. The end-diastolic volume (*EDV*) is equal to the cube of the end-diastolic dimension $(Dd)^3$ and end-systolic volume (*ESV*) is equal to the cube of the end-systolic dimension $(Ds)^3$.

This method, as described by Pombo and associates,[5] equates left ventricular stroke volume with the difference in cubes of the end-diastolic and end-systolic dimensions.

$$\text{Stroke volume } (SV) = EDV - ESV$$
$$\text{or } SV = (Dd)^3 - (Ds)^3$$

and

$$\text{Ejection fraction} = \frac{SV}{EDV} \text{ or } \frac{(Dd)^3 - (Ds)^3}{Dd^3}$$

Another method for determining ejection fractions has been described by Fortuin and co-workers and utilizes regression equations.[6]

$$EDV = 59\ Dd - 153$$
$$ESV = 47\ Ds - 120$$

Although this method has been reported to give more accurate results, especially in patients with low stroke volume, others have disputed these claims.[9]

Initial correlations between the ultrasonic diastolic left ventricular dimension and the angiographic end-diastolic volume were satisfactory.[7] Squaring the ultrasonic measurements improved the correlation value, and cubing the ultrasonic diastolic left ventricular dimension improved the *r* value from 0.7880 to 0.8950. Similar findings were reported with systolic measurements.[7] Ultrasonic stroke volume correlations with angiographic stroke volumes were initially disappointing.[7] However, when stroke volume, as determined by ultrasound, was compared with stroke volume, as determined by the Fick or indicator dilution techniques, better correlation was obtained with an *r* value of 0.9620.[2] It should be noted that the technique of recording interventricular septal echoes and posterior wall endocardial echoes were better standardized in the latter study. In addition, ultrasonic measurements were recorded simultaneously with stroke volume or cardiac output determinations measured by indicator dilution or Fick method.[2]

Several studies have reported on the validity of the ventricular internal dimensions as a method of calculating ventricular volumes, stroke volume, and ejection fraction.[3-7] Although it is generally believed that the ultrasonic left ventricular internal dimension approximates the short axis, in point of fact it may represent a dimension lying between the short and long axes of the ventricle.[13] It is possible, therefore, that volumes determined by ultrasound may overestimate a large ventricle because it is more spherical and underestimate a small left ventricle because it is more oblong. In addition, Teicholz[14] found no correlation between the echocardiographically determined left ventricular volume and the angiographically determined volume in patients with asynergy of the left ventricle.

Despite the glowing reports in the literature attesting to the value of ultrasonic determination of left ventricular internal dimensions, the technique is difficult. The technical failure rate varies between 18% and 40%.[5,15] In patients with gross obesity, emphysema, or chest deformity, satisfactory recordings may not be obtained. Since a small portion of the posterior left ventricular wall can be evaluated by ultrasound, large anterior akinetic or dyskinetic areas may be missed. In three patients with diaphragmatic infarction, the stroke volume was somewhat greater with measurements obtained with ultrasound than that obtained by the indicator dilution method.[15]

LEFT VENTRICULAR WALL THICKNESS AND MASS

Several investigators have studied left ventricular wall thickness by echocardiography.[16-18] It appears that wall thickness increases with age and that systolic measurements exceed diastolic measurements by approximately 5 to 7 mm.[18] The correlation between wall thickness as determined by ultrasound correlates well with values calculated by angiographic methods and with autopsy specimens.[18]

Troy and associates[19] studied twenty-four patients with valvular and/or myocardial disease and found a good correlation between ultrasonically determined left ventricular mass as compared to angiographically determined left ventricular mass. The *r* value was 0.883. The technique for studying left ventricular wall thickness and mass is identical to that described in the section on volume determinations. Particular attention should be paid to obtaining clear endocardial and epicardial echoes (Fig. 6-4). In order to define the strong pericardial echo, the attenuation or gain setting has to be changed in the latter half of the sweep across the screen, decreasing the number of recordable echoes (Fig. 6-4). Wall thickness *(d)*, or *WTd*, represents the end-diastolic wall thickness and wall thickness *(s)*, the end-systolic wall thickness (Fig. 6-4). Note that the wall thickens from end-diastole to end-systole.

In order to determine the mass of the left ventricular myocardium, two basic measurements are required: (1) the end-diastolic diameter of the left ventricular cavity *(Dd)*, measured as the distance from the left side of the ventricular septal echo to the endocardial echo of the posterior wall at the time of inscription of the *R* wave, and (2) the thickness of the wall echo at end-diastole *(WTd)*, measured as the distance between endocardium and epicardium of the posterior wall. Therefore, the total volume of the left ventricle (cavity plus muscle) can be expressed as:

$$\text{Volume } LV\ (C + M) = (Dd + WTd)^3$$

where

$$C = \text{cavity}$$
$$M = \text{muscle}$$

The volume of the *left ventricular myocardium* would be equal to the total volume of the left ventricle minus the ventricular cavity volume:

$$\text{Volume } LVM = (Dd + WTd)^3 - (Dd)^3$$

In order to calculate *left ventricular mass*, left ventricular myocardial volume is multiplied by 1.05, the specific gravity of heart muscle. Thus:

$$\text{Left ventricular mass} = LVM \text{ Vol} \times 1.05$$

One potential serious limitation of this technique is that if the endocardium or pericardium were markedly thickened, determination of myocardial wall thickness would be falsely increased.

Although determinations of left ventricular mass and the percent of systolic wall thickening may be useful, it is not entirely clear that these measurements offer any advantage over stroke volume and ejection fraction determinations in the evaluation of left ventricular performance.

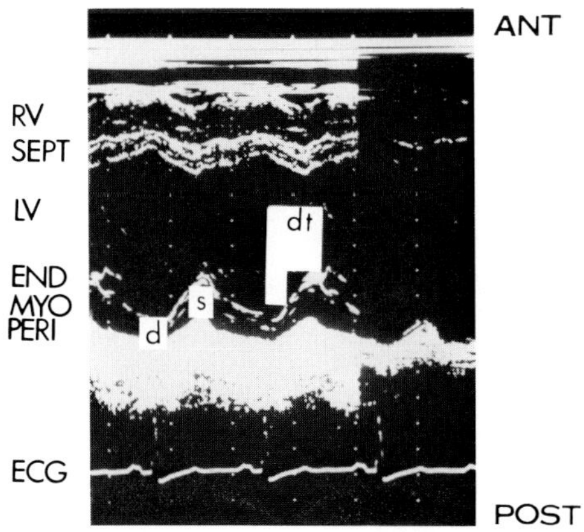

Fig. 6-4. Echocardiogram obtained from a patient with chronic aortic and mitral insufficiency. Simultaneous electrocardiogram *(ECG)* and time-distance markers are displayed. The distance between each dot on the vertical axis represents 1 cm and the interval between each dot on the horizontal axis represents 0.5 second. From anterior to posterior are seen the right ventricle *(RV)*, interventricular septum *(SEPT)*, left ventricular cavity *(LV)*, and endocardium *(END)*, myocardium *(MYO)*, and pericardium *(PERI)*. In the right third of the Polaroid picture, the attenuation or gain setting has been changed to identify the strong pericardial echo. Diastolic wall thickness *(d)* and systolic wall thickness *(s)* are measured from endocardium to pericardium during end-diastole and during maximal shortening, respectively. The duration of shortening *(dt)* is measured from the time from initial anterior movement of the posterior wall to the peak of anterior wall motion.

MEASUREMENT OF MEAN RATE OF CIRCUMFERENTIAL FIBER SHORTENING

The mean velocity of circumferential fiber shortening (VCF), previously determined by cineangiographic methods,[20] is directly related to cardiac muscle function and may provide more reliable information about ventricular performance than the determination of ejection fraction alone. Based on the previously described formulas used for determination of ejection fraction, mean rate of circumferential fiber shortening can be calculated as follows: Internal circumference at end-diastole *(Cd)* can be determined by $Cd = \tilde{\Pi}\ Dd$ and at end-systole *(Cs)*, $Cs = \tilde{\Pi}\ Ds$.

The mean velocity of circumferential shortening (VCF) in centimeters per second (cm/sec) is equal to the change in circumference during systole divided by the duration of shortening:

$$VCF = \frac{Cd - Cs}{dt} = \frac{(Dd - Ds)}{dt}$$

However, since VCF is affected by heart size, the equation is divided by *Cd,* which allows for comparison of a mean VCF among different patients.[21] Thus:

$$VCF = \tilde{\Pi}\frac{(Dd - Ds)/dt}{\tilde{\Pi}\ Dd}$$

or

$$\frac{Dd - Ds/dt}{Dd}$$

dt can be determined directly from the echocardiogram by measuring the time from initial anterior movement of the posterior wall to the peak of anterior wall motion (Fig. 6-4).[21] In another report[9] *dt* or ejection time was defined as the length of time from the peak of the QRS complex to the maximum anterior excursion of the left ventricular posterior wall less 50 msec for preejection period when no appreciable fiber shortening takes place.

In patients with normal left ventricular function, the average mean VCF determined by ultrasound was 1.29 ± 0.23 circumferences per second, while in patients with reduced left ventricular performance the value was less than average, 0.75 circumference per second.[9] Mean VCF by ultrasound correlated well with mean VCF by cine angiographic methods ($r = 0.81$, $P \langle\ 0.0001$).[9] Fortuin and co workers,[21] applying mean VCF as determined by ultrasound, were able to separate those patients with congestive heart failure from normal persons. In addition, patients with mitral stenosis had reduced values whereas those patients with idiopathic hypertrophic subaortic stenosis had increased values as compared to normal individuals.

Based on the two reported series[9,21] ultrasound determination of the mean rate of circumferential fiber shortening does not offer a distinct advantage over determination of ejection fraction as indices of left ventricular function.

LEFT VENTRICULAR WALL MOTION

Kraunz and Kennedy[22] studied the posterior wall motion in twenty-five healthy adult males at rest and following exercise. A characteristic posterior wall motion curve was obtained in all individuals. Fig. 6-5 demonstrates the normal posterior wall motion at rest and exercise with the normal measurements listed in Table 7. Point *A* in Fig. 6-5 corresponds to the onset of atrial contraction. The line from *B* to *C* describes wall motion during the period of isovolumetric contraction. During systolic ejection *(CD)* anterior wall motion occurs. Isovolumetric relaxation is represented by the period from point *D* to *E*. The posterior wall motion returns almost to its baseline position *F*, and the line from *E* to *F* describes the wall motion in early diastole. The total amplitude of excursion of the posterior wall motion (PWE)[22] or systolic endocardial excursion (SEE)[23] was measured as the vertical distance between the *C* and *D* points. By drawing a tangent to the steepest point of the systolic limb of the curve and measuring the slope in centimeters per second, the maximal posterior wall velocity (PWVM)[22] or the maximal systolic endocardial velocity (SEVM)[23] was

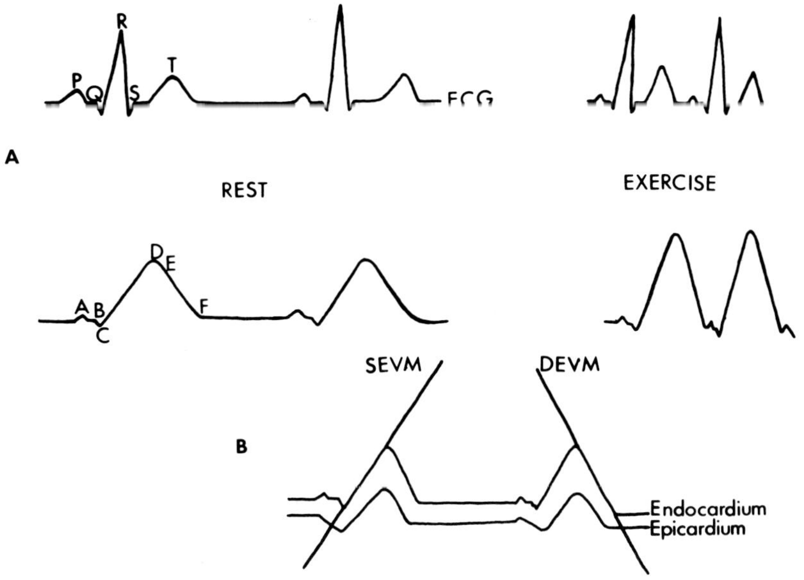

Fig. 6-5. A, Demonstration of normal posterior wall motion and excursion (pericardium) at rest and exercise (Kraunz and Kennedy[22]). **B,** Normal posterior wall motion (endocardium) at rest (Fogelman[23]). Endocardial slopes are steeper than epicardial or pericardial slopes. For abbreviations see text.

TABLE 7. Posterior left ventricular wall motion obtained at rest and on exercise in normals and in patients with angina pectoris*

Data of Kraunz and Kennedy[22]

	REST	EXERCISE
Heart rate (beats/min)	66 ± 8	107 ± 17
Posterior wall (PWE) (cm)	0.72 ± 0.18	0.96 ± 0.25
Maximum velocity (PWVM) (cm/sec)	41 ± 1.1	9.2 ± 2.8
Mean posterior wall velocity (PWV) (cm/sec)	2.7 ± 0.58	5.2 ± 1.3

Data of Fogelman, Abbasi, Pearce, and Kattus[23]

	REST		IMMEDIATELY AFTER EXERCISE	
	NORMAL	ANGINA	NORMAL	ANGINA
Heart rate (beats/min)	69	63	74	90
Systolic endocardial excursion (SEE) (cm)	1.4 ± 0.3	1.4 ± 0.3	1.5 ± 0.3	1.5 ± 0.3
Maximal systolic endocardial velocity (SEVM) (cm/sec)	6.6 ± 1.0	6.5 ± 1.3	7.2 ± 1.4	7.2 ± 2.2
Maximal diastolic endocardial velocity (DEVM) (cm/sec)	17 ± 3	15 ± 4	21 ± 3	8.2 ± 32
Mean systolic endocardial velocity (SEV) (cm/sec)	4.7 ± 0.6	4.4 ± 0.8	5.0 ± 0.6	5.3 ± 1.6
Mean early diastolic endocardial velocity (DEV) (cm/sec)	9.3 ± 1.6	8.4 ± 0.8	10 ± 2	5.7 ± 2.2

*All values are mean ± standard deviation.

determined (Fig. 6-5). Similarly, the maximal diastolic endocardial velocity (DEVM)[23] was determined by drawing a tangent to the steepest point of the diastolic limb of the curve and measuring the slope in centimeters per second (Fig. 6-5). The mean posterior wall velocity (mean PWV)[22] or mean systolic endocardial velocity (SEV)[23] was measured as the slope of the line extending from the onset of anterior displacement of the posterior wall[22] or endocardial displacement[23] to peak of the echogram *(C-D)*. Fogelman and associates[23] measured the mean early diastolic endocardial velocity (DEV) as the slope of the line extending from the peak of the echogram to the end of the rapid posterior motion of the endocardium in early diastole *(D-F)*.

Considerable differences are apparent in values obtained between the two series published (Table 7). It should be noted that measurements obtained by Kraunz and Kennedy[22] applied to the pericardium, whereas the measurements obtained by Fogelman and co-workers[23] were limited to movement of the endocardium.

On the basis of Fogelman's observations,[23] the following conclusions could be drawn:

1. Posterior wall movement of the heart was more rapid during early diastolic relaxation then during systolic contraction.
2. Exercise increased the rate of systolic motion, a finding that is compatible with Kraunz and Kennedy's observations.[22]
3. In patients with angina pectoris, no significant difference was observed with regard to systolic endocardial excursion (SEE) and maximal systolic endocardial velocity (SEVM) at rest and during exercise as compared to normal controls.
4. In eight patients with typical ischemic findings, manifested by anginal pain and/or associated S-T segment depression, there was a marked and significant decrease in maximal diastolic endocardial velocity (DEVM) and mean early diastolic endocardial velocity (DEV) below the control resting values.

Although this interesting phenomenon observed by Fogelman and others[23] has not been adequately explained, it appears that during the ischemic state impaired early diastolic relaxation may occur. The alternate hypothesis, namely an abnormal response to exercise associated with the aging phenomenon, seems less likely.

Inoue and co-workers[24] evaluated the left ventricular posterior wall motion in eleven patients with acute myocardial infarction. Five patients had posterior wall excursions less than 0.6 cm and four patients had mean posterior wall velocities of less than 2.0 cm/sec. These findings were ascribed to a decreased left ventricular stroke volume and a reduction in myocardial contractility. The mechanism of production of the bulges was thought to result from myocardial asynergy or abnormal ventricular motion. The conclusions drawn by Inoue and his colleagues[24] may not be entirely justified, since they studied the epicardium and interpreted their findings in relation to myocardial abnormalities. Similarly, Wharton and co-workers[25] studied the epicardium in eight patients with acute myocardial infarction and concluded that maximum posterior wall velocity decreased by 26% and posterior wall excursion decreased by 46% during the first 36-hour period after infarction.

In addition, atrial pacing by increasing the heart rate actually resulted in a reduction of both maximal posterior wall velocity and posterior wall excursion,[26] suggesting that the opposite effects of exercise are probably caused by other factors and are not related to the increased heart rate.

Twenty-four patients with heart failure of diverse etiology studied by Carson and Kanter[27] had a slower rate of backward diastolic wall motion at rest than did normal subjects. From their published echocardiogram it is not clear whether endocardium or epicardium is the posterior wall echo.

It is evident from the numerous reports that there is lack of standardization concerning the technique of obtaining the posterior left ventricular wall echo. In addition, as mentioned previously, chordal echoes may be erroneously misinterpreted as representing endocardial echoes. From a practical point, the technique of recording endocardial and left ventricular wall echoes during exercise in the supine position is extremely difficult to obtain because of hyperventilation. It is almost impossible to perform an adequate study in the upright position during bicycle or treadmill exercise because of the inability to hold the transducer stationary and because of the constant angulation of the transducer that is necessary to focus on the posterior left ventricular wall at all times. In order to overcome this problem, investigators have recently devised a technique that allows the transducer to be mounted on an aluminum platform held to the chest wall.[28] With the aid of a remote control system that is also connected to two hydraulic pistons mounted on the platform, the transducer can be moved and angulated. The apparatus allows the transducer to be adjusted constantly and to be held stationary despite movement of the patient during tilting and exercise. This promising technique should allow investigators a unique opportunity of employing a noninvasive method in evaluating left ventricular function in the exercising patient.

Despite the numerous reports[22-29] confirming the reliability of posterior wall velocity as an index of left ventricular contractility, a recent report has cast doubt on this assumption.[30] Karliner and coworkers[30] compared mean posterior wall velocity as obtained by echocardiography with externally recorded systolic time intervals in thirty-nine patients with coronary heart disease and in twenty of the patients with the ejection fraction obtained from biplane left ventricular cine angiograms. Mean posterior wall velocity correlated poorly with ejection fraction and with the ratio of the preejection period to the left ventricular ejection time.

McDonald and co-workers[31] studied the septal and posterior left ventricular wall motion on twenty individuals with normal hearts. Careful attention was paid to obtaining echoes of good quality from the endocardial surfaces of the left side of the interventricular septum and of the posterior left ventricular wall. In order to achieve the ideal direction of the transducers, identification of the posterior mitral valve anterior to the posterior left ventricular wall was mandatory. On closer analysis during preejection systole, slight movement either toward or away from the transducer was observed, but for the most part the posterior left ventricular wall endocardial echo remained stationary.

After injecting indocyanine green dye into the left ventricular cavity, a cloud of echoes is produced that completely fills the left ventricular cavity, clearly delineating the endocardial surfaces of the left ventricular septum and posterior left ventricular wall.[32] This technique allows true confirmation of endocardial septal and posterior left ventricular wall echoes. Thus the classic descriptions of movement of the posterior left ventricular wall echoes at rest, during exercise,[22] in patients with angina pectoris[23] or myocardial infarction,[29] and after pharmacologic interventions[33] may be misleading since the techniques were not standardized.

MITRAL VALVE FLOW AND CHANGES IN MOTION OF THE ANTERIOR MITRAL VALVE LEAFLET AS DETERMINANTS OF LEFT VENTRICULAR FUNCTION

The typical mitral valve orifice as determined by echocardiographic studies has three distinctive components[34] (Fig. 6-6). The first component is diamond shaped, and it is during this part of the cardiac

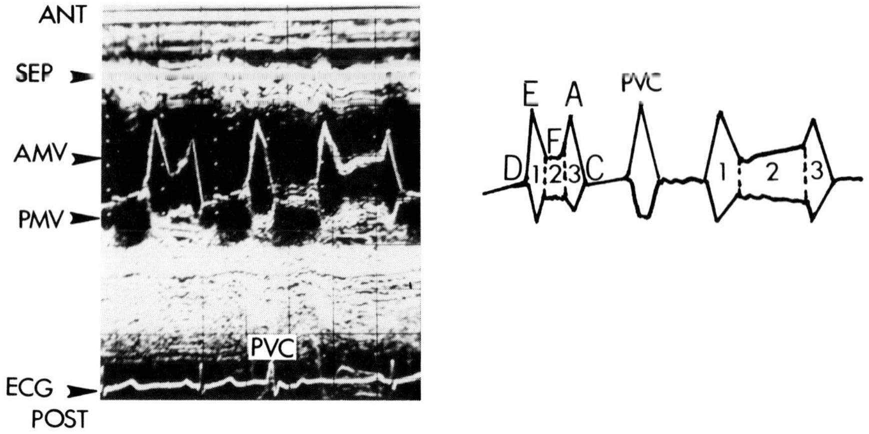

Fig. 6-6. Normal mitral echogram before, during, and after a premature ventricular contraction *(PVC)*. The three distinctive components of the mitral valve orifice are clearly seen in the idealized diagram on the right before and after the PVC. Note that mitral valve orifice begins at the *D* point (when both anterior [*AMV*] and posterior mitral valve [*PMV*] leaflets begin to separate) and ends at the *C* point (when both AMV and PMV meet in systole). Mitral valve orifice is increased following a PVC analogous to the increased stroke volume following a PVC.

cycle that rapid filling of the ventricle occurs. Following the rapid filling phase, the valves assume a semiclosed position, producing a low-amplitude, rectangular configuration or second component. With the onset of atrial contraction the third component is produced; it is short and diamond shaped. The sum of the products of the maximal amplitude and duration of the individual components resulted in a mitral valve index.[34] In thirteen patients the mitral valve index correlated with the stroke volume, the latter measurement determined by the Fick method.

In patients with significantly elevated left ventricular end-diastolic pressure, a reduced atrial component or an inapparent A wave of the mitral echogram may be recorded (Fig. 6-7).

In addition, delay between atrial relaxation and ventricular systole may occur in these patients, giving a rounded appearance to the terminal part of the A wave (Fig. 6-7). This pause or delay has been found to occur between the peak of the A wave and the onset of rapid systolic rise in left ventricular pressure.[35]

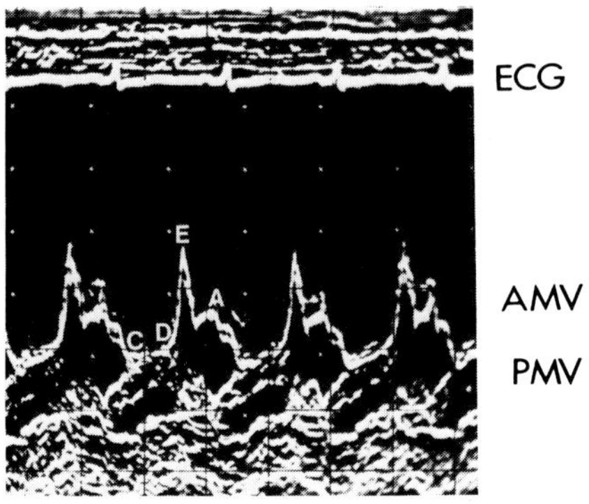

Fig. 6-7. Mitral valve echogram from a patient with ischemic heart disease, papillary muscle dysfunction, and severe ventricular dysfunction. Cardiac index measured 2 L/min/m^2 and LVEDP 30 mm Hg. The inapparent A wave and closure of the mitral valve *A-C* is prolonged. Rate of diastolic closure slope is increased measuring 185 mm/sec.

SUMMARY

Of fundamental importance in determining left ventricular function by ultrasound is the ability to record clear endocardial echoes from the left side of the septum and posterior left ventricular wall. Techniques and formulas for determining left ventricular volume measurements, stroke volume, ejection fraction, left ventricular wall mass, and rate of circumferential fiber shortening have been reviewed. Controversy still persists as to the method of recording left ventricular wall motion and its usefulness as an index of left ventricular function. Echocardiographic evaluation of left ventricular function offers the investigator physiologic and useful information, and it allows the clinician a more rational approach to a problem with regard to functional evaluation and therapy. In the field of coronary artery disease, where this technique would be of the most value, problems have been encountered. Hopefully, with newer engineering developments and techniques, the ability to obtain adequate recordings will improve. In addition, because of the tremendous enthusiasm generated by the initial promising results, reports containing conflicting data have appeared. In the future more attention should be paid to the control and design of studies. Nevertheless, as more functional information is obtained, echocardiography will be recognized as a safe and reliable method of assessing the function of the left ventricle.

REFERENCES

1. Feigenbaum, H., Zaky, A., and Nasser, W. K.: Use of ultrasound to measure left ventricular stroke volume, Circulation **35:**1092-1099, 1967.
2. Feigenbaum, H., and others: Left ventricular stroke volume measured by ultrasound (abstract), Circulation **40**(Suppl. III):79, 1969.
3. Popp, R. L., and Harrison, D. C.: Ultrasonic cardiac echography for determining stroke volume and valvular regurgitation, Circulation **41:** 493-502, 1970.
4. Murray, J. A., Johnston, W., and Reid, J. M.: Echocardiographic determination of left ventricular performance (abstract), Ann. Intern. Med. **72:**777, 1970.
5. Pombo, J. R., Troy, B. L., and Russell, R. O., Jr.: Left ventricular volumes and ejection fraction by echocardiography, Circulation **43:**480-490, 1971.
6. Fortuin, N. J., and others: Determination of left ventricular volumes by ultrasound, Circulation **44:**575-584, 1971.
7. Feigenbaum, H., and others: Ultrasound measurements of the left ventricle: a correlative study with angiocardiography, Arch. Intern. Med. **129:**461-467, 1972.
8. Cahill, N. S., and others: Left ventricular echocardiograms as a non-invasive functional index following acute myocardial infarction (abstract), Am. J. Cardiol. **31:**124, 1973.
9. Cooper, R. H., and others: Comparison of ultrasound and cineangiographic measurements of the mean rate of circumferential fiber shortening in man, Circulation **46:**914-923, 1972.
10. Feigenbaum, H.: Clinical applications of echocardiography, Progr. Cardiovasc. Dis. **14:**531-558, 1972.
11. Dodge, H. T., and others: The use of biplane angiocardiography for the measurement of left ventricular volume in man, Am. Heart J. **60:**762-766, 1960.
12. Sandler, H., and Dodge, H. T.: The use of single plane angiocardiograms for the calculation of left ventricular volume in man, Am. Heart J. **75:**325-334, 1968.
13. Feigenbaum, H.: Echocardiography, ed. 1, Philadelphia, 1972, Lea & Febiger, p. 114.
14. Teicholz, L. E., and others: Problems in echocardiographic volume determinations: echo-angiographic correlations (abstract), Circulation **46**(Suppl. II):75, 1972.
15. Pombo, J. F., and others: Comparison of stroke volume and cardiac output determinations by ultrasound and dye dilution in acute myocardial infarction, Am. J. Cardiol. **27:**631-635, 1971.
16. Feigenbaum, H., and others: Left ventricular wall thickness measured by ultrasound, Arch. Intern. Med. **121:**391-395, 1968.
17. Sjögren, A. L., Hytönen, I., and Frick, M. H.: Ultrasonic measurements of left ventricular wall thickness, Chest **57:**37-40, 1970.
18. Sjögren, A. L.: Left ventricular wall thickness determined by ultrasound in 100 subjects without heart disease, Chest 341-346, 1971.
19. Troy, B. L., Pombo, J., and Rackley, C. E.: Measurement of left ventricular wall thickness and mass by echocardiography, Circulation **45:**602-611, 1972.
20. Karliner, J. S., and others: Mean velocity of fiber shortening, Circulation **44:**323-333, 1971.
21. Fortuin, N. J., Hood, W. P., and Craige, E.: Evaluation of left ventricular function by echocardiography, Circulation **46:**26-35, 1972.
22. Kraunz, R. F., and Kennedy, J. W.: Ultrasonic determination of left ventricular wall motion in normal man, Am. Heart J. **79:**36-43, 1970.
23. Fogelman, A. M., and others: Echocardiographic study of the abnormal motion of the posterior left ventricular wall during angina pectoris, Circulation **46:**905-913, 1972.
24. Inoue, K., and others: Ultrasonic measurement

of left ventricular wall motion in acute myocardial infarction, Circulation **43**:778-785, 1971.
25. Wharton, C. F. P., Smithen, C. S., and Sowton, E.: Changes in left ventricular wall movement after acute myocardial infarction measured by reflected ultrasound, Br. Med. J. **4**:75-77, 1971.
26. Smithen, C., Wharton, C. F. P., and Sowton, E.: Changes in left ventricular wall movement following exercise, atrial pacing and acute myocardial infarction measured by reflected ultrasound (abstract), Am. J. Cardiol. **29**:293, 1972.
27. Carson, P., and Kanter, L.: Left ventricular wall movement in heart failure, Br. Med. J. **4**:77-79, 1971.
28. Redwood, D. R. and others: Echocardiography during upright exercise (abstract), Am. J. Cardiol. **31**:153, 1973.
29. Ratshin, R. A., Rackley, C. E., and Russel, R. O.: Serial evaluation of left ventricular volumes and posterior wall movement in the acute phase of myocardial infarction using diagnostic ultrasound (abstract), Am. J. Cardiol. **29**:286, 1972.
30. Karliner, J., and others: Posterior wall velocity: an unreliable index of left ventricular contractility (abstract), Circulation **46**:45, 1972.
31. McDonald, L. G., Feigenbaum, H., and Chang, S.: Analysis of left ventricular wall motion by reflected ultrasound: application to assessment of myocardial function, Circulation **46**(Suppl. II):14-25, 1972.
32. Feigenbaum, H., and others: Identification of ultrasound echoes from the left ventricle by use of intracardiac injections of indocyanine green, Circulation **41**:615-621, 1970.
33. Kraunz, R. F., and Ryan, T. J.: Ultrasound measurements of ventricular wall motion following administration of vasoactive drugs, Am. J. Cardiol. **27**:464-473, 1971.
34. Fischer, J. C., and others: Echocardiographic determination of mitral valve flow (abstract), Am. J. Cardiol. **29**:262, 1972.
35. Feigenbaum, H., and others: Effect of elevated atrial component of left ventricular pressure on mitral valve closure (abstract), Am. J. Cardiol. **25**:95, 1970.

7

Echocardiography in congenital heart disease

MORRIS N. KOTLER, M.B., BCH., M.R.C.P. (Edin.)

Precise anatomic information in infants with complex congenital heart lesions requires cardiac catheterization and angiocardiography. These procedures may carry a risk even if performed in highly specialized centers. The advantages of utilizing a noninvasive procedure that may yield reliable anatomic information are obvious. Recently, echocardiography has been employed in the study of a variety of complex congenital heart lesions. The results are extremely promising and the information obtained is most helpful in the management of patients with congenital heart disease.

Echocardiographic technique differs slightly in newborns and infants as compared to adults. Infants generally have to be sedated with the aid of a sugar nipple. A distinct advantage of the neonate over the adult is that the transducer can be placed over the noncalcified sternum. The normal dimensions of the cardiac chambers and structures in neonates and infants are listed in Table 8. It should be noted that the left atrial dimension is usually measured between the posterior aortic wall and posterior left atrial wall at end-systole. Similarly, the aortic root is equivalent to the distance between the anterior and posterior aortic wall at the level of the aortic valve at end-diastole. Aortic valve opening refers to separation of the aortic valve cusps with the onset of left ventricular ejection.

The findings of Konecke and Feigenbaum differ somewhat from Meyer and Kaplan[1] and Hagan and Deely,[2] but it should be remembered that infants were included with neonates and that the cutoff point used weight and height rather than age. For a further detailed analysis of normal echocardiographic findings in relation to body surface area in infants and chil-

TABLE 8. Echocardiographic findings in normal neonates

	Meyer and Kaplan[1]		*Hagan and Deely*[2]		*Konecke and Feigenbaum**[3]	
	RANGE	MEAN	RANGE	MEAN	RANGE	MEAN
AGE (HOURS)	5-125	44	12-72			
WEIGHT (KG)	2.3-4.9	3.2				
NUMBER OF PATIENTS	50		200		24	
Left ventricle cavity						
End-diastolic (cm)	1.2-2.0	1.6	1.6-2.1	1.8	1.3-3.2	2.4
End-systolic (cm)			1-1.5	1.35		
Outflow tract (cm)	0.7-1.2	1.0				
Left ventricular wall thickness						
Systolic (mm)			2.8-5.0	3.7		
Diastolic (mm)			1.5-3.3	2.5	.5-7	6
Right ventricle cavity						
End-diastolic (cm)	1.0-1.7	1.3	0.93-1.63	1.25	0.3-1.3	.8
End-systolic (cm)			0.73-1.13	0.97		
Right ventricular wall thickness						
Systolic (mm)			3.3-6.1	4.6		
Diastolic (mm)			2-4.2	2.7		
Septal wall thickness (mm)			2.3-3.3	2.7	4-6	5
Left atrium (cm)	0.6-1.3	0.9	0.4-0.88	0.61	0.7-2.4	1.7
Aortic root (cm)			0.83-1.13	1.0	0.7-1.5	1.2
Aortic valve opening (cm)					0.5-1.0	0.8
Mitral valve						
Velocity (mm/sec)	36-80	53	51-105	74		
Excursion (cm)	0.6-1.2	1.0	0.87-1.21	1.0		
Tricuspid valve						
Velocity (mm/sec)	34-56	43	50-100	68		
Excursion (cm)	0.8-1.4	1.1	0.9-1.33	1.09		

*The normal values are based on body surface area (BSA) and included twenty-four infants with BSA of 0.5 m^2 or less.

dren, the reader is referred to the work reported upon by Konecke and Feigenbaum.[3]

Conventional placement of the transducer suffices in most instances; occasionally, it may have to be positioned in the xiphoid notch in neonates or infants with enlarged hearts.

Since all the structures in neonates and infants are smaller than in adults, it is not surprising that cardiac echoes are recorded within 5 to 6 cm from the skin surface. The scale has to be expanded and the depth compensation control has to be adjusted so that maximum gain at 3 to 4 cm is achieved. This produces the strongest echoes from the mitral valve and left ventricular wall. Similarly, for identification of the ventricular septum and tricuspid valve, the gain and control can be adjusted for near echoes.

The concept of mitral and posterior aortic root wall and septal and anterior aortic wall continuity is especially important in congenital heart disease. Normal mitral valve and posterior aortic wall continuity is demonstrated in Fig. 7-1. In addition, the interventricular septum is contiguous with the anterior aortic wall. The tricuspid valve, obtained by angulating the transducer medially and toward the spine, is contiguous with the anterior aortic wall. The tricuspid valve is usually recordable without much difficulty in neonates and

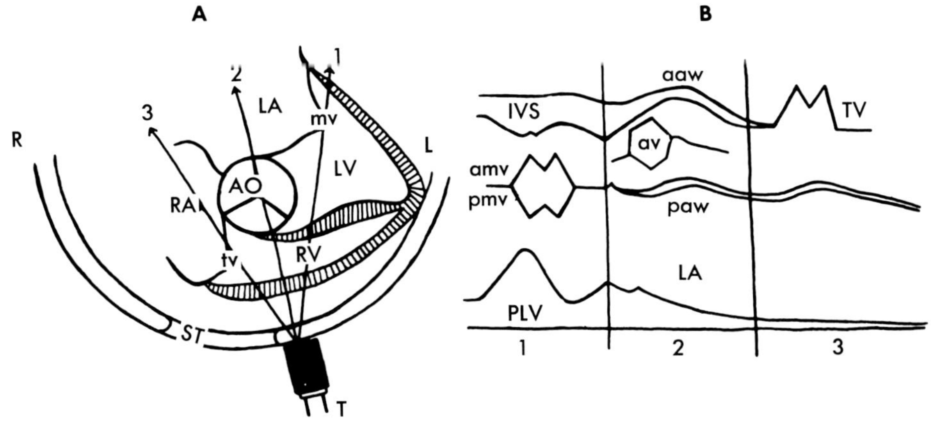

Fig. 7-1. Diagrammatic representation of a transverse section of the heart illustrating the location of intracardiac structures by angulating the transducer from positions 1, 2, and 3, **A,** Positions *1, 2,* and *3* indicate location of mitral valve *(mv),* aortic root *(AO),* and tricuspid valve *(tv). LA,* Left atrium; *RA,* right atrium; *LV,* left ventricle; *RV,* right ventricle; *ST,* sternum; *T,* transducer; *R* and *L,* right and left sides of the chest. In **B,** a diagrammatic representation of the echocardiogram in positions *1, 2,* and *3* is shown. As the transducer is angulated from position 1 to position 2, the interventricular septum *(IVS)* merges into the anterior aortic wall *(aaw),* which eventually becomes contiguous with the tricuspid valve *(TV)* in position 3. The anterior mitral valve *(amv)* is contiguous with the posterior aortic wall *(paw)* as the transducer is angulated from position 1 to 2. *PLV,* Posterior left ventricular wall; *LA,* left atrium.

infants. The pulmonary valve can also be recorded by positioning the transducer one interspace above the usual aortic valve recording level and angulating it laterally.[4]

HYPOPLASIA OF THE LEFT VENTRICLE

Included in this category of congenital malformations are severe hypoplasia of the left ventricle (consisting of a slit-like ventricular cavity), atresia of aortic and/or mitral valves, and severe hypoplasia of the ascending aorta.[5,6] Hypoplastic left ventricle should be differentiated from noncardiac conditions such as septicemia.[1] The clinical manifestations of hypoplastic left ventricle include tachypnea, cyanosis, and congestive heart failure with weak peripheral pulses.

The echocardiographic features of six patients with autopsy-proved aortic atresia and hypoplastic left ventricle were absence or gross distortion of the mitral valve echo, small to absent aortic root, and a small posterior left ventricular chamber in the presence of an enlarged anterior right ventricle.[7] The left ventricular chamber measured less than 0.9 cm (end-diastolic dimension) and the mean right ventricular chamber measured 2.5 cm. In some patients the left ventricular outflow tract could not be identified, although an aortic root was present.[8]

The tricuspid valve echo in patients with aortic atresia is easily identifiable.[1] Recently, Meyer and Kaplan have updated their experience by reporting on fourteen patients with aortic atresia and hypoplastic left ventricle.[1] The three echocardiographic features were so characteristic that the authors believed that cardiac catheterization and angiography could be avoided, and the last eight patients with aortic atresia were diagnosed by echocardiography alone.[1] In each instance the diagnosis was subsequently confirmed at autopsy.

Additional congenital malformations included in the hypoplastic left heart syndrome are mitral atresia, mitral stenosis, and cor triatriatum. In two cases of mitral atresia studied by Lundström,[9,10] an echo from the anterior mitral leaflet could not be obtained (although an echo resembling movement of the annulus was recorded). The movement was of small amplitude (3 to 3.5 mm), and its pattern consisted of anterior movement during ventricular systole and of posterior movement during ventricular diastole. In one of the patients studied, this echo was clearly distinguished from the echo obtained from the interventricular septum. Lundström postulated that this abnormal echo represented the atretic mitral region.[9] In both patients the movement of the anterior leaflet of the tricuspid valve was easily observed and appeared normal.

Congenital mitral stenosis is usually associated with other abnormalities of the cardiovascular system[11] but may occur as an isolated heart malformation. In a study of seven patients with congenital mitral stenosis combined with other cardiovascular malformations, Lundström found good correlation between the echocardiographic findings and the findings at cardiac catheterization, surgery, and autopsy.[12] Preoperative assessment of the severity of mitral stenosis and postoperative assessment after mitral valvotomy by echocardiography correlated well with the clinical and cardiac catheterization findings.

The echocardiographic features of congenital mitral stenosis were similar to those of acquired mitral stenosis, with reduced diastolic closure slopes the most diagnostic feature. However, in only two of the seven cases reported by Lundström was significant decrease in the amplitude of movement of the anterior leaflet of the mitral valve observed, and in both instances short fused chordae tendineae were found.

In one patient with cor triatriatum studied by echocardiography, an unusual echo situated posteriorly to the normal appearing mitral valve echo was described.[9] The distinctive features were a slight movement during systole but a more pronounced movement during ventricular diastole, especially during atrial systole. Lundström postulated that this abnormal echo originated from the membrane dividing the left atrium. In a patient with a supravalvular ring in the left atrium, an abnormal echo situated in the left atrium was observed.[9] However, its pattern was not that distinctive to enable accurate diagnosis of supravalvular ring in the left atrium.

HYPOPLASIA OF THE RIGHT VENTRICLE

Chesler and associates[13] described six cases of hypoplasia of the right heart and recently updated their findings in a further report on eleven patients.[6] The abnormal anterior motion of a single atrioventricular valve leaflet and the absence of a septal echo were the characteristic features observed (Fig. 7-2).

In this anomaly there is no tricuspid valvular tissue, and the increased motion of the single atrioventricular valve is recorded from the mitral valve. Usually there is associated pulmonary stenosis or atresia, and in the former situation the pulmonary artery arises from a hypoplastic basal infundibular chamber. Therefore a small anterior ventricular chamber or right ventricle is common in patients with tricuspid atresia and can measure less than 0.6 cm in the newborn. The left ventricle may be larger than normal, measuring 2.3 cm. In addition, the left ventricular outflow tract with posterior aortic wall-mitral valve continuity is present.[1] This is in contrast to aortic atresia in which the tricuspid valve or anterior atrioventricular wall echo is continuous with the anterior margin of the aortic root.

The tricuspid valve motion is easily demonstrated in every normal newborn,[1]

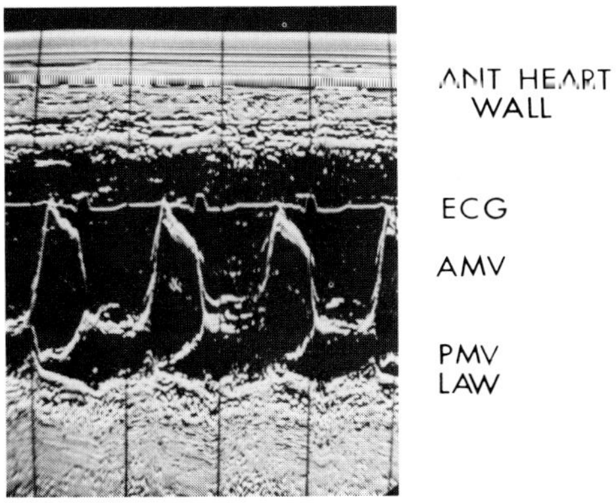

Fig. 7-2. Echogram of a patient with tricuspid atresia showing marked anterior movement of the mitral valve *(AMV)*. No definite septal echoes or tricuspid valve motion could be demonstrated. *PMV,* Posterior mitral valve echo; *LAW,* left atrial wall.

although it may be more difficult to record in normal older children and adults.[6]

SINGLE VENTRICLE

One of the most useful applications of echocardiography has been to locate the ventricular septum. Besides evaluating normal and abnormal motion of the septum,[14] recent investigators have measured septal thickness in relation to posterior left ventricular wall thickness and found abnormal ratios to be highly diagnostic of hypertrophic cardiomyopathy with or without outflow obstruction.[15]

In single ventricle, the ventricular septum is absent and the inability to locate the ventricular septum has been an important feature in the echocardiographic diagnosis of single ventricle. Usually single

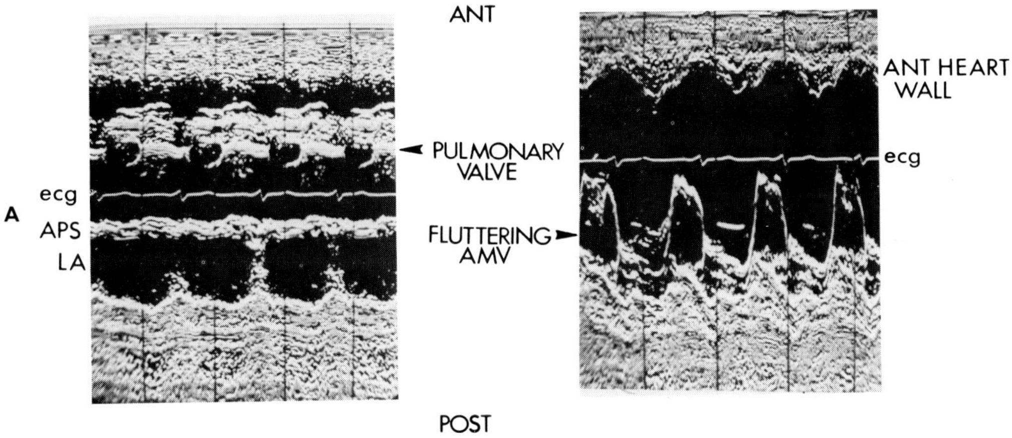

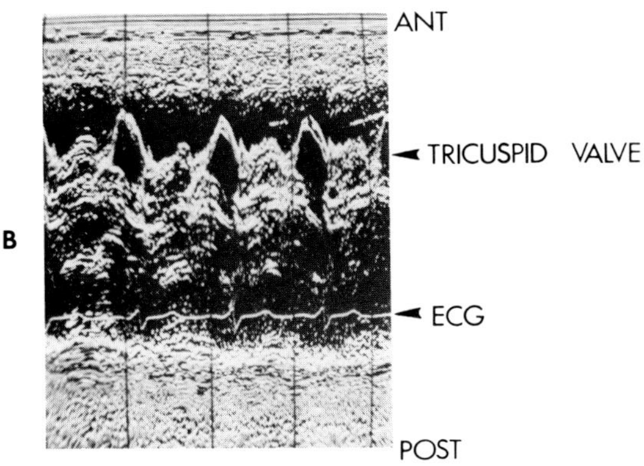

Fig. 7-3. A, Echocardiogram of an 18-year-old patient with single ventricle, transposition of the great vessels, pulmonary hypertension, and insufficiency of the pulmonary valve. *Left,* From anterior to posterior are seen pulmonary valve, enlarged pulmonary trunk, atriopulmonic sulcus *(APS),* and left atrium *(LA). Right,* Excessive posterior systolic movement of the anterior heart wall and significant anterior movement of the anterior mitral valve leaflet *(AMV)* are seen. Septal echoes could *not* be recorded. The AMV demonstrates evidence of flutter in diastole as a result of insufficiency of the pulmonary valve. **B,** Echogram of the triscuspid valve of the same patient with single ventricle. No evidence of flutter in diastole could be demonstrated.

ventricle can exist with or without a rudimentary chamber representing the infundibulum or conus of the right ventricle. In most instances, the great vessels are transposed (Fig. 7-3, *A*) but on occasion they may be normally related. The most common arrangement of the atrioventricular valves in single ventricle is a separate mitral and tricuspid valve (Fig. 7-3). However, in those patients with a single atrioventricular valve, excessive anterior excursion of the valve may be recorded.

Although the diagnosis of single ventricle cannot readily be differentiated from malformations such as the hypoplastic right ventricle, Meyer and Kaplan[1] have demonstrated in the latter condition continuity of one atrioventricular valve and the aortic root. They could not demonstrate continuity with an atrioventricular valve and the pulmonary root echo in neonates with single ventricle.[1] On occasion, in patients with corrected or L-transposition of the great arteries, the septum is perpendicular to the chest wall and may not be recorded during routine echocardiography since the transducer beam is parallel to the septum.[1] This may pose a problem in the differential diagnosis of single ventricle.

TETRALOGY OF FALLOT

Chung and associates studied seventeen patients with diagnosis of tetralogy of Fallot proved by ultrasound.[16] The most characteristic abnormality was discontinuity between the ventricular septum and anterior aortic margin, with aortic overriding occurring in fifteen of the seventeen patients studied. In this condition the aortic root was found to be enlarged.[16,17]

In five patients, an abnormal mitral valve motion during systole was characterized by flattening, sagging, or gradual posterior motion. In addition, a narrowed right ventricular outflow tract was demonstrated. It is anticipated that accurate anatomic relationships, particularly of the aortic root and right ventricular outflow tract, may be demonstrated with the technique of compound-B ultrasonography.[10]

DOUBLE OUTLET RIGHT VENTRICLE

It may be difficult clinically to differentiate tetralogy of Fallot from double outlet right ventricle (origin of both great vessels from the right ventricle). In double outlet right ventricle, the only outlet for the left ventricle is through the ventricular septal defect. Since routine closure of the ventricular septal defect may be associated with a catastrophic outcome, correct diagnosis is essential. Furthermore, the aortic and pulmonary valves tend to lie at the same level and the anterior mitral leaflet is separated by muscular tissue from the aortic root. Selective left ventricular angiography performed in the lateral view demonstrates mitral-semilunar valve discontinuity.[19]

Chesler and associates[20] demonstrated mitral-semilunar valve discontinuity in five patients with double outlet right ventricle. The degree of separation determined by ultrasound (measured as the posterior border of the adjacent great vessel lying anterior to the mitral valve echo) correlated well with angiographic assessment. Unfortunately, mitral semilunar valve discontinuity has been demonstrated in patients with tetralogy of Fallot[16] and with grossly enlarged left ventricles (Fig. 7-4) and is not specifically characteristic of the double outlet right ventricle alone.

TRANSPOSITION OF THE GREAT ARTERIES

Gramiak and colleagues[21] studied eleven patients with transposition of the great arteries by echocardiography. The echocardiographic features consisted of an anteriorly situated outflow vessel when the transducer was medially angulated. With normally situated arteries the left ventricular outflow artery is situated more

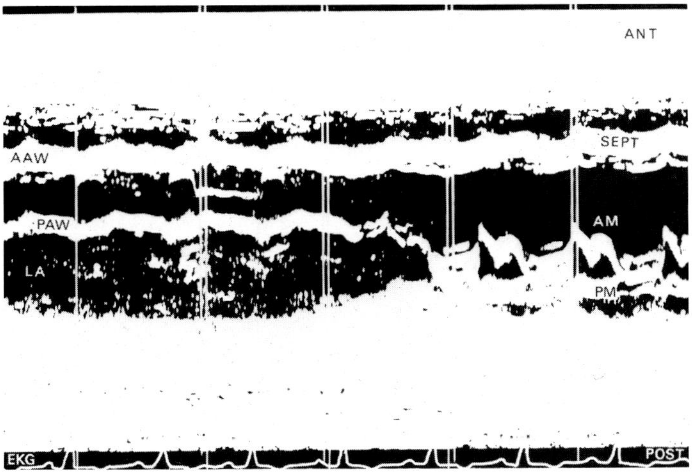

Fig. 7-4. M-mode scan obtained when the transducer and ultrasonic beam moves from the left atrium *(LA)* to the left ventricle in a patient with congestive cardiomyopathy and gross left ventricular dilation. Posterior margin of aorta *(PAW)* is situated anterior to *closed* position of mitral valve, which occurs when anterior mitral leaflet *(AM)* meets posterior mitral leaflet *(PM)* in systole immediately after the QRS complex. *AAW,* Anterior aortic wall; *SEPT,* septum; *ANT,* anterior; *POST,* posterior.

posteriorly. The space anterior to the aortic root represents the right ventricular outflow tract, while the space behind the aortic root is the left atrium. The pulmonary valve and pulmonary root, situated anteriorly with respect to the aorta, may be detected in normal individuals by angling the transducer laterally (Fig. 7-5). Lateral angulation of the transducer in patients with transposition of the great arteries reveals a posteriorly situated pulmonary outflow artery in most instances. Less commonly, the two arteries may have a side-to-side relationship. The technique depends upon the method of angulation of the transducer and not upon specific echocardiographic differentiating features between the aorta and pulmonary arteries and thus may be of limited value. However, superimposition of the great arteries without intervening crista was recorded in fourteen infants with transposition of the great arteries.[22] In addition, in thirteen of fourteen patients the semilunar valves were recorded simultaneously.[22]

ATRIAL SEPTAL DEFECT

Diamond and his associates[14] studied thirty-nine adult patients with atrial septal defect. An increased right ventricular dimension (RVD) or RVD index and an abnormal septal motion were observed (Fig. 7-6). These patients could be differentiated from normal individuals, those with other types of left-to-right shunting, or those with uncomplicated right ventricular pressure overload (pulmonic stenosis). However, patients with volume overload of the right ventricle and tricuspid regurgitation could not be differentiated from the group with atrial septal defects. Popp and associates[23] originally described the abnormal septal motion in which the pattern and direction of movement are similar to those exhibited by the left ventricular wall echo.

It should be noted that the septal movement immediately below the anterior aortic wall may be abnormal. Therefore, it is important that the transducer be angulated away from the anterior mitral valve before any valid conclusion can be drawn about

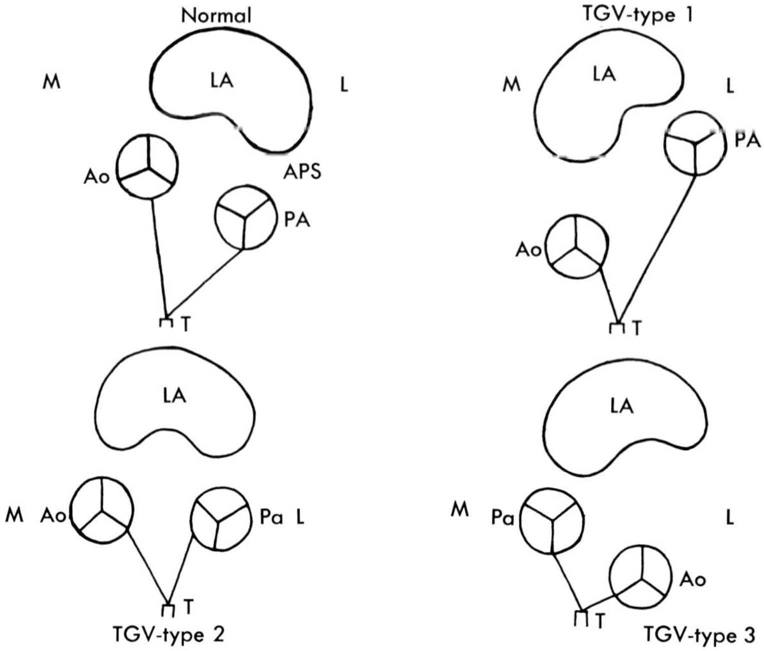

Fig. 7-5. Schematic diagrams of the relationship of the great vessels in normal individuals and in transposition of the great vessels (TGV). In normal persons (upper left) the aorta *(Ao)* is in a posterior and medial position, whereas the pulmonary artery *(PA)* is lateral and in an anterior position. In TGV-type 1 (the most common arrangement, upper right), the Ao is in an anterior and medial position, whereas the PA is in a lateral and posterior position. In TGV-type 2 (lower left) the aorta is directly to the right and medially so that the vessels are side by side. In TGV-type 3 (rarest of the types) the Ao is in an anterior and lateral position whereas the PA is in a posterior and medial position. *APS,* Atriopulmonic sulcus; *LA,* left atrium; *T,* transducer; *M,* medial; *L,* lateral.

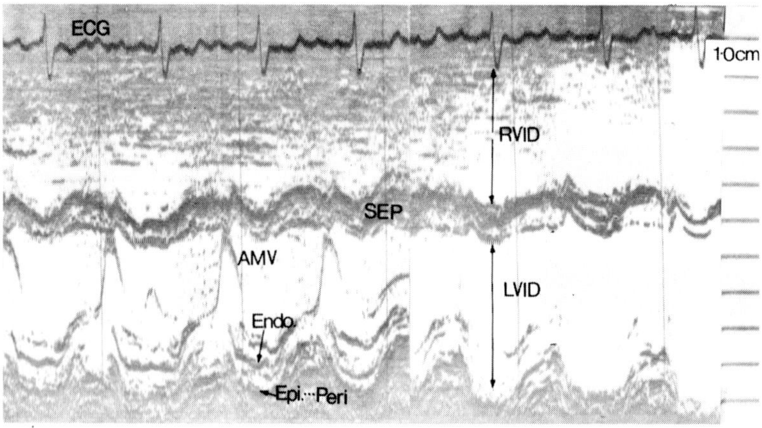

Fig. 7-6. Atrial fibrillation echocardiogram from a patient with an ostium secundum atrial septal defect and atrial fibrillation. The distance between the anterior right ventricular wall and the septum *(SEP)* is increased *(RVID)*. The septal motion is abnormal (type A) and is consistent with a volume overload of the right ventricle. Both the left ventricular posterior wall endocardium *(Endo)* and the septum *(SEP)* move in the same anterior direction during systole. *AMV,* Anterior mitral valve leaflet; *LVID,* left ventricular diameter; *Endo,* endocardium; *Epi,* epicardium; *Peri,* pericardium.

septal motion.[23] In addition, if clear right ventricular wall echoes were not clearly identified, the location of the right ventricular epicardium was estimated to be 0.5 cm posterior to the chest wall echoes.[14]

Several theories have been proposed as to the mechanism of the abnormal septal movement.[24] One theory proposed that abnormal septal motion may be the result of right bundle conduction disturbance. However, many patients with either incomplete or complete right bundle branch block have normal septal motion. An unlikely theory states that the abnormal plane of the septum parallels that of the chest wall in patients with dilated right ventricle. Meyer and colleagues[24] proposed that in right ventricular volume overload the dilated right ventricle displaces the left ventricle posteriorly. Because of this increased right ventricular stroke volume, the anterior movement of the heart exceeds the normal posterior motion of the septum, resulting in a net anterior motion of the septum. Despite these attractive hypotheses, proof is lacking. Recently Brown and associates[25] have challenged the original findings of right ventricular volume overload. Based on new echocardiographic criteria involving careful examination of diastolic movement of the septum, more accurate correlations were obtained.[25]

In a study of eleven patients with atrial septal defect, Kamigaki and Goldschlager[26] observed abnormal motion of the valve leaflets. The most striking abnormality observed was a reduction in velocity of opening of the mitral valve primarily involving the posterior leaflet. In addition, reduced amplitude of motion was recorded. Various contributing factors may include left ventricular disease, effects of left-to-right shunt with altered flow patterns at the site of the mitral valve and thickening of the

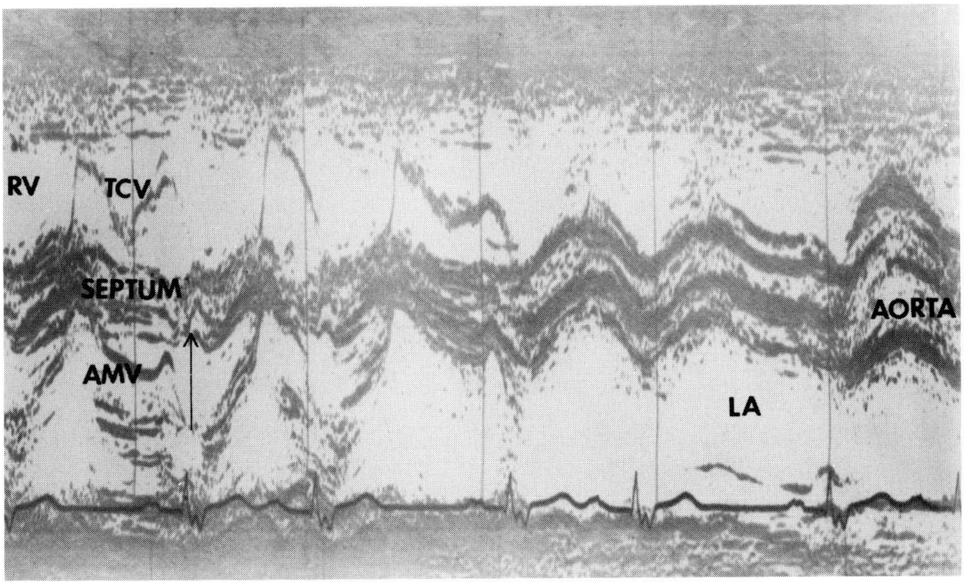

Fig. 7-7. Echocardiogram from a patient with an ostium primum septal defect. The vertical arrow represents the distance between the endocardial surface of the septum and the closed position of the mitral valve during early systole. This measurement is the left ventricular outflow tract and is narrowed in primum defects. Prolonged mitral-septal apposition in early diastole, abnormal (type A) septal motion, and an increased right ventricular dimension are shown. *RV,* Right ventricle; *AMV,* anterior mitral valve; *LA,* left atrium.

valve, and the effect of paradoxic motion of the interventricular septum.

Although Diamond and his associates[14] could not differentiate primum defects from secundum defects based on their echocardiographic findings, Gramiak and Nanda[27] have presented evidence that ostium primum defects can be detected by echocardiography. The echocardiographic features in five adult patients with ostium primum septal defects included narrowing of the left ventricular outflow tract, prolonged mitral-septal apposition in diastole, in addition to the usual anterior systolic motion of the septum and the enlarged right ventricular chamber (Fig. 7-7).

In total anomalous pulmonary venous drainage, abnormal septal motion and an increased right ventricular dimension were characteristic echocardiographic features.[28] In addition to these above findings, reduction in the left atrial dimension has been described in infants.[29] The finding of a small left atrium was helpful in distinguishing total anomalous pulmonary venous drainage from atrial septal defect.[29]

False positive or abnormal septal motion has been observed in normal individuals. In addition, normal septal motion has been reported in patients with atrial septal defects.[14,30,31] Echocardiography in atrial septal defects may be helpful, but cardiac catheterization is essential prior to any contemplated surgical procedure.

EBSTEIN'S ANOMALY OF THE TRICUSPID VALVE

In Ebstein's anomaly there is malformation and downward displacement of the tricuspid valve with resultant reduction in size of the right ventricular cavity. The functioning valvular tissue is usually composed of the anterior valve leaflet alone. The right atrium is enlarged, and frequently a right-to-left shunt at the atrial level is present. The overall appearance, as viewed from the right atrium, is that of a large, single, concave, sail-like valve sweeping out into the right ventricular cavity from an abnormal downward position on the ventricular wall. This results in a transection of the right ventricle, the proximal portion becoming "atrialized" and the distal portion representing the small, narrow, functioning right ventricle.

The echocardiographic features of Ebstein's anomaly are quite distinctive, and the most striking abnormality is the large amplitude of anterior movement of the tricuspid valve during diastole[32] (Fig. 7-8). In seven patients with Ebstein's anomaly studied by ultrasound, the large amplitude of movement of the tricuspid valve as compared to mitral valve movement was characteristic. In most instances, the movement of the tricuspid valve was recorded further to the left of the sternum than normal. Delayed closure of the tricuspid valve (0.04 to 0.10 second) after mitral valve closure has been described.[33] In addition, the delayed component of the

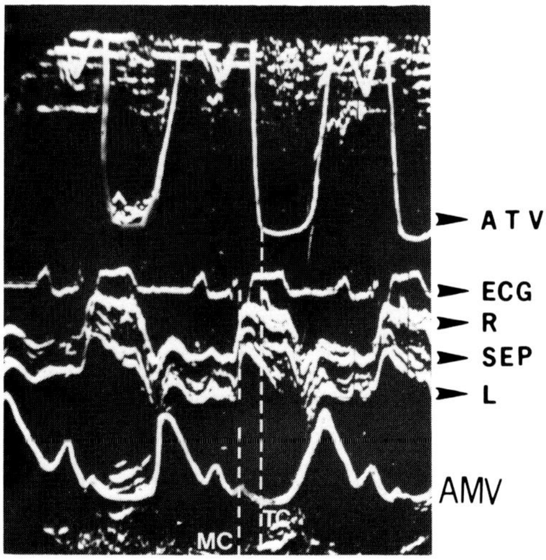

Fig. 7-8. Echocardiogram from a patient with Ebstein's anomaly of the tricuspid valve. Mitral and tricuspid valves were retouched for clarification. The significant anterior movement of the tricuspid valve *(ATV)* as compared to the mitral valve *(AMV)* is shown. Type B septal motion is present with flattening of the septal echoes *(SEP)* during ventricular ejection. Tricuspid valve closure *(TC)* follows mitral valve closure *(MC)* by 40 msec. *R,* Right side of septum; *L,* left side of septum.

widely split first sound was thought to result from closure of the abnormally large anterior leaflet of the tricuspid valve.[33] Other echocardiographic findings include abnormal type B septal motion and an enlarged right atrium or atrialized ventricle. Lundström described a very shallow E to F slope during diastole,[10] although normal diastolic closure rates can occur.

SUMMARY

Echocardiography in the diagnosis of congenital heart disease is helpful if used in conjunction with the clinical, electrocardiographic, and radiologic findings. In most instances echocardiography should not be regarded as a substitute for cardiac catheterization. As a rapid screening technique, the greatest value of ultrasound is its ability to identify both right and left ventricular cavities and ventricular septum. The role of echocardiography in the study of single ventricle, hypoplastic right heart syndrome, double outlet right ventricle, tetralogy of Fallot, transposition of the great vessels, and atrial septal defect has been reviewed. Echocardiography allows accurate diagnosis of the hypoplastic left heart syndrome, congenital mitral stenosis, and Ebstein's anomaly of the tricuspid valve. It is hoped that with improved noninvasive techniques including compound-B ultrasonography and real-time, multitransducer scanning, more accurate diagnoses of congenital heart disorders can be obtained.

Acknowledgments

The help of Mrs. Patricia Tocci is gratefully acknowledged in the preparation of Chapters 6 and 7. I wish to thank Dr. Norman Sarachek and Dr. Nathaniel Reichek for providing me with Figs. 6-1 and 7-6.

REFERENCES

1. Meyer, R. A., and Kaplan, S.: Non-invasive techniques in pediatric cardiovascular disease, Progr. Cardiovasc. Dis. **15:**341-367, 1973.
2. Hagan, A. D., and others: Echocardiographic criteria for normal newborn infants, Circulation **48:**1221-1226, 1973.
3. Feigenbaum, H.: Echocardiography, ed. 1, Philadelphia, 1972, Lea & Febiger, 1972, pp. 215-218.
4. Gramiak, R., Nanda, N. C., and Shah, P. M.: Echocardiographic detection of the pulmonary valve, Radiology **102:**153-157, 1972.
5. Elliot, R. S., and others: Mitral atresia: a study of 32 cases, Am. Heart J. **70:**6-22, 1965.
6. Chesler, E., and others: Echocardiography in the diagnosis of congenital heart disease, Pediatr. Clin. North Am. **18:**1163-1189, 1971.
7. Meyer, R. A., and Kaplan, S.: Echocardiography in the diagnosis of hypoplasia of the left or right ventricles in the neonate, Circulation **46:**55-64, 1972.
8. Meyer, R. A., Schwartz, D. C., and Kaplan, S.: The diagnosis of aortic atresia by echocardiography (abstract), Am. J. Cardiol. **29:**280, 1972.
9. Lundström, N. R.: Ultrasound cardiographic studies of the mitral valve region in young infants with mitral atresia, mitral stenosis, hypoplasia of the left ventricle and cor triatriatum, Circulation **45:**324-334, 1972.
10. Lundström, N. R., and Edler, I.: Ultrasound cardiography in infants and children, Acta Paediatr. Scand. **60:**117-128, 1971.
11. Van Der Horst, R. L., and Hastreiter, A. R.: Congenital mitral stenosis, Am. J. Cardiol. **20:**773-783, 1967.
12. Lundström, N. R.: Echocardiography in the diagnosis of congenital mitral stenosis and in evaluation of the results of mitral valvotomy, Circulation **46:**44-54, 1972.
13. Chesler, E., and others: Ultrasound cardiography in single ventricle and the hypoplastic left and right heart syndromes, Circulation **42:**123-129, 1970.
14. Diamond, M. A., and others: Echocardiographic features of atrial septal defect, Circulation **43:**129-136, 1971.
15. Henry, W. L., Clark, C. E., and Epstein, S. E.: Asymmetric septal hypertrophy: echocardiographic identification of the pathognomonic anatomic abnormality of IHSS, Circulation **47:**225-233, 1973.
16. Chung, K. J., and others: Echocardiographic findings in tetralogy of Fallot (abstract), Am. J. Cardiol. **31:**126, 1973.
17. Gramiak, R., and Shah, P. M.: Cardiac ultrasonography: a review of current applications, Radiol. Clin. North Am. **9:**469-490, 1971.
18. King, D. L.: Cardiac ultrasonography, Radiology **103:**387-392, 1972.
19. Hallerman, F. J., and others: Mitral-semilunar valve relationships in the angiography of cardiac malformations, Radiology **94:**63-68, 1970.
20. Chesler, E., and others: Echocardiographic recognition of mitral-semilunar valve discontinuity: an aid to the diagnosis of origin of both great ves-

sels, from the right ventricle, Circulation **43:**725-732, 1971.
21. Gramiak, R., and others: Echocardiographic diagnosis of transposition of the great vessels, Radiology **106:**187-189, 1973.
22. Dillon, J. C., and others: Echocardiographic manifestations of transposition of the great vessels (abstract), Am. J. Cardiol. **31:**128, 1973.
23. Popp, R. L., and others: Estimation of right and left ventricular size by ultrasound: a study of echoes from the interventricular septum, Am. J. Cardiol. **24:**523-530, 1969.
24. Meyer, R. A., and others: Ventricular septum in right ventricular volume overload, Am. J. Cardiol. **30:**349-353, 1972.
25. Brown, O. R., Popp, R. L., and Harrison, D. C.: Improved diagnosis of atrial septal defect and analogous conditions by cardiac echography (abstract), Circulation **46**(Suppl. II):37, 1972.
26. Kamigaki, N., and Goldschlager, N.: Echocardiographic analysis of mitral valve motion in atrial septal defect, Am. J. Cardiol. **30:**343-348, 1972.
27. Gramiak, R., and Nanda, N. C.: Echocardiographic diagnosis of ostium primum septal defect (abstract), Circulation **46**(Suppl. II):37, 1972.
28. Tajik, A. J., Gau, G. T., and Schattenberg, T. T.: Echocardiogram in total anomalous pulmonary venous drainage: report of a case, Mayo Clin. Proc. **47:**247-250, 1972.
29. Glaser, J., Whitman, V., and Liebman, J.: The differential diagnosis of total anomalous pulmonary venous drainage in infancy by echocardiography (abstract), Circulation **46**(Suppl. II):38, 1972.
30. Tajik, A. J., and others: Normal ventricular septal motion in atrial septal defect: an echocardiographic observation, Mayo Clin. Proc. **47:** 635-638, 1972.
31. Tajik, A. J., and others: Echocardiographic pattern of right ventricular diastolic volume overload in children, Circulation **46:**36-43, 1972.
32. Kotler, M. N., and Tabatznik, B.: Recognition of Ebstein's anomaly by ultrasound (abstract), Circulation **44:**34, 1971.
33. Crews, T. L., and others: Auscultatory and phonocardiographic findings in Ebstein's anomaly: correlation of the first heart sound with ultrasonic records of tricuspid valve movement Br. Heart J. **34:**681-687, 1972.

8 Doppler echocardiography

STEVE L. JOHNSON, M.D., AND DONALD W. BAKER, B.S.

The first clinical application of a continuous-wave Doppler flowmeter in cardiology was described by Satomura[1] in 1957. Subsequent articles by Yoshida, Nimura, and other Japanese workers[2-6] have described the high-pitched clicks generated by rapid valve leaflet motion and the low-pitched sounds generated by wall motion. The major application of this work was in timing the events of the cardiac cycle both in normal individuals and in disease states. This work was recently extended by Kostis and associates.[7] They used the mitral opening click for timing the opening snap, S-3 gallop, and wide splitting of the second heart sound. The aortic cusp opening click was used to time ejection clicks and systolic clicks, and a signal obtained from the atrial wall was used to time the S-4 gallop. Other intracardiac applications of continuous-wave Doppler have included the study of cardiac arrhythmias,[1] bubble detection (especially during hyperbaric decompression and neurosurgical operations),[9-13] and the detection of a pseudoaneurysm of the left ventricle.[14]

Continuous-wave Doppler signals from the proximal aorta and subclavian, brachial, and carotid arteries have also been used to study cardiac disease, including the diagnosis of idiopathic hypertrophic subaortic stenosis,[15] detection of aortic stenosis, and the estimation of the severity of aortic insufficiency.[16-18] Kalmanson and co-workers have recently described the measurement of jugular venous flow with a directional continuous-wave Doppler flowmeter. The applications include the study of arrhythmias, diagnosis of atrial septal defects, and the estimation of left-to-right shunt size.[19-21]

One of the major limitations of the continuous-wave Doppler flowmeter for intracardiac work has been the lack of spatial resolution, since the device records a composite velocity along the entire length of the beam. To overcome this disadvantage, work was begun in the late 1960's on the development of range-gated pulse Doppler flowmeters, both at the University of Washington School of Medicine[22,23] and at other institutions.[24-26] A recently described application of the pulse Doppler flowmeter was the velocity measurement of the posterior heart wall.[27] An adaptation of the range-gated Doppler flowmeter to visualize peripheral vessels—a technique called "ultrasonic arteriography"[28-30]—has recently been used by Gould and colleagues to determine the patency of saphenous vein coronary bypass grafts.[31]

Recently, an echocardiographic laboratory has been established at the University of Washington School of Medicine to develop range-gated pulse Doppler flowmeter applications in cardiology. To date, over 200 patient studies have been performed.

TECHNIQUE

The transcutaneous range-gated pulse Doppler flowmeter system (Figs. 8-1 and 8-2) has a small (½ × 1½ inch) hand-held transducer. One half of the split circular, disk-shaped, piezoelectric crystal transmits short (1.0- to 1.5-μsec), high-frequency (3.0 MHz) pulses of ultrasonic energy, at a pulse repetition rate (PRF) that varies between 2 and 15 kHz, depending on the depth of penetration. A lens mounted on the face of the transducer generates a collimated beam. In the case of moving blood, the transmitted ultrasound pulses are reflected from the blood cells (scattering elements) and returned to the other half of the piezoelectric crystal. The range-gate feature allows the system to record only the velocity of the blood cells within a small teardrop-shaped sample volume 2 × 4 mm in size. The return signal is amplified by a wide-band receiver. The Doppler shift frequency is detected by a phase detection circuit whose dual outputs are 90 degrees out of phase to provide directionality. The range delay circuit, with its range-gate adjustment knob, in combination with the sample-and-hold amplifiers and bandpass filters, results in an output signal in which the frequency spectrum is proportional to the velocity spectrum within the teardrop-shaped sample volume. The output signal is the summation of the Doppler

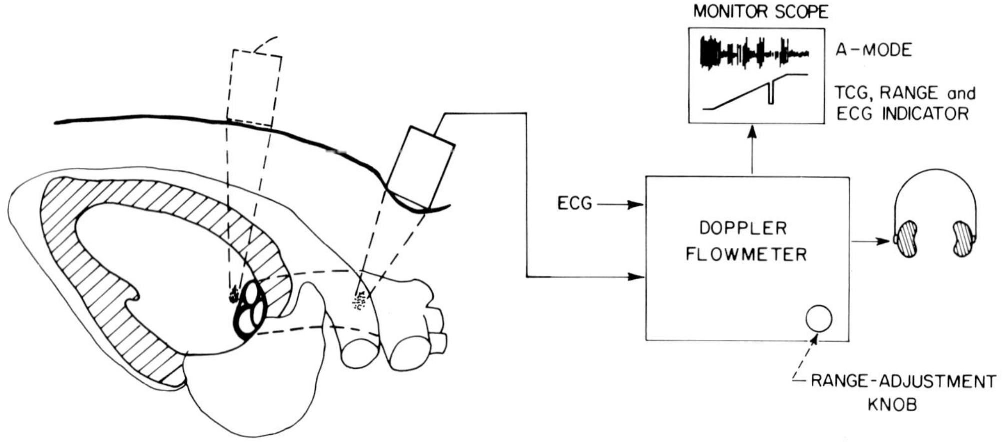

Fig. 8-1. Schematic diagram of the range-gated pulse Doppler flowmeter system. *ECG,* Electrocardiogram; *TCG,* time-compensated gain.

shift signals from each blood cell. Since blood velocities may vary throughout the sample volume, the output wave-form is usually a spectrum of frequencies rather than a single frequency.

Since the output signal is in the audio range, it can be detected by loudspeaker or earphone output. A zero-crossing frequency meter can also be used to display the signal on a strip-chart recorder. The signal can also be recorded on magnetic tape for later processing with a spectral analyzer.

The audio signal contains detailed information concerning blood flow. In laminar flow with a flat velocity profile, all blood cells passing through the sample volume theoretically would have the same velocity amplitude and direction. The output signal in this situation has a very narrow frequency bandwidth and the sound is similar to a pure tone (Fig. 8-3, *A*). In the case of turbulent flow, each blood cell theoretically has a different velocity amplitude and direction, and the resulting output signal has a very wide frequency bandwidth that has a very harsh, "noisy" sound (Fig. 8-3, *B*). In general, the development of turbulence in the heart and great vessels depends upon the flow

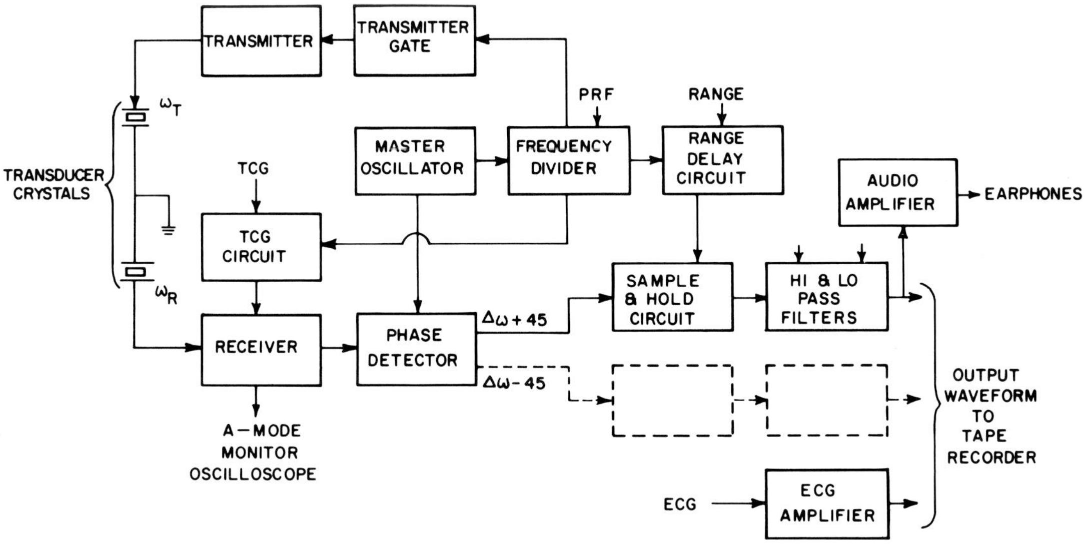

Fig. 8-2. Block diagram of the Doppler flowmeter circuits. The master oscillator frequency is 3.0 MHz. The pulse repetition frequency (PRF) can be manually varied from 5 to 16 kHz in five steps, depending on the depth of penetration required. The phase difference output from the quadrature phase detector circuit is two signals 90 degrees apart, which permits directional flow to be obtained from the output of a zero-crossing frequency meter (not shown on the diagram). The sample and hold amplifiers sample these signals during a 1-μsec interval that is suitably delayed after each pulse by the range delay circuit. This results in a staircase-like signal whose amplitude is proportional to the phase (or frequency) of the Doppler shift signal at one point along the beam. The low-pass filter removes the PRF transients and the high-pass filter removes the low-frequency motion signals. The most commonly used output is earphones and loudspeaker. The two phase-difference signals are also the input for a zero-crossing frequency meter (not shown on the diagram), and the ouput, which is proportional to directional flow, is displayed on a large monitor oscilloscope. The two phase-difference signals, electrocardiogram, and a voice channel are also recorded on a 4-track magnetic tape unit for off-line computer analysis. *TCG,* Time-compensated gain; *ECG,* electrocardiogram; *PRF,* pulse repetition frequency.

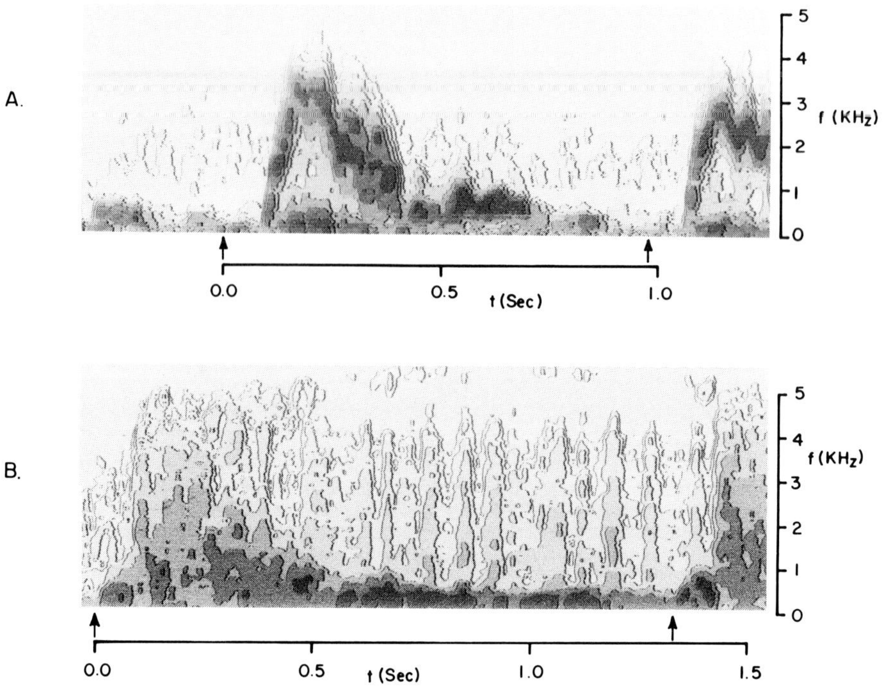

Fig. 8-3. Spectrograms of proximal aortic flow recorded with the transducer in the suprasternal notch, using a Sona-graph, Model 6061-A, spectral analyzer manufactured by Kay Electric Co. The contours indicate the relative intensity of the sound energy. In **A** is shown an example of non-turbulent flow in a normal subject, and in **B** is an example of turbulent flow in a patient with severe aortic stenosis. (From Johnson, S. L., and others: Doppler echo-cardiography: the localization of cardiac murmurs, Circulation **48:**810-822, 1973. By permission of The American Heart Association, Inc.)

velocity and geometry. Turbulence is more common in large tubes and when there is an abrupt change in tube diameter, as, for example, when the narrow jet of aortic stenosis enters a dilated aortic root.

The range-gated pulse Doppler system also requires an input electrocardiogram for accurate interpretation of the audio flow signals, since interpretation often depends on timing of the sound within the cardiac cycle. For example, normal left ventricular inflow from the mitral valve occurs during diastole, whereas normal left ventricular outflow through the aortic valve occurs during systole. The precise localization of the sample volume within the heart and great vessels is also of crucial importance in the successful utilization of this system. Anatomic localization of the sample volume requires a thorough knowledge of standard echocardiography. Without the data on ultrasonic anatomy that standard echocardiography supplies, accurate Doppler echocardiography would not be possible.

Sample volume localization is accomplished by several techniques. The A-mode monitor scope (Fig. 8-4) displays the raw video A-mode Doppler signal from the receiver on the upper channel and the receiver time-compensated-gain (TCG) characteristics on a lower channel. A negative pulse indicating range distance from the transducer face to the sample volume is superimposed on the TCG display. The range pulse is secondarily modulated with

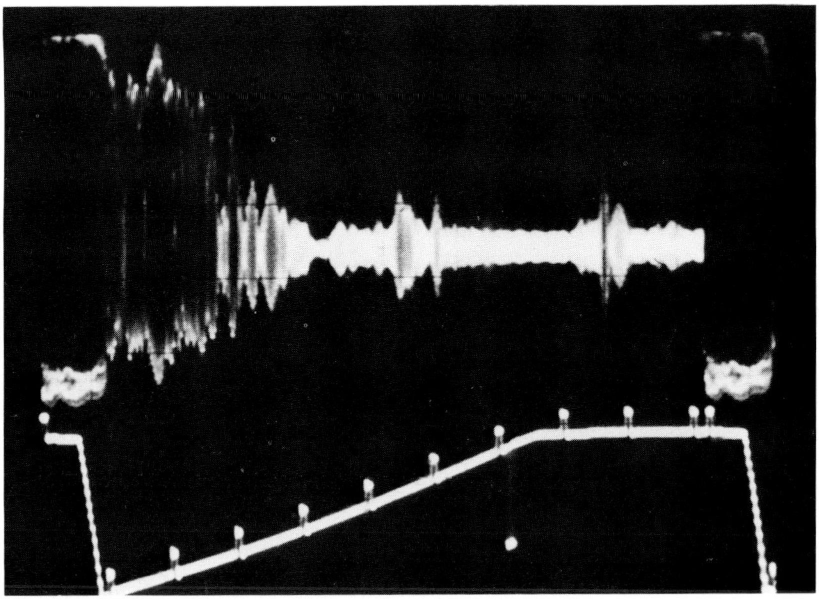

Fig. 8-4. A-mode monitor oscilloscope display. The top channel is the raw video signal from the receiver, and the bottom channel is the output of the time-compensated gain circuit, with superimposed positive range distance pips and the negative range-gate pulse, which shows the location of the sample volume along the beam. The range-gate pulse is also modulated with the electrocardiogram to provide information on the timing of the cardiac cycle.

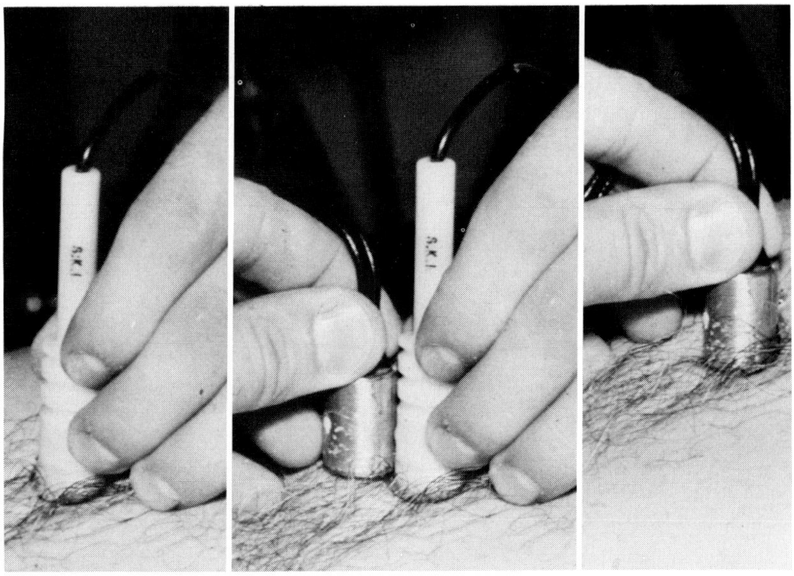

Fig. 8-5. Three-panel photograph illustrating the technique of using the standard pulse-echo transducer for localization of the sample volume within the heart. The structure of interest is first located with the pulse-echo transducer (left panel). The Doppler transducer is then positioned adjacent and parallel, and the range gate is set to the proper distance (middle panel). The pulse-echo transducer is then moved into position (right panel). This technique is a temporary expedient and probably will not be required when a new T-M–mode display for receiver output has been developed.

the electrocardiogram (ECG) to provide cardiac cycle information on the oscilloscope face. One-centimeter range marks are also superimposed on the TCG display. Another anatomic localization technique (Fig. 8-5) uses the standard pulse echo transducer. The area of interest—for example, the aortic valve orifice—is first localized with the pulse-echo transducer. The Doppler transducer is then aligned adjacent and parallel to this transducer. When the pulse echo transducer is removed, the Doppler transducer is slipped into the same position, and the range adjustment knob is then set to the area of interest.

The examination protocol begins with a brief review of the patient's chart and a cardiac physical examination with emphasis on cardiac murmurs. If there is a murmur, an abbreviated phonocardiogram is obtained with simultaneous electrocardiogram, external carotid pulse tracing, and one-channel phonocardiogram. The next step is a complete standard echocardiographic examination that includes visualization of the aortic root, aortic valve, mitral valve, left atrium, posterior left ventricular wall, interventricular septum, and tricuspid valve. If there are right-sided abnormalities, an attempt is made to locate the pulmonic valve. The final step is the Doppler examination described in the following section.

NORMAL INTRACARDIAC FLOW

The Doppler transducer is initially positioned within the suprasternal notch (Fig. 8-6). By manipulation of transducer orientation and the range adjustment knob, the sample volume is placed in the proximal aorta. On the raw video A-mode display, the posterior and sometimes the anterior aortic root walls are easily recognized as large, thick echoes with much smaller echoes generated from within the lumen. The range distance varies from about 3.5 to 7 cm. The audio signal from normal flow peaks early in systole, has a relatively narrow frequency bandwidth, and has a good signal-to-noise ratio. The detection of turbulent flow in the proximal aorta may be a useful screening test for outflow tract obstruction (aortic stenosis, idiopathic hypertrophic subaortic stenosis, aortic sclerosis) or increased ejection velocity, such as may occur with anemia.

The sample volume is then positioned in the right pulmonary artery, which can be confirmed by positioning the range-gate pulse between the two large echoes from the anterior and posterior walls of the right pulmonary artery, as seen on the raw video A-mode display. The range-

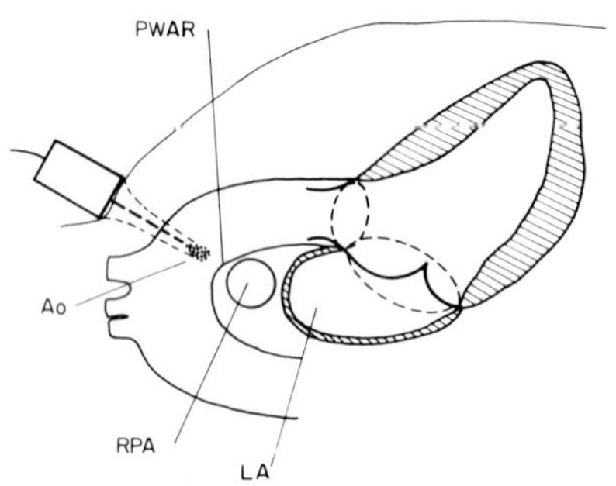

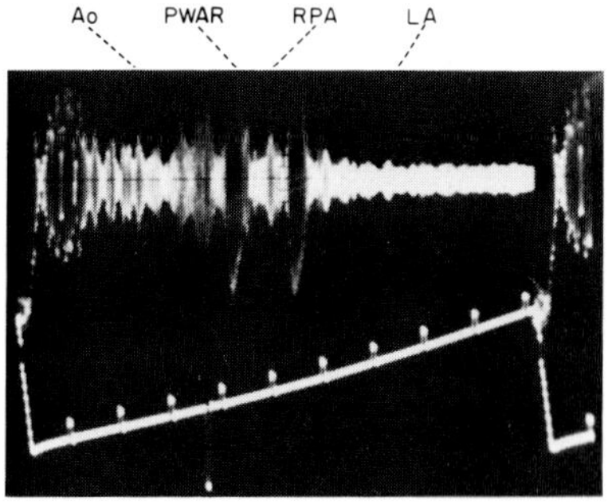

Fig. 8-6. Proximal aortic flow from the suprasternal notch showing sample volume position. On the right is a photograph of the face of the A-mode monitor oscilloscope. The range gate pulse is located within the proximal aorta. *Ao,* Aorta; *PWAR,* posterior wall aortic root; *RPA,* right pulmonary artery; *LA,* left atrium.

gate distance is usually about 6 to 8 cm. The audio signal from normal right pulmonary artery flow has low intensity, a lower signal-to-noise ratio than aortic flow, and a narrow frequency bandwidth. The detection of turbulence in the right pulmonary artery is also a useful screening test for the detection of left-to-right shunts or obstruction in the right ventricular outflow tract.

The remainder of the Doppler examination is performed from the precordial ultrasonic window. The sites are almost identical to those used in standard echocardiography. From the precordium the sample volume is next placed within the aortic valve orifice (Fig. 8-7). The normal flow signal peaks in early systole and has a low intensity, because of the almost perpendicular orientation of the beam. Localization is confirmed by hearing the brief, high-pitched clicks generated by the opening and closing motions of the aortic valve cusps as they pass through the sample volume. The diameter of the ejection flow column through the aortic valve orifice can be semiquantitatively measured by slowly moving the sample volume through the flow. In normal individuals, flow sounds can be detected throughout almost the entire diameter of the aortic valve orifice, but in aortic stenosis the flow column is transformed into a narrow jet. There are a number of potential errors with this technique for measuring jet diameter, including the change in distance between the jet and the skin surface during the respiratory cycle and the anteroposterior motion of the aortic root with the cardiac cycle. These errors can be partially controlled by very slowly ranging the sample volume through the jet and by listening to the flow sound at only one point during the cardiac cycle (early systole).

The sample volume is next placed in the left ventricular outflow tract (Fig. 8-8), just proximal to the aortic valve. The audio signal is similar to that recorded in the aortic valve orifice, but the high-pitched clicks from the aortic valve cusps are either absent or of very low intensity. If the sample volume is moved too far down into the left ventricular outflow tract, the high-pitched clicks generated by the anterior leaflet of the mitral valve can be detected. In the outflow tract, the harsh diastolic

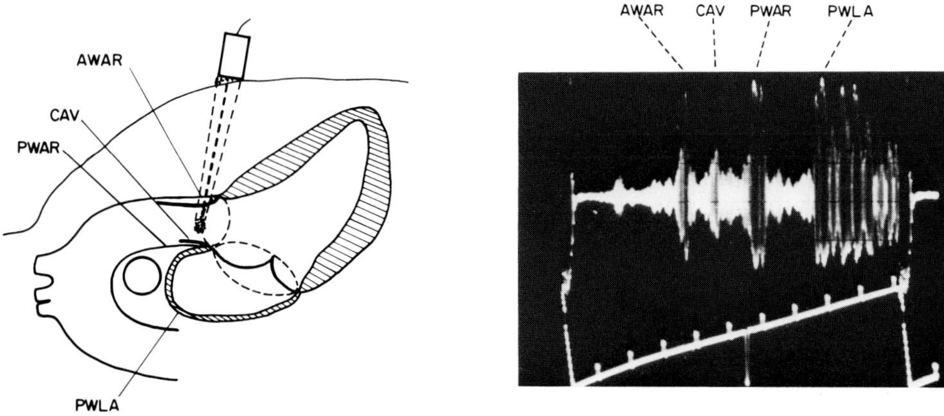

Fig. 8-7. Aortic valve orifice flow from the anterior precordium showing sample volume position. *AWAR,* anterior wall aortic root; *CAV,* cusps of aortic valve; *PWAR,* posterior wall aortic root; *PWLA,* posterior wall left atrium. (From Johnson, S. L., and others: Doppler echocardiography: the localization of cardiac murmurs, Circulation **48:**810-822, 1973. By permission of The American Heart Association, Inc.)

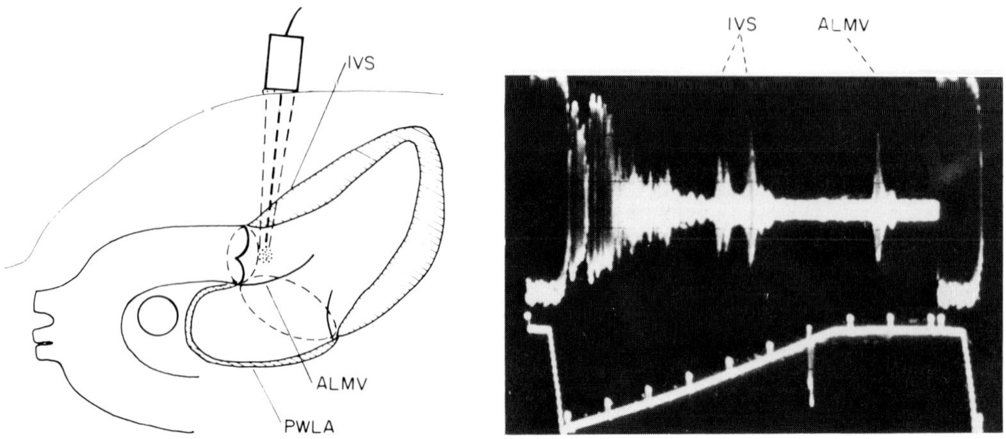

Fig. 8-8. Flow in left ventricular outflow tract showing sample volume localization. *IVS,* Intraventricular septum; *ALMV,* anterior leaflet mitral valve; *PWLA,* posterior wall left atrium.

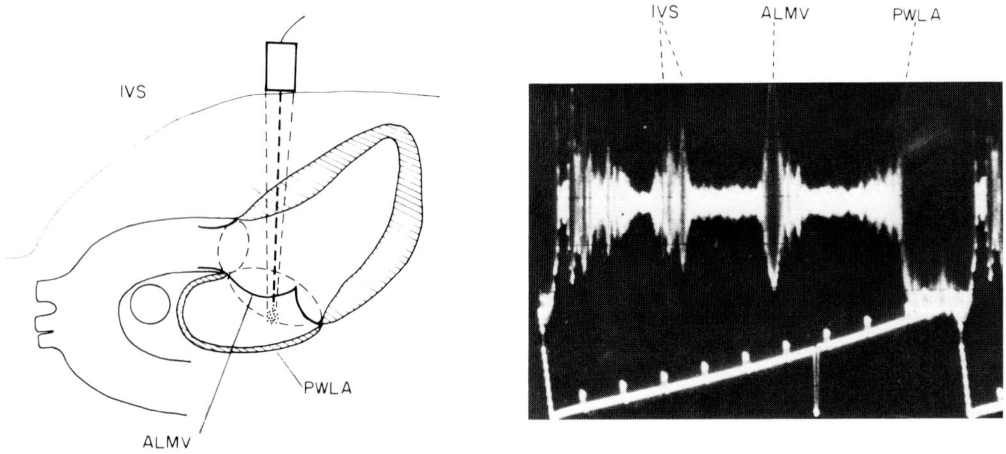

Fig. 8-9. Sample volume localization for the detection of mitral insufficiency. *IVS,* Intraventricular septum; *ALMV,* anterior leaflet mitral valve; *PWLA,* posterior wall left atrium.

murmur of aortic insufficiency may be heard. In idiopathic hypertrophic subaortic stenosis, the obstruction may result in a small, harsh systolic jet.

The sample volume is next positioned within the mitral valve orifice or in the left ventricular inflow tract. Normal flow at this point is diastolic, with low intensity and narrow bandwidth. The flow signal may be bifid, with a late diastolic peak due to an A-wave kick. High-pitched, brief opening and closing clicks are usually heard at the onset and termination of diastole and are generated by motion of the mitral valve leaflets passing through the sample volume. At this location the harsh diastolic jet of mitral stenosis can be heard.

To observe flow in the left atrium, just proximal to the mitral valve orifice, the sample volume is positioned with the aid of the pulse echo transducer. The beam should pass through the anterior leaflet of the mitral valve and then into the left atrium and should have a superior orienta-

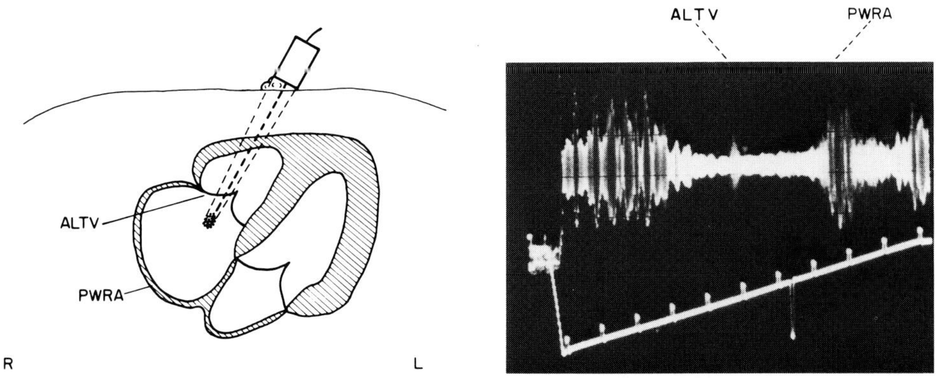

Fig. 8-10. Sample volume localization for the detection of tricuspid insufficiency (cephalad perspective, transverse cross-section of the heart). *ALTV,* Anterior leaflet tricuspid valve; *PWRA,* posterior wall right atrium.

tion to avoid the posterior leaflet of the mitral valve (Fig. 8-9). With the Doppler transducer in place, the sample volume is ranged through the anterior leaflet of the mitral valve and into the left atrium. Normally there is little or no flow at this location during systole, but with mitral regurgitation, there may be a harsh systolic jet. This procedure is repeated along three separate vectors in an attempt to examine flow at mid-orifice and at the medial and lateral commissures.

The next step is to examine flow within the right heart, especially in those patients with increased turbulence in the right pulmonary artery or in patients in whom abnormalities have been noted on the preceding echocardiographic examination. The sample volume is placed within the orifice of the tricuspid valve or distal to this point in the right ventricular inflow tract. Normal flow in the right ventricular inflow tract is primarily diastolic and similar to that recorded in the mitral valve orifice. A brief, high-pitched click at the onset and termination of diastole can often be heard. This is usually generated by the motion of the anterior leaflet of the tricuspid valve through the sample volume. In tricuspid stenosis a harsh diastolic murmur can be heard at this site. The sample volume is then advanced through the tricuspid valve orifice into the right atrium (Fig. 8-10). In normal subjects there is little or no flow during systole, but in tricuspid regurgitation a harsh systolic sound may be heard.

Examination of the right ventricular outflow tract hinges on detection of the pulmonic valve cusps. This valve can often be more easily detected with the Doppler flowmeter than by standard echocardiography. The first step is to find flow in the pulmonary artery and then move the sample volume back along the outflow tract until the high-pitched brief clicks of the pulmonic valve cusps are detected (Fig. 8-11). For confirmation, the Doppler transducer can be replaced with the pulse echo transducer along the same beam vector to obtain a T-M mode picture of the pulmonic valve. Flow signals from the right ventricular outflow tract have a relatively high intensity because of the short range distance and the acute angle between beam and flow. Normal flow through the pulmonic valve orifice peaks early in systole and has a relatively narrow bandwidth. Once the orifice is localized, the sample volume can be moved back along the outflow tract to listen for the harsh jet of pulmonic insufficiency or a jet from a high ventricular septal defect. The sample volume is then moved distally from the valve orifice into the pulmonary artery to check for turbulence, which can occur in right ventricular outflow tract obstruction, such as pulmonic stenosis.

CLINICAL APPLICATIONS

Aortic stenosis

In aortic stenosis, turbulent flow can be detected in the proximal aorta. This is not a specific finding, since turbulence can also occur in idiopathic hypertrophic subaortic stenosis and aortic valve sclerosis and with high ejection velocities such as may occur with anemia. More specific information can be obtained by ranging the sample volume through the aortic valve orifice. In aortic stenosis a small harsh-sounding jet can be detected within the orifice. As described previously, a

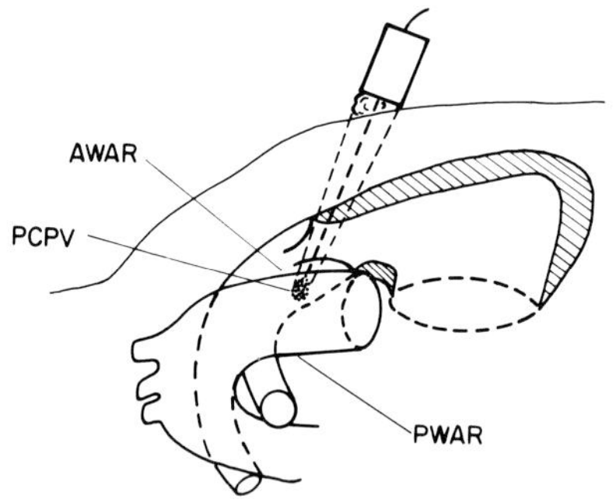

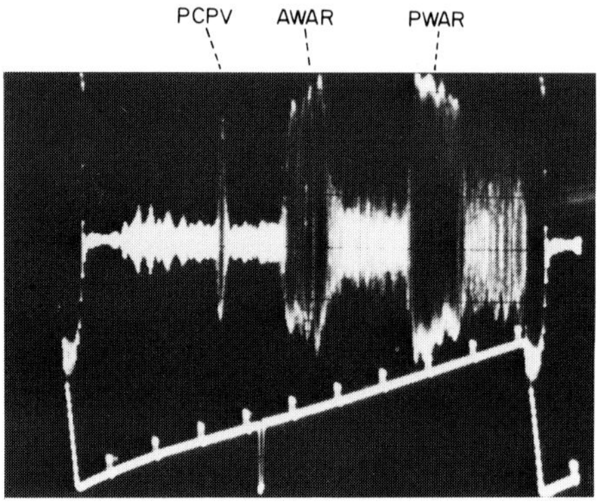

Fig. 8-11. Pulmonary artery flow showing sample volume localization. As shown, the beam often passes through both the pulmonary artery and the aorta. *PCPV,* Posterior cusp pulmonic valve; *AWAR,* anterior wall aortic root; *PWAR,* posterior wall aortic root.

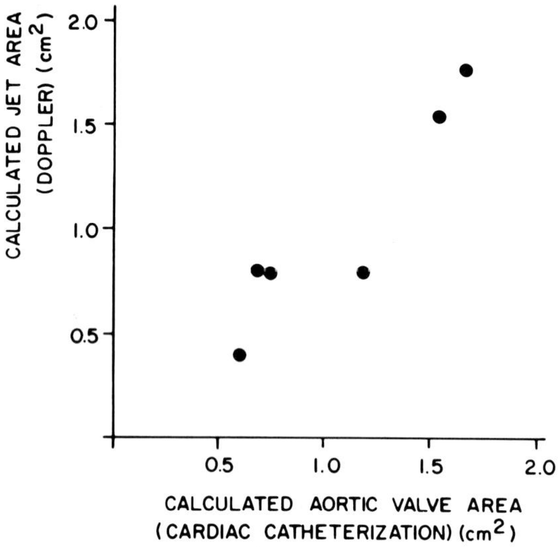

Fig. 8-12. Initial results using the Doppler technique to measure the aortic valve jet diameter in six patients with aortic stenosis. The jet area is calculated with the assumption of a jet of circular cross-section.

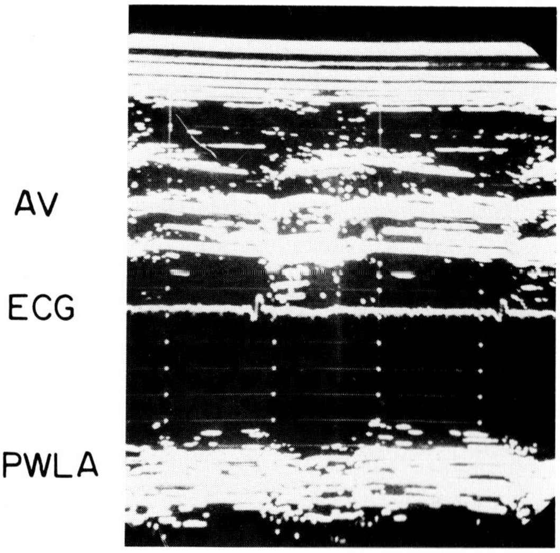

Fig. 8-13. Aortic valve echocardiogram in patient A. J., who had with aortic stenosis. *AV,* Aortic valve; *ECG,* electrocardiogram; *PWLA,* posterior wall left atrium.

semiquantitative measurement of the jet diameter can be made. Preliminary results (Fig. 8-12) suggest that the method is reasonably accurate with mild or absent stenosis and with severe stenosis. The diameter of the jet is underestimated with severe stenosis.

Case 1

Patient A. J. was a 49-year-old white male with known rheumatic heart disease and severe, persistent congestive heart failure. Clinical findings on admission suggested that he had aortic stenosis, aortic insufficiency, mitral stenosis, pulmonary hypertension, and a large right ventricle. The aortic valve echocardiogram (Fig. 8-13) showed increased echo intensity and an aortic valve opening of 10 to 14 mm, both of which suggested aortic stenosis. The echoes from the anterior leaflet of the mitral valve were thickened, and the E-F slope was 7 mm/sec, compatible with severe mitral stenosis. The left atrial dimension was 78 mm and the right ventricular dimension was increased (RVD = 32 mm). On Doppler examination

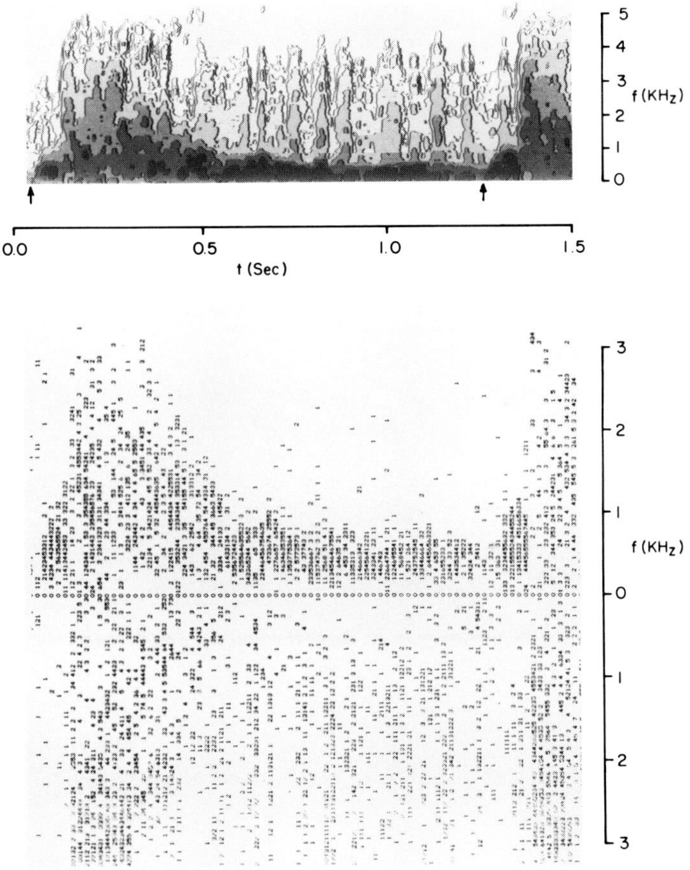

Fig. 8-14. Spectrogram of proximal aortic flow in patient A. J. The upper diagram is a spectrogram obtained with a Kay Sona-graph. The arrows indicate the onset of the Q wave of the electrocardiogram. The lower diagram is the computer print-out from a spectral analysis program using a fast Fourier transform technique. The numbers (n) indicate the sound power levels, using the equation: Sound power = 2^n. This output is directional, unlike the spectrogram generated by the Kay Sonagraph. The wide frequency bandwidth during both systole and diastole is characteristic of turbulent flow.

there was marked turbulence in the proximal aorta (Fig. 8-14) and a 10 mm harsh turbulent jet in the aortic valve orifice (Fig. 8-15), which supported the diagnosis of aortic stenosis. There was also a harsh, turbulent diastolic murmur of aortic insufficiency in the left ventricular outflow tract and a harsh pencil-thin jet in the left ventricular inflow tract caused by mitral stenosis. No mitral regurgitation was detected in the left atrium, and there was no tricuspid regurgitation in the right atrium. A harsh diastolic jet of pulmonic insufficiency was detected in the right ventricular outflow tract just proximal to the pulmonic valve, suggesting the presence of pulmonary hypertension. The impression following the ultrasound examination was severe aortic stenosis, severe mitral stenosis, aortic insufficiency, and pulmonic insufficiency secondary to pulmonary hypertension. At cardiac catheterization, the pulmonary artery pressure (PA = 70/25) and the left atrial pressure (LA = 25/22[25]) were both elevated. The mean gradient across the mitral valve was 11.8 mm Hg, and the calculated mitral valve orifice was 0.85 cm^2. The mean aortic valve gradient was 32 mm Hg with a calculated orifice area of 0.73 cm^2.

COMMENT: In this complex patient, there was good agreement between the aortic valve area calculated from the Doppler jet diameter (0.79 cm^2) and the valve area calculated at cardiac catheterization (0.73 cm^2).

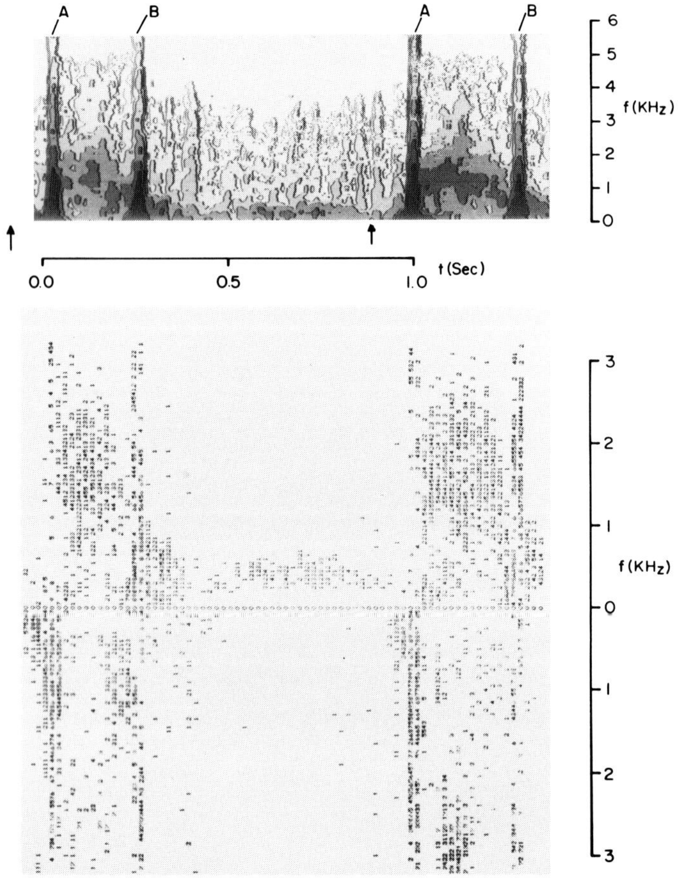

Fig. 8-15. Spectrograms of the harsh, turbulent jet within the aortic valve orifice in patient A. J. *A* is the opening click of an aortic valve cusp and *B* is the closing click. Note the wide-frequency bandwidth sound on both sides of the zero line, compatible with turbulent flow.

Aortic insufficiency

In aortic insufficiency, a harsh turbulent diastolic jet can be detected in the left ventricular outflow tract just below the aortic valve cusps, and in some patients the jet can be detected just above the anterior leaflet of the mitral valve. This test is probably more sensitive and specific than the detection of high-frequency fluttering of the anterior leaflet of the mitral valve, especially in patients who have thickening of the anterior leaflet, a not uncommon finding in patients with rheumatic heart disease.

Case 2

H. L. was a 39-year-old man with a 1-year history of progressive dyspnea on exertion and an intermittent burning sensation in the substernal area. On admission he had a sustained left ventricular impulse, S-4 gallop, gr 2/4 ejection murmur in the aortic area with radiation into the neck, and a gr 2/6 diastolic blow along the left sternal border. The electrocardiogram was within normal limits. The aortic valve echocardiogram showed multiple echoes of increased intensity (Fig. 8-16). A clear view of the aortic cusp opening was not obtained. There was fluttering of the anterior leaflet of the mitral valve (Fig. 8-17). On Doppler examination there was moderate turbulence in the proximal aorta, and a harsh 15 mm jet was detected within the aortic valve orifice. There was also a loud, harsh diastolic jet of aortic insufficiency in the left ventricular outflow tract (Fig. 8-18). The cardiac catheterization findings revealed aortic stenosis and moderate aortic insufficiency.

COMMENT: In this patient the aortic insufficiency was detected by both the high-frequency fluttering of the anterior leaflet of the mitral valve and by the Doppler flowmeter.

Mitral regurgitation

Mitral regurgitation is one of the most difficult murmurs to detect by Doppler flowmeter, but it is also one of the most useful. Great care must be taken to ensure that the sample volume is located in the

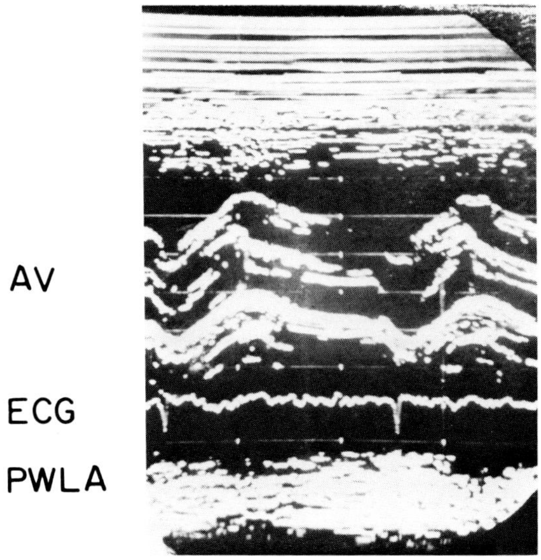

Fig. 8-16. Aortic valve echocardiogram in patient H. L., who had mild aortic stenosis and aortic insufficiency. There is a suggestion of the definable aortic valve opening between two cusps, especially in the first beat, but it is not clear cut. *AV,* Aortic valve; *ECG,* electrocardiogram; *PWLA,* posterior wall left atrium.

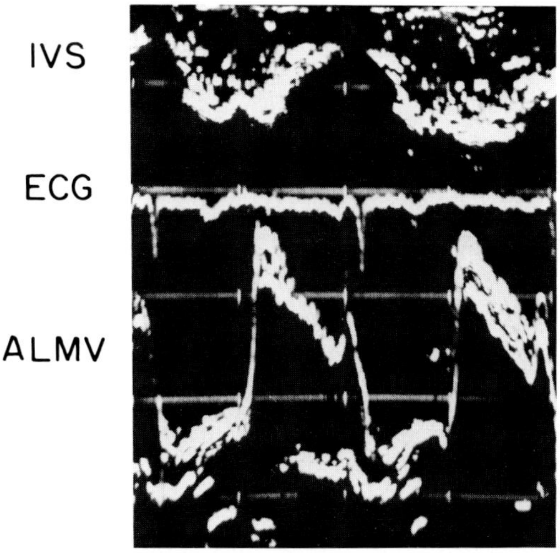

Fig. 8-17. High-frequency fluttering of the anterior leaflet of the mitral valve in patient H.L. *IVS,* Intraventricular septum; *ECG,* electrocardiogram; *ALMV,* anterior leaflet mitral valve.

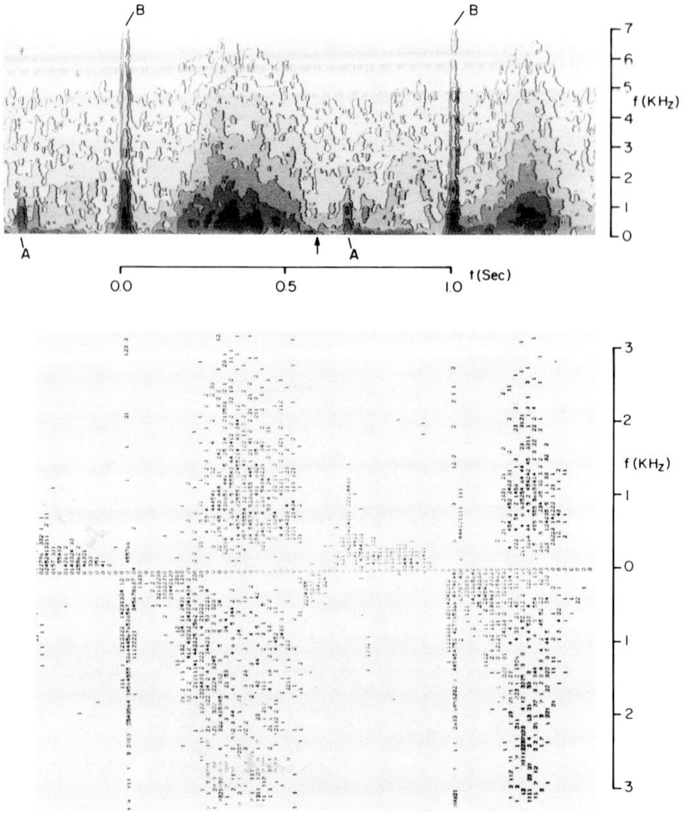

Fig. 8-18. Spectrogram of the harsh, diastolic jet of aortic insufficiency, detected in the left ventricular outflow tract of patient H.L. The variation in sound intensity results from the movement of the sample volume in and out of the jet during the respiratory cycle. *A* is the opening click of the aortic valve cusp and *B* is the closing click. Note the broad bandwidth sound in the computer spectrogram, which indicates turbulent flow.

left atrium, behind the mitral valve orifice, and not in the left ventricular outflow tract.

Case 3

M. K. was 58-year-old male with a known apical holosystolic murmur. Two weeks prior to admission he had sudden onset of acute pulmonary edema. On admission there were basilar rales, the liver was down two fingerbreadths, and there was a gr 4/6 holosystolic murmur at the apex. The murmur could also be heard in the aortic area with radiation into the neck. One observer detected a faint thrill in the second right interspace. There was also a gr 1/6 aortic insufficiency murmur along the left sternal border. The pulse tracing revealed a normal carotid pulse. The electrocardiogram showed sinus tachycardia and the chest x-ray revealed pulmonary edema with a small heart size. Echocardiograms of the aortic valve revealed no increase in echo intensity, and the aortic valve opening was 17 mm, suggesting that there was no aortic stenosis. The mitral valve findings, compatible with mitral regurgitation, included an anterior leaflet amplitude of 25 mm with a wide opening between the anterior and posterior leaflets during diastole. There was no evidence suggesting prolapse or a flail valve leaflet. The left atrial dimension was 45 mm. On Doppler examination there was no turbulence in the proximal aorta and no jet in the aortic valve orifice, which provided additional evidence for the absence of aortic

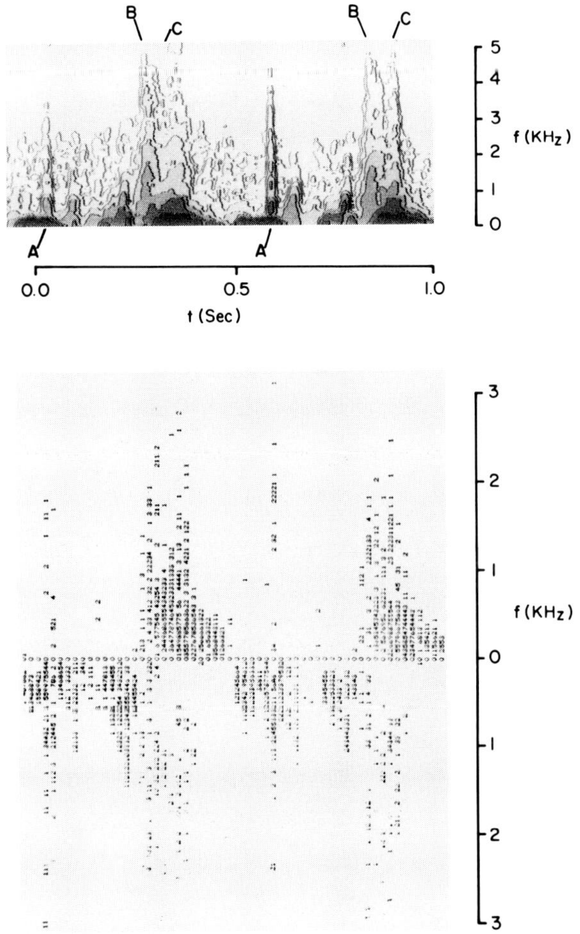

Fig. 8-19. Spectrogram of left atrial flow, just proximal to the mitral valve orifice, in patient M.K., who had mitral regurgitation. *A* is the opening click and *B* the closing click of the anterior leaflet of the mitral valve. *C* is the harsh, early systolic broad-spectrum sound of mitral regurgitation, which was recorded well only during early systole.

stenosis. An aortic insufficiency murmur was detected in the left ventricular outflow tract, and with the sample volume in the left atrium proximal to the mitral valve orifice a loud, harsh, early systolic murmur of mitral regurgitation was detected (Fig. 8-19). At cardiac catheterization, there was no pressure gradient between the left ventricle and aorta, and the left ventricular angiocardiogram showed moderate mitral regurgitation with a regurgitant fraction of 31%.

COMMENT: In this case, a Doppler examination was useful in pinpointing the location of the systolic murmur. The findings of a faint thrill along the upper right sternal border combined with a systolic murmur in the aortic area with radiation into the neck suggested that there might be aortic stenosis in addition to the mitral regurgitation.

Tricuspid regurgitation

Tricuspid regurgitation is detected with the transducer positioned along the lower left sternal border with the beam pointed medial and the sample volume in the right atrium just distal to the tricuspid valve orifice.

Case 4

P. S. was a 5-year-old boy admitted for cardiac evaluation with a tentative diagnosis of Ebstein's anomaly. Physical findings on admission included a gr 3/6, harsh pansystolic murmur at the lower left sternal border that did not increase with inspiration. The V wave in the jugular venous pulse was not increased, and there were no liver pulsations. On echocardiographic examination, the tricuspid valve orifice was found to be displaced to the left and there was also a large right atrium. The excursion of the anterior tricuspid valve leaflet was increased, and the leaflet motion had an unusual pattern (Fig. 8-20). On Doppler examination a very loud, harsh systolic jet of tricuspid regurgitation was present in the right atrium (Fig. 8-21). At cardiac catheterization, the diagnosis of Ebstein's anomaly was confirmed. The right atrial pressures were normal.

COMMENT: In this case the tricuspid regurgitation was not detected at cardiac catheterization.

Pulmonic stenosis

In pulmonic stenosis, a very loud, harsh (turbulent) flow sound can be detected in the pulmonic artery, distal to this obstruction. The murmur is similar to that found in aortic stenosis.

Case 5

K. M. was a 9-year-old boy with suspected pulmonic stenosis who was admitted for cardiac catheterization. On physical examination he

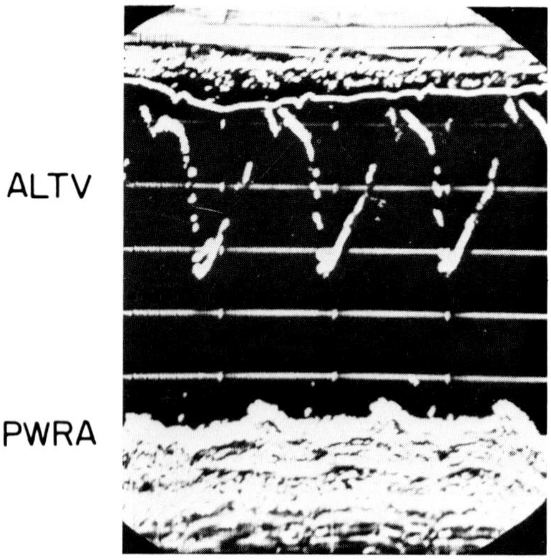

Fig. 8-20. Tricuspid valve echocardiogram in patient P.S., who had Ebstein's anomaly. *ALTV,* Anterior leaflet tricuspid valve; *PWRA,* posterior wall right atrium.

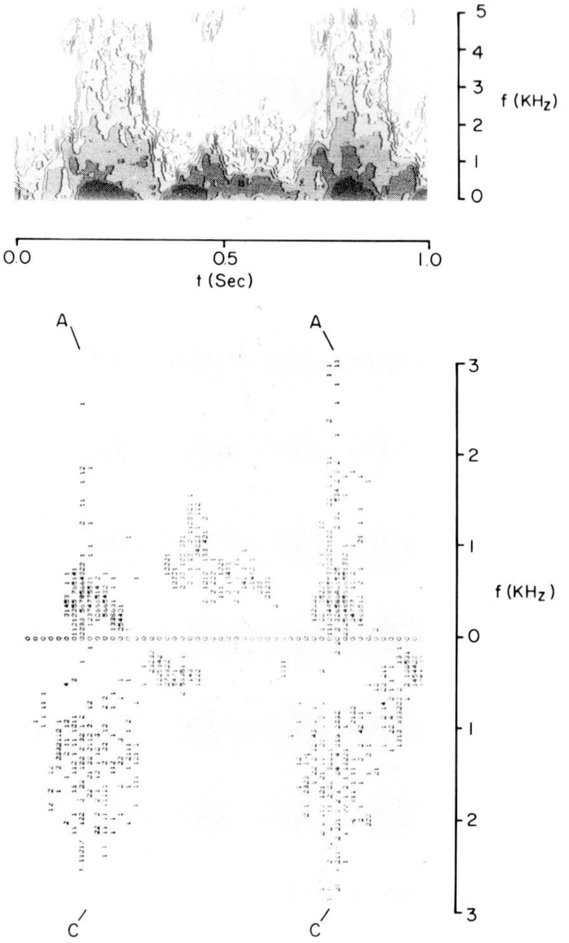

Fig. 8-21. Spectrogram of right atrial flow, just proximal to the tricuspid valve orifice, in patient P.S., who had Ebstein's anomaly and tricuspid insufficiency. *A* is the closing click and *B* the opening click of the anterior leaflet of the tricuspid valve. *C* is the harsh, early systolic, wide-frequency bandwidth sound of tricuspid insufficiency. The recording of the jet only in early systole was probably caused by anterior motion of the jet out of the sample volume during systole. On auscultation the jet was holosystolic.

had a gr 5/6 systolic murmur in the pulmonic area with wide radiation. The electrocardiogram showed right ventricular hypertrophy, and the chest film revealed a prominent right ventricle and pulmonary artery segment. On Doppler examination, with the sample volume in the pulmonary artery, there was a brief, harsh jet during systole, followed by high-intensity, low-pitched turbulence during diastole (Fig. 8-22). This flow sound can be easily distinguished from normal pulmonary artery flow (Fig. 8-23). At cardiac catheterization the mean gradient across the pulmonic valve was 96 mm Hg, and the calculated pulmonic valve orifice area was 0.50 cm^2/m^2. Angiocardiography showed thickened leaflets in the dome-shaped pulmonic valve, poststenotic dilation of the pulmonary artery, and marked right ventricular hypertrophy with a normal sized infundibulum during diastole. These findings were confirmed at operation.

COMMENT: The downstream turbulence generated in pulmonic and aortic stenosis leads to identical Doppler flow sounds. The high-

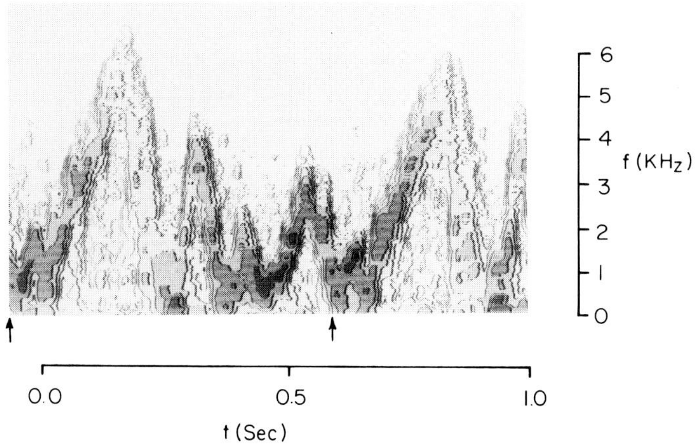

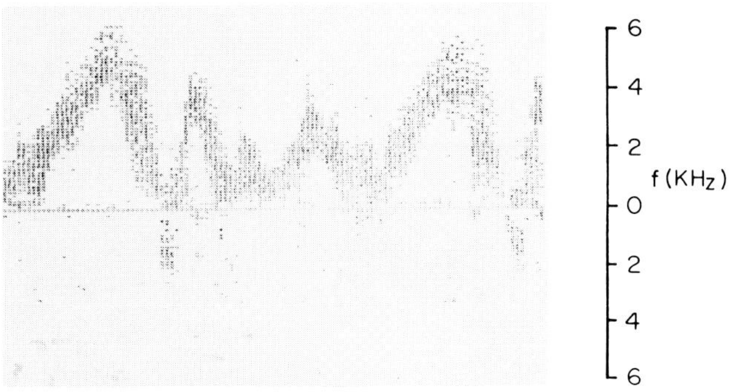

Fig. 8-22. Spectrogram of pulmonary artery flow in patient K.M., who had severe pulmonic stenosis. The transducer was placed high along the left sternal border, with the beam angled inferiorly, so that systolic outflow was positive. The high-intensity diastolic sounds are probably caused by eddies and vortices created by the systolic jet. The arrows indicate the Q wave of the electrocardiogram. (From Johnson, S. L., and others: Doppler echocardiography: the localization of cardiac murmurs, Circulation **48**:810-822, 1973. By permission of The American Heart Association, Inc.)

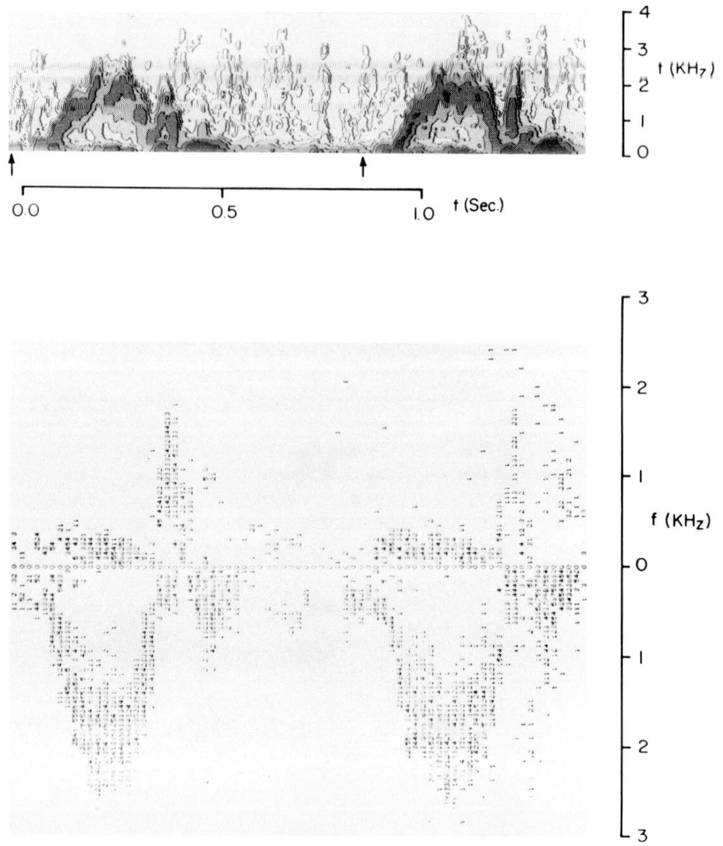

Fig. 8-23. Spectrogram of pulmonary artery flow in a normal subject. The transducer was positioned anterior to the pulmonic valve and directed superiorly, so that systolic flow is negative, as shown in *A* in the computer spectrogram. There is also reverse flow *(B)* in early diastole.

intensity, low-pitched "noisy" flow sounds heard during diastole may be secondary to eddy or vortex formation.

SUMMARY

Doppler echocardiography is a noninvasive technique for studying blood flow within the heart and great vessels. The technique has become feasible with the recent development of a range-gated pulse Doppler flowmeter with a small sample volume (2 × 4 mm) whose position along the ultrasonic beam can be controlled by a range adjustment knob. The characteristics of the output signal can be used to differentiate laminar from turbulent flow. The most useful output at present is an audio signal picked up with a pair of earphones. The entire system can be viewed as a noninvasive technique for intracardiac phonocardiography. The precise localization of the sample volume within the heart is critical and depends heavily upon standard echocardiographic techniques. Doppler echocardiography is not a stand-alone technique, and the operator must be well versed in standard echocardiography. Current applications include the detection of turbulence in both the proximal aorta and in the right pulmonary artery, which are useful screening tests for upstream obstruction or increased blood velocity. Semiquantitative measurement of jet diameter can be used to estimate the severity of aortic stenosis. Doppler echocardiography is also useful in the detection of valvular insufficiency, such as aortic, mitral, tricuspid, and pulmonic insufficiency. Right ventricular outflow tract obstruction, such as pulmonic valve stenosis, can be recognized by the characteristic turbulent flow sound heard in the pulmonary artery. The technique of range-gated Doppler echocardiography is relatively new, so additional applications are sure to follow.

REFERENCES

1. Satomura, S.: Ultrasonic Doppler method for the inspection of cardiac function, J. Acoust. Soc. Am. **29:**1181, 1957.
2. Yoshida, T., and others: Analysis of heart motion with ultrasonic Doppler method and its clinical application, Am. Heart J. **61:**61-75, 1961.
3. Yoshida, T., and others: Studies of the time of valvular movements in mitral valvular disease with ultrasonic Doppler method, Jap. Heart J. **1:**261-274, 1960.
4. Yoshida, T.: Studies of cardiac function by the ultrasonic Doppler method. In Luisada, A., editor: Examination of the cardiac patient, New York, 1965, McGraw-Hill Book Co., pp. 4-425.
5. Nimura, Y., and others: Analysis of the cardiac cycle of the left side of the heart in cases of left ventricular overloading or damage with the ultrasonic Doppler method, Am. Heart J. **75:**49-65, 1968.
6. Yoshida, T.: Ultrasonic Doppler method for analyzing heart motion, Jap. Circ. J. **27:**1-11, 1963.
7. Kostis, J. B., Fleischmann, D., and Bellet, S.: Use of the ultrasonic Doppler method for timing of valvular movement, Circulation **40:**197-207, 1969.
8. Bellet, S., and Kostis, J.: Study of the cardiac arrhythmias by ultrasonic Doppler method, Circulation **38:**721-736, 1968.
9. Spencer, M. P., and Campbell, S. D.: Development of bubbles in venous and arterial blood during hyperbaric decompression, Bull. Mason Clin. **22:**26-32, 1968.
10. Spencer, M. P., and others: Experiments on decompression bubbles in the circulation using ultrasonic and electromagnetic flowmeters, J. Occup. Med. **2:**238-244, 1969.
11. Edmonds-Seal, J., and Maroon, J. C.: Air embolism diagnosed with ultrasound, Anaesthesia **24:**438-440, 1969.
12. Carden, E., and Doll, W.: A Doppler flowmeter for detecting air and other emboli, incorporating a simple method of screening against interference, Anesthesiology **33:**551-552, 1970.
13. Maroon, J. C., Edmonds-Seal, J., and Campbell, R. L.: An ultrasonic method for detecting air embolism, J. Neurosurg. **31:**196-201, 1969.
14. Fallah-nejad, M., Abelson, D. M., and Blakemore, W. S.: Left ventricular pseudoaneurysm, Chest **61:**90-92, 1972.
15. Joyner, C. R., Jr., Harrison, F. S., Jr., and Gruber, J. W.: Diagnosis of hypertrophic subaortic stenosis with a Doppler velocity flow detector, Ann. Intern. Med. **74:**692-696, 1971.
16. Benchimol, A., and others: Telemetry of arterial flow in man with a Doppler ultrasonic flowmeter, Am. J. Cardiol. **22:**75-84, 1968.
17. Pedoe, D. S. T.: The use of Doppler ultrasound blood velocity measurements in the diagnosis of aortic incompetence, Oxford Med. School Gazette **24:**1971.
18. Pedoe, D. S. T.: Blood velocity measurements in aortic regurgitation using heated thin film and ultrasonic techniques, Br. Heart J. **33:**611, 1971.
19. Kalmanson, D., and others: Arch. Mal. Coeur Vaisseaux **61:**291, 1968.
20. Kalmanson, D., Veyrat, C., and Chiche, P.: Venous return disturbances induced by arrhythmias, Cardiovasc. Res. **4:**279-290, 1970.
21. Kalmanson, D., and others: Non-invasive technique for diagnosing atrial septal defect and assessing shunt volume using directional Doppler ultrasound, Br. Heart J. **34:**981-991, 1972.
22. Baker, D. W.: Pulsed ultrasonic Doppler bloodflow sensing, I.E.E.E. Trans. Sonics Ultrasonics **SU-17:**170-185, 1970.
23. Jorgensen, J. E., Campau, D. N., and Baker, D. W.: Physical characteristics and mathematical modelling of the pulsed ultrasonic flowmeter, Med. Biol. Eng. **11:**404-421, 1973.
24. Wells, P. N. T.: A range-gated ultrasonic Doppler system, Med. Biol. Eng. **7:**641-652, 1969.
25. Light, L. H.: Progress in blood velocity measurement, Br. J. Radiol. **43:**227, 1970.
26. Peronneau, P., and others: Vélocimétre sanguin par effet Doppler à emission ultra-sonore pulsée. L'Onde Electrique **50:**369-389, 1970.
27. Kostis, J. B., and others: Use of range-gated, pulsed ultrasonic Doppler technique for continuous measurement of velocity of the posterior heart wall, Chest **62:**597-604, 1972.
28. Hokanson, D. E., and others: Ultrasonic arteriography: a new approach to arterial visualization, Biomed. Eng. **6:**420, 1971.
29. Hokanson, D. E., and others: Ultrasonic arteriography; a noninvasive method for arterial visualization, Radiology **102:**435-436, 1972.
30. Mozersky, D. J., and others: Ultrasonic arteriography, Arch. Surg. **103:**663-667, 1971.
31. Gould, K. L., and others: A noninvasive technique for determining patency of saphenous vein coronary bypass grafts, Circulation **46:**595-600, 1972.

9 Cardiac ultrasonography

DONALD L. KING, M.D.

Ultrasonic imaging of the heart is a new application of diagnostic ultrasound in comparison to its use for abdominal and pelvic ultrasonography. It is only now coming into clinical use as a result of the development of electronic scanning instruments. The slow development of cardiac ultrasonography has been caused in part by the technical difficulties presented by the constant, comparatively rapid movement of cardiac structures. This results in a marked blurring of the ultrasonic image when it is made by a conventional abdominal contact scanner. The complexities of visualizing intracardiac anatomy in cross-section have also been a barrier to rapid development. Cross-sectional representation of the heart, inherent with ultrasonic imaging, is unfamiliar to most physicians, even those working in the field of cardiology. Furthermore, the geometry of anatomic relationships in the heart does not lend itself well to cross-sectional representation except in a comparatively few specific planes.

Choice and recognition of these planes for imaging has required the development of new skills in addition to a new understanding of cross-sectional anatomy of the heart. With these developments cardiac ultrasonography is rapidly improving and will almost certainly become a widely used and valuable clinical diagnostic procedure. Because of its noninvasive nature and highly favorable benefit-to-risk ratio, ultrasonic imaging of the heart may eventually become the principal means for visualization of intracardiac morphology and function.

Following Howry's development of compound scanning, Holmes,[1] in 1954, suggested its use synchronized with the

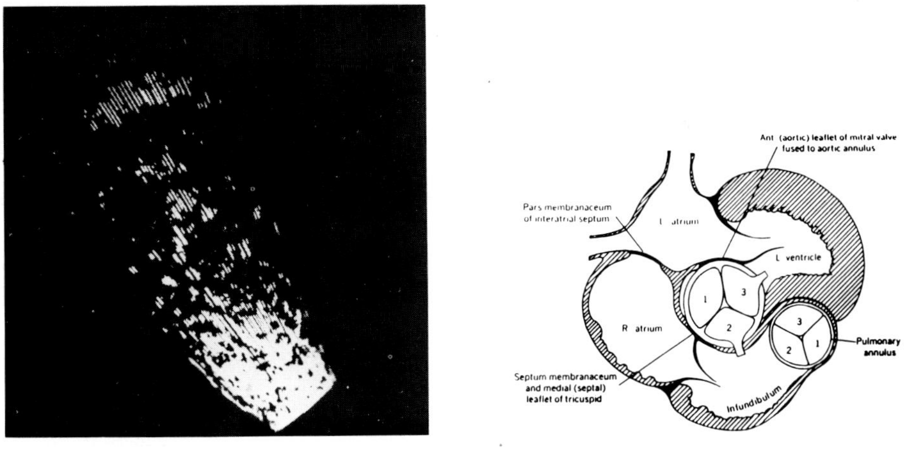

Fig. 9-1. Cross-section of the base of the heart by Asberg and Hertz. (From Hertz, C. H.: Med. Elec. Bio. Eng. **2**:39-45, 1964.)

patient's electrocardiogram to permit imaging of the heart during various phases of the cardiac cycle. At this time Edler and Hertz were developing the one-dimensional technique, echocardiography or ultrasound cardiography, for recording cardiac motion as a function of time. A decade later Hertz, Olofsson, and Asberg[2,4] developed an ultrasonic mirror system for two-dimensional imaging of the heart. The mirror system was immersed in water and motor-driven to sweep the ultrasound beam rapidly back and forth across the heart ten times per second. The images, each approximately 0.1 second in duration, were recorded on cine film. An example of an early image obtained with this system is shown in Fig. 9-1.

At the same time Ebina, Kikuchi, Tanaka, and associates[5-7] developed a similar motorized water-path scanning system in which a focused transducer was used. The transducer, placed very close to the chest wall, was rapidly and continuously moved through a 60-degree sector scan without being synchronized to the cardiac cycle. The display oscilloscope was put into operation for 30 msec at a selected phase of each cardiac cycle by use of the electrocardiogram. Echo signals were thus

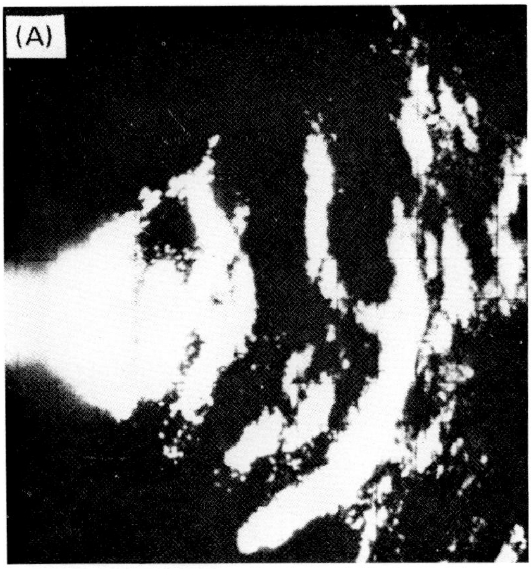

Fig. 9-2. Ultrasonotomogram of the heart through the long axis of the left ventricle made by a motor-driven sector scan. (From Kikuchi, Y., and Okuyama, D.: Jap. Elec. Eng., pp. 53-60, Oct. 1970.)

positionally patched in a random manner over twenty to thirty successive heart cycles. The result was a stationary image of a complete sector scan of the heart at one phase of the cardiac cycle (Fig. 9-2). A sequence of these images at nine different points throughout the cardiac cycle could thus be obtained and a motion picture of the beating heart produced by animation of a series of these images on cine film.

In 1970 King described the stop-action technique for cardiac ultrasonography.[8] This technique utilizes a commercially available hand-operated compound contact scanner synchronized to the cardiac cycle by the electrocardiogram. In this technique the scanning transducer in direct contact with the skin is freely movable in a plane across the precordium. A variable combination of linear, arc, and sector motions appropriate for recording any variation of intracardiac anatomy could be used. Echo signals from a sufficient variety of positions in the heart are integrated into a static, two-dimensional image on the storage display oscilloscope. Recording is carried out over a 5- or 6-minute sequence of cardiac cycles. An

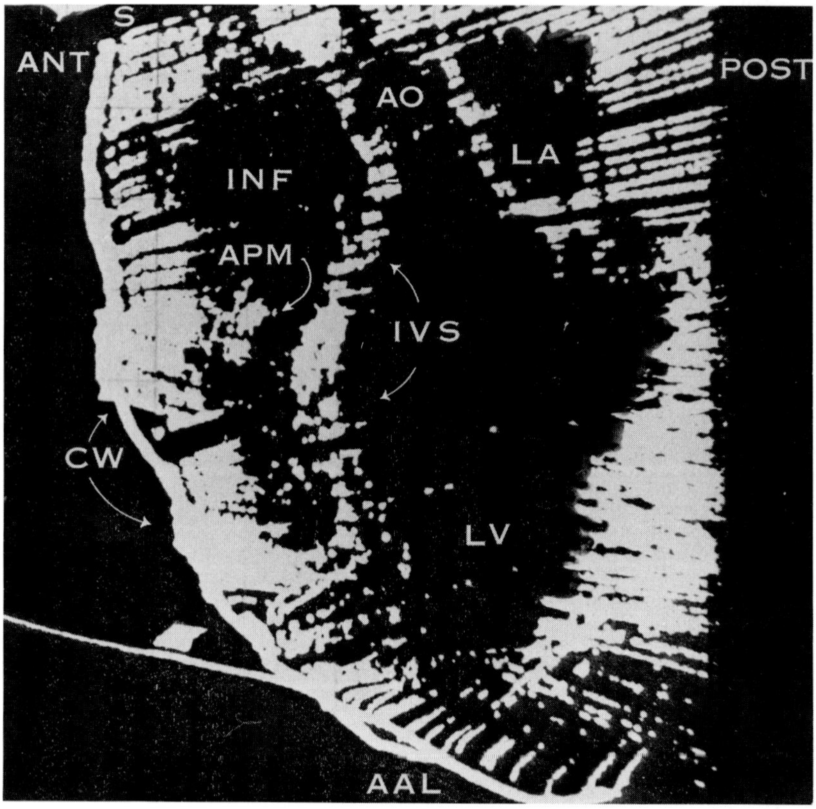

Fig. 9-3. Cross-section through the long axis of the left ventricle made by the stop-action technique using an ECG-gated hand-operated contact scanner. (From King, D. L.: Radiology **103:**387-392, 1972.)

The following abbreviations are used in Figs. 9-3 to 9-26: *AAL,* Anterior axillary line; *AAR,* anterior aortic root wall; *AMV,* anterior mitral valve; *ANT,* anterior; *AO,* aorta; *APM,* anterior papillary muscle; *AV,* aortic valve; *CT,* chordae tendineae; *CW,* chest wall; *INF,* infundibulum; *IVS,* interventricular septum; *LA,* left atrium; *LT,* left; *LV,* left ventricle; *MV,* mitral valve; *PA,* pulmonary artery; *PAR,* posterior aortic root wall; *PE,* pericardial effusion; *PM,* papillary muscle; *PMV,* posterior mitral valve; *POST,* posterior; *PPM,* posterior papillary muscle; *PV,* pulmonary valve; *PW,* posterior wall; *RT,* right; *RV,* right ventricle; *RVO,* right ventricular outflow tract; *S,* sternum or skin; *VS,* ventricular septum; *VSD,* ventricular septal defect.

early example of this technique is shown in Fig. 9-3. Images such as these are able to show the size and shape of the cardiac chambers in systole and diastole, the appearance of the heart valves, particularly the aortic and mitral valves, and the orientation of the great vessels.

ANATOMY

An understanding of cross-sectional anatomy of the heart is best achieved by study of heart specimens, angiocardiograms, and anatomic texts.[9] An appreciation of the wide anatomic variation among normal and abnormal individuals is gained through extensive clinical experience. Skillful echocardiography is an essential means for determining the location of specific intracardiac structures and for gaining a three-dimensional concept of in vivo anatomic relationships.

The "ultrasonic window" to the heart is generally the left third, fourth, and fifth rib interspaces. Its boundaries may be determined by moving the transducer laterally in each interspace and noting the point at which the lung echoes obliterate the intracardiac echoes. With cardiac enlargement this area increases in a lateral and cephalad direction. With emphysema it diminishes in a caudad and medial direction. The last recording area to be obliterated by hyperinflation of the lungs is immediately adjacent to the lower left sternal margin and the xiphoid process.

For ultrasonic examination, it is essential to understand cardiac anatomy and the relationship of intracardiac structures in terms of surface landmarks. Beneath the chest wall left of the sternum lies the anterior wall of the heart. Medially it is the anterior wall of the right ventricle, while laterally it becomes the anterior wall of the left ventricle. The right ventricle may be thought of as a flattened, V-shaped bellows. The right horizontal limb of the V, the inflow tract, begins at the tricuspid valve, beneath the sternum, and runs leftward toward the cardiac apex. The left vertical limb, the outflow tract, is directed toward the left clavicle and terminates at the pulmonary valve (Fig. 9-4).

The ultrasonic anteroposterior diameter or thickness of the right ventricular chamber depends not only on its intrinsic size but on the position and direction of the ultrasound beam at the time the measurement is made. Diagonal diameters will be spuriously increased while those taken close to the left edge of the outflow tract may appear narrow. The posterior wall of the right ventricle is the interventricular septum. The septum bulges convexly in a right anterior direction because of the high pressure of the left ventricle. As a

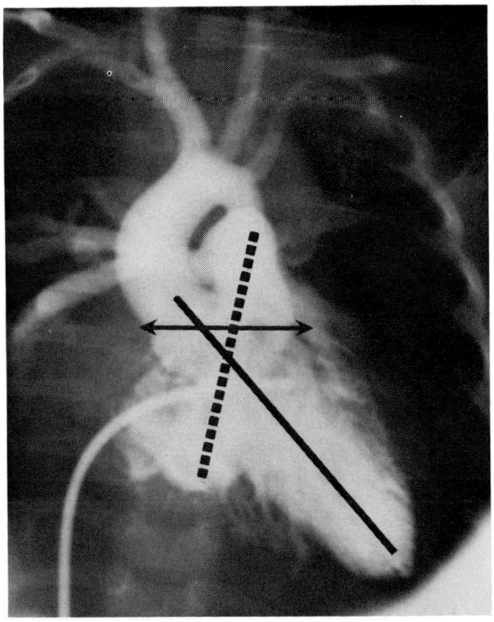

Fig. 9-4. Anteroposterior projection of a left ventricular angiocardiogram. Shunting of contrast from left to right through a ventricular septal defect has also visualized the right ventricular outflow tract and pulmonary artery. The superimposed lines show the approximate direction of the long axis of the left ventricle (solid line), the axis of the right ventricular outflow tract (broken line), and the direction of a transverse cross-section through the origins of the great arteries (horizontal arrows).

result the low-pressure right ventricle is flattened over the convexity of the left ventricle. The curved septum courses from the base of the heart between the tricuspid and mitral valves obliquely leftward and anteriorly toward the pulmonary valve and cardiac apex.

The left ventricle posterior to the septum is roughly cone shaped. The apex of the cone points anteriorly, leftward, and caudad. The long axis of the left ventricle (Fig. 9-4) extends from the midportion of the base to the apex. The base of the cone, made up of the aortic and mitral orifices, is directed toward the posterior right shoulder. The aortic orifice lies to the right anteriorly and cephalad in the base of the ventricle. The fibrous mitral ring is contiguous with the posterior margin of the aortic root and lies posterior, caudad, and to the left of it. The anterior mitral leaflet arising from the anterior portion of the mitral ring is contiguous with the posterior wall of the aortic root and extends downward from it toward the cardiac apex. As a consequence, the anterior leaflet divides the basilar portion of the left ventricle into an anterior outflow tract and a posterior inflow tract. The plane of the anterior mitral leaflet in its midposition is roughly parallel to the anterior chest wall. Posterior to the inflow tract lies the posterior mitral leaflet and the posterior free wall of the left ventricle. The left atrium lies above, or cephalad, and to the right of the mitral valve orifice, directly behind the aortic root. The mitral orifice occupies the left caudal aspect of the left atrium.

Depicting these relationships is an anatomic drawing of the heart sectioned through the long axis of the left ventricle (Fig. 9-5). The perspective is rightward from the left shoulder. The left lateral wall of the ventricle has been removed. The remaining visible right wall of the left ventricle is the interventricular septum. Its upper portion, dividing the left ventricle from the upper right ventricular outflow tract, has been sectioned. Immediately posterior to the right ventricular outflow tract in this plane of cross-section lies the aortic root, its orifice anterior and slightly superior to the mitral orifice. The parallel anterior and posterior walls of the aortic root are directed anteriorly and cephalad from the base of the ventricle at an angle to the left ventricular long axis. The oval left atrium lies adjacent to the posterior wall of the aortic root and above the mitral orifice. Ultrasonographic cross-sections through the same plane of the left ventricle (Fig. 9-6) are similar in appearance and represent the anatomic cross-section as if one were viewing en face only the cut surfaces of the heart. Echo signals (white) arising from the skin, anterior chest wall, and anterior wall of the heart merge indistinguishably. The blood-filled arteries and cardiac chambers are echo-free (black), while their margins are defined by echoes arising from the blood-muscle interface. The posterior heart walls also are indistinguishable from the adjacent lung. Intracardiac anatomy surrounded by blood—that is, the interventricular septum, aortic walls, aortic and mitral valves and their associated chordae tendineae, and papillary muscles—may be visualized as discrete structures. The cone-shaped left ventricle appears roughly triangular in the ultrasonographic cross-section. The same plane passing obliquely through the upper right ventricular outflow tract produces an oval cross-section of that structure. The upper interventricular septum separating the two ventricles curves from the anterior heart wall posteriorly and cephalad, becoming continuous with the anterior wall of the aortic root. The posterior wall of the aortic root is seen to be continuous with the anterior mitral leaflet. On some cross-sections the chordae tendineae can be shown connecting the leaflets to the papillary muscles.

With normal anatomic development, the right ventricular outflow tract–pulmonary

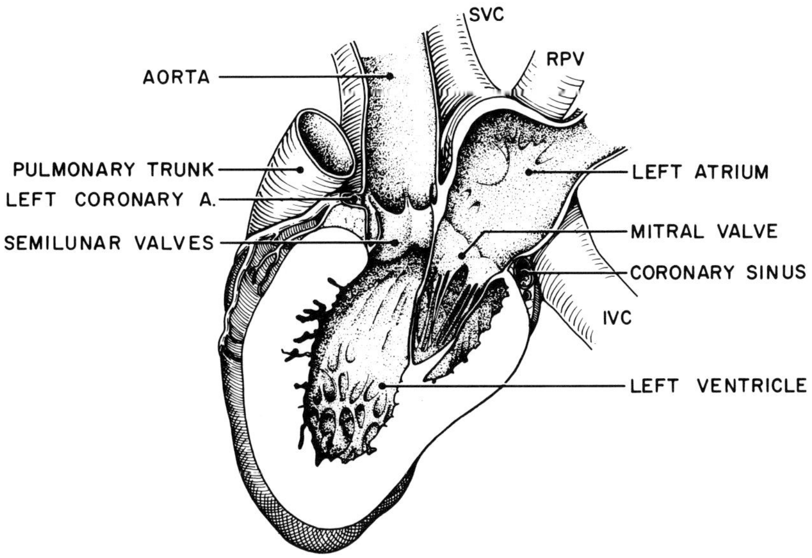

Fig. 9-5. Anatomic drawing of a heart sectioned through the long axis of the left ventricle. The left side has been removed to view the remaining structures from the left. This cross-section obtained sonographically is most useful for evaluating left ventricular size and function. (Compare with Figs. 9-3 and 9-6.)

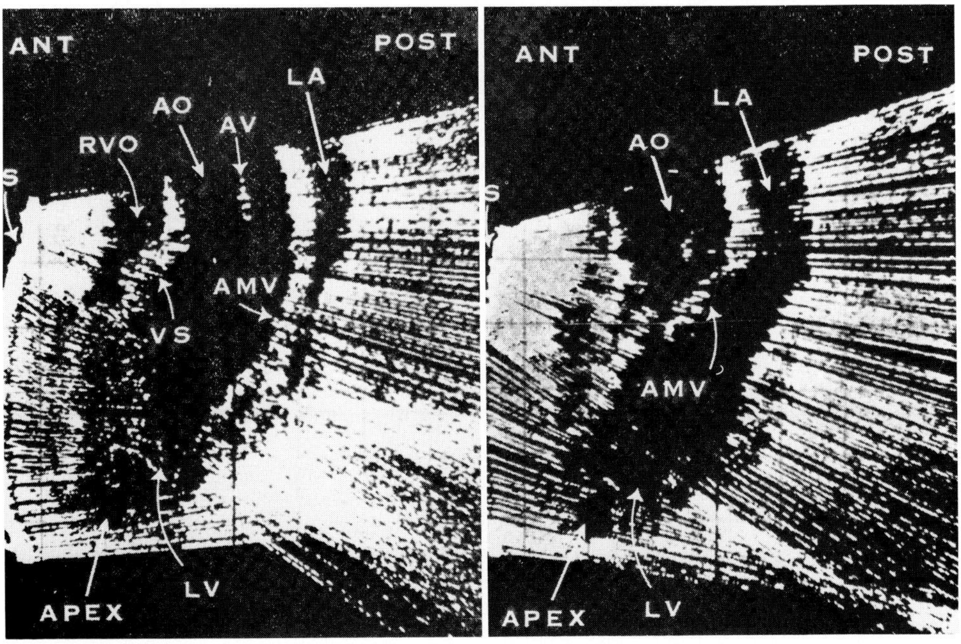

Fig. 9-6. Normal long axis cross-sections on the same patient made by the stop-action technique. *Left,* The imaging interval was set to record late diastole. The anterior mitral valve leaflet is shown just prior to complete closure. *Right,* The imaging interval was set to record early diastole. The anterior mitral valve leaflet is shown in its extreme anterior, open position. (From King, D. L.; Cardiac ultrasonography; cross-sectional imaging of the heart, Circulation **47:**843-847, 1973. By permission of The American Heart Association, Inc.)

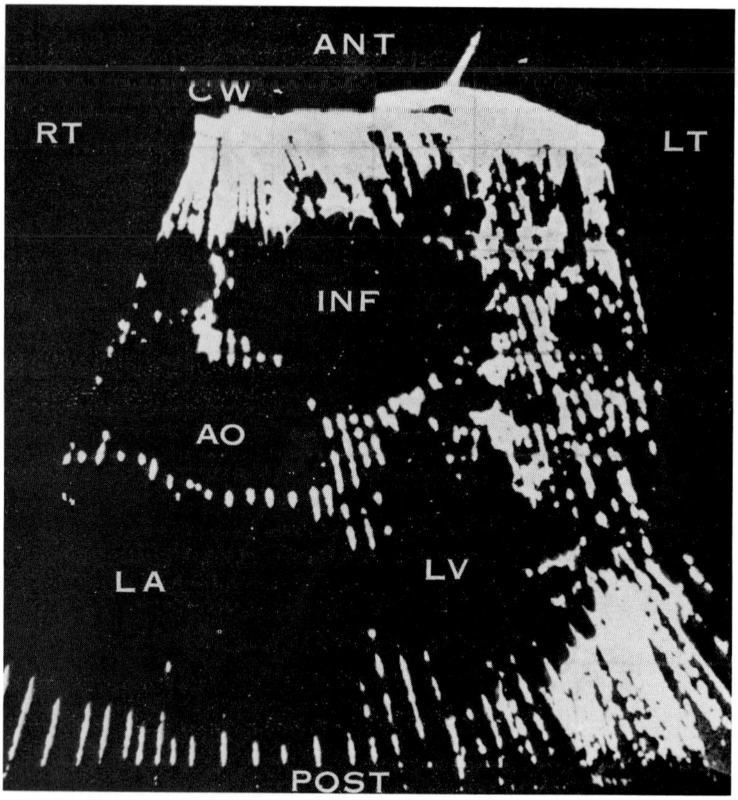

Fig. 9-7. A transverse cross-section along the third left intercostal space through the aortic root at the level of the aortic valve. The right ventricular outflow tract is anterior and left of the aortic root. (From King, D. L.: Radiology **103:**387-392, 1972.)

trunk follows a curvilinear course in an anteroposterior direction over the cephalad surface of the left ventricle to the left of the aortic root (Fig. 9-4). A transverse cross-section in the second or third left intercostal space at the level of the aortic valve will show the right ventricular outflow tract anteriorly and displaced to the left. The aortic root will be seen lying deeper, posteriorly and to the right, or medially (Fig. 9-7). Depending upon variations in the position and angulation of the scanning plane and variations in the size and rotation of the heart, the left atrium and upper portion of the left ventricle will also appear in these cross-sections.

STOP-ACTION IMAGING

Instrumentation for stop-action cardiac ultrasonography includes a conventional contact scanner, an electrocardiogram, and a QRS trigger circuit. The R wave of the patient's electrocardiogram activates the trigger circuit and serves as a timing signal. The output signal of the trigger circuit controls the operation of the ultrasonic scanner, turning it on for an appropriate short recording interval and then off again. The duration of the output or unblanking signal is variable but is usually maintained at 8 to 10 msec. The elapsed time, or delay, between the R wave and the recording interval is varied by a delay control. Adjustment of the delay control permits selection of any portion of the cardiac cycle for imaging, such as end-systole or end-diastole. Echoes received during the selected interval are recorded, while all others received during the remainder of the cardiac cycle are eliminated. In this manner all points within the heart recorded over a long series of cardiac cycles are at the same state of contraction.

A single, unblurred "line" of the echo data is recorded from within the heart during each cardiac cycle. The position of the "line" in the image corresponds to the direction of the sound beam during that cardiac cycle. By asynchronous movement of the position and angulation of the transducer between recording intervals, additional "lines" are accumulated in phase on subsequent cardiac cycles. The lines are retained and integrated upon the recording storage oscilloscope until the cross-section is complete and the image photographed.

The most critical technical step for stop-action cardiac ultrasonography is selection of a satisfactory imaging plane. The examiner must know which plane of cross-section he wishes to visualize. He must then adjust the position, tilt, and angulation of the scanning apparatus to coincide with the desired plane through the heart. To correctly adjust the scanner in each case, the examiner must determine the size and position of the heart and must localize several important intracardiac landmarks. This is best accomplished by means of echocardiography. The aortic root and mitral valve are located by their characteristic patterns of motion. The position of optimum recording most directly over each structure is marked on the chest wall. The cardiac apex is also located by palpation and echocardiography. In this manner the direction of the long axis of the left ventricle is approximated (Fig. 9-4). With the scanner in normal mode of operation, its plane is adjusted to include the long axis, aortic root, mitral valve, and apex. The scanner is then switched from normal to stop-action mode of operation, the delay control having been previously adjusted to image the desired portion of the cardiac cycle. The image is integrated one "line" per cardiac cycle over a period of several minutes. By trial and error slight adjustments of the scanning plane and instrument sensitivity permit creation of an optimal cross-sectional image.

In some situations cross-sections other than the left ventricular long axis cross-section may be desirable. A minor axis cross-section of the left ventricle may be made perpendicular to and through the midpoint of the left ventricular long axis. This is a somewhat less useful cross-section since the medial and lateral margins of the left ventricle (the septum and free wall) are roughly parallel to the sound beam and are therefore difficult to image. Cross-sections through the long axis of the right ventricular outflow tract may also be made. Its direction is somewhat more difficult to define. This may be done by rapidly scanning in the normal mode of operation. Another useful cross-section has been one directed transversely through the origins of the aorta and pulmonary trunk roughly perpendicular to the patient's sagittal and coronal planes. This cross-section, in the second or third intercostal space, demonstrates the orientation of the great arteries. In congenital heart disease special cross-sections must be devised to demonstrate specific structural abnormalities.

Certain technical limitations apply to cardiac ultrasonography as they do to echocardiography. The ultrasound beam may be transmitted into the heart only through the "ultrasonic window." This is the area of the precordium through which the ultrasound beam may pass unimpeded by interposed lung or bone. In infants and children cardiac imaging is considerably easier than in adults because of incomplete ossification of the sternum. The air containing lung and calcified bone will not adequately transmit the sound waves. The area of the ultrasonic window varies with the position of the heart, increasing with cardiac enlargement and decreasing with emphysema. As a result there is a limitation to the variety of positions from which the heart may be imaged. A further limitation is imposed by the orientation of intracardiac anatomy and the necessity for the sound beam to impinge on a structure at normal or near-normal incidence to produce a recordable echo. Because of this some structures may be imaged in certain planes but not in others. Not all structures may be imaged in any one plane.

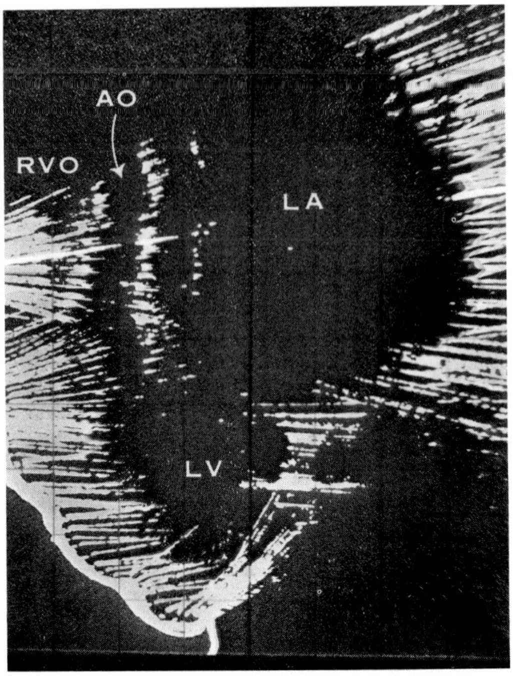

Fig. 9-8. Long axis cross-section of a patient with chronic, marked mitral regurgitation. The left atrium is shown to be markedly enlarged in relationship to the left ventricle. Cross-section was obtained at end-systole.

APPLICATION

By means of cardiac ultrasonography, it is possible to evaluate the relative size and shape of the heart chambers (Fig. 9-8). Although the right ventricle and right and left atria cannot always be visualized in their entirety, sufficiently large portions can usually be seen to estimate their size both absolutely and in relationship to the size of the left ventricle. Cross-sections made through the long axis of the left ventricle at end-systole and at end-diastole may be utilized to calculate left ventricular volumes (Fig. 9-9). By use of the area-length method,[10] volumes calculated in this manner are comparable to those calculated from single plane right anterior oblique angiocardiograms. Such cross-sections have the advantages of being noninvasive, of not altering the patient's physiologic status, and of being repeatable without risk. Visualization of the left ventricle may also in some instances reveal areas of dyskinesia or akinesia along the posteroinferior free wall. It is also possible to image some ventricular aneurysms in this way. A cross-section of the left ventricle in a patient with idiopathic hypertrophic subaortic stenosis (Fig. 9-10) shows the diminished left ventricular chamber size and marked hypertrophy of the interventricular septum.

Ultrasonography of normal and abnormal valves, particularly the aortic and mitral valves in various phases of their motion, may be useful in demonstrating morphologic abnormalities of these structures. Fig. 9-11 is a demonstration of "doming" of the mitral valve caused by mitral stenosis. In other instances it may be possible to show failure of apposition or prolapse of the leaflets. It may also be possible to directly measure the cross-sectional area of the mitral orifice in certain instances. Atrial myxomas prolapsing into the mitral orifice may also be seen.

Evaluation of patients for congenital heart disease is a particularly useful application of cardiac imaging.[11] In patients with transposition of the great arteries

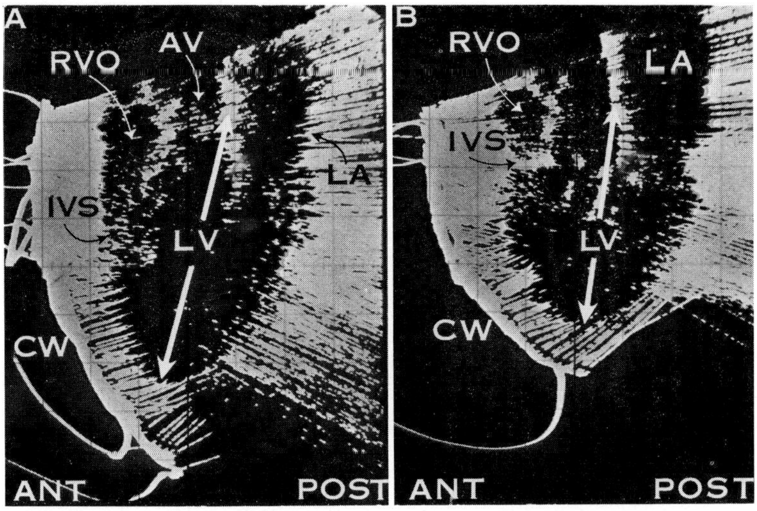

Fig. 9-9. Long axis cross-sections of the left ventricle in **A,** diastole and **B,** systole. The cross-sectional area of the left ventricle may be measured by planimeter and the major axis measured directly. Volume is then calculated using the area-length formula. Note the volume change of the left atrium of this patient with mitral regurgitation. (From King, D. L., and others: Radiology **104:**201-202, 1972.)

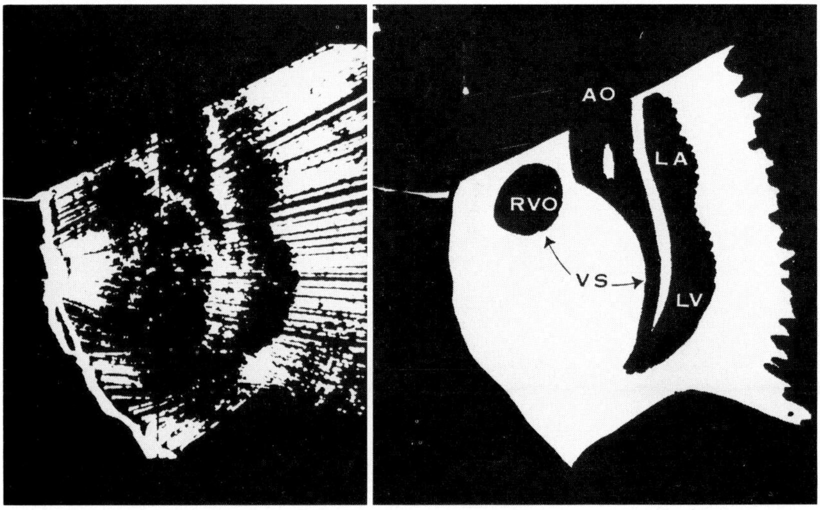

Fig. 9-10. Idiopathic hypertrophic subaortic stenosis. Asymmetrical septal hypertrophy is seen encroaching upon the left ventricular outflow tract, markedly reducing the size of the left ventricle.

there is a failure to develop normal spiraling of the aorta and pulmonary artery. Instead of crossing, the axes of the ventricular outflow tracts and great arteries are more or less parallel. In addition, the aorta is variably rotated anteriorly and the pulmonary trunk rotated posteriorly. When parallel alignment of their axes (Fig. 9-12) is demonstrated on longitudinal cross-section or an abnormal right-left

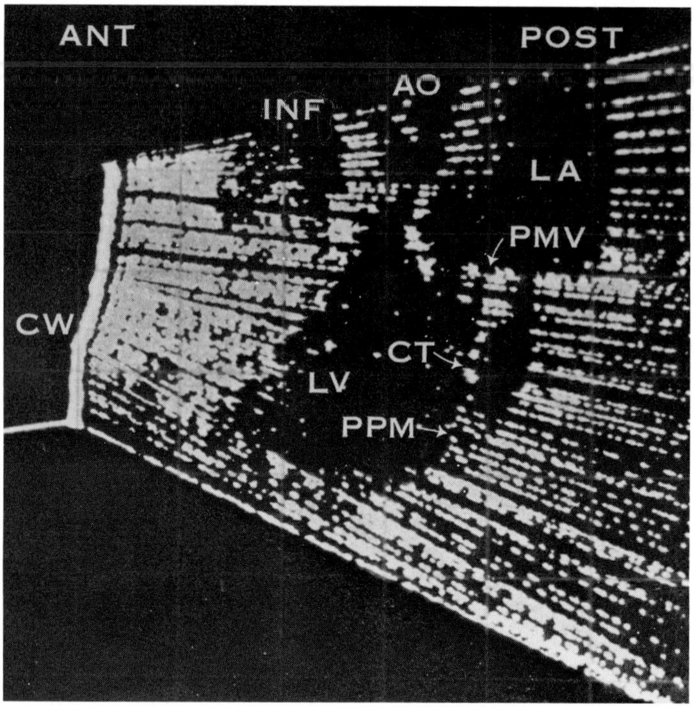

Fig. 9-11. Mitral stenosis. This cross-section, made in early diastole, passes through the aortic root and mitral valve. The fused, dome-shaped mitral leaflets are seen curving toward each other. (Compare with Fig. 9-6.) Thickened, fused chordae tendineae extend from the posterior mitral valve leaflet to the posterior papillary muscle. (From King, D. L.: Radiology **103:**387-392, 1972.)

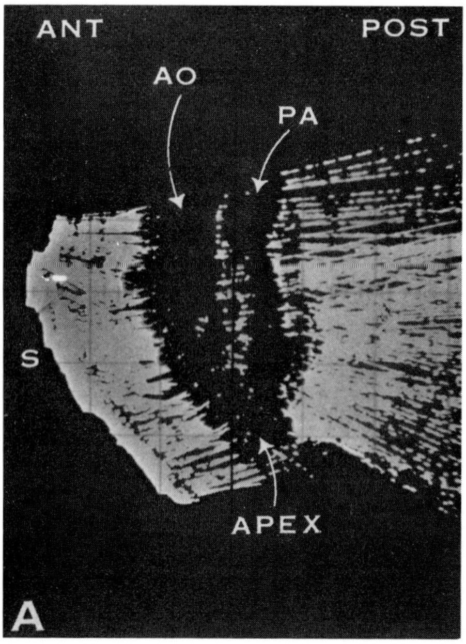

Fig. 9-12. Transposition of the great arteries produces a parallel alignment of the axes of the ventricular outflow tracts and great arteries rather than the normal crossed, spiral relationship. This feature is visualized when the plane of cross-section passes through both axes. Other congenital anomalies such as truncus arteriosus may also be visualized by cardiac sonography. (From King, D. L., Steeg, C. N., and Ellis, K.: Radiology **107:**181-187, 1973.)

relationship of the arteries (Fig. 9-13) is demonstrated on transverse cross-section, a diagnosis of transposition of the great arteries may be suspected.[12] In some cases of transposition, an associated stenosis of the pulmonary orifice may also be suspected on the basis of the ultrasonogram. It is also possible to demonstrate truncus arteriosus as well as instances of hypoplastic left heart.

In tetralogy of Fallot long axis cross-sections can demonstrate the abnormally large aortic root, the ventricular septal defect, and overriding of the aorta. They may also reveal a narrowing of the infundibulum or right ventricular outflow tract (Fig. 9-14). Overriding of the ventricular septum may also be shown in certain other instances, such as double-outlet right ventricle with transposition of the great arteries (Fig. 9-15). Visualization of overriding of the aorta and of discontinuity between the anterior aortic root wall and ventricular septum, as in these two examples, represents one type of sonographic appearance of ventricular septal defect.[13] High membranous defects, the most common type, are located immediately below the level of the aortic valve (Fig. 9-16). Muscular septal defects more caudad in the septum appear significantly below the level of the aortic valve toward the cardiac apex (Fig. 9-17). In both the membranous and muscular types the alignment between the upper septum and the anterior aortic root wall appears normal.

DYNAMIC IMAGING (SONOCARDIOGRAPHY)

Dynamic imaging of the heart adds the dimension of time to cardiac ultrasonog-

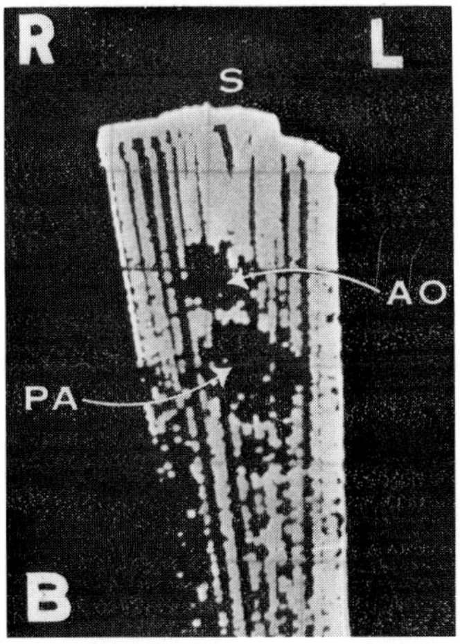

Fig. 9-13. Transverse cross-section through the origins of the great arteries in a patient with D-transposition. The anterior artery is to the right at this level rather than to the left indicating a diagnosis of transposition of the great arteries. (From King, D. L., Steeg, C. N., and Ellis, K.: Radiology **107:**181-187, 1973.)

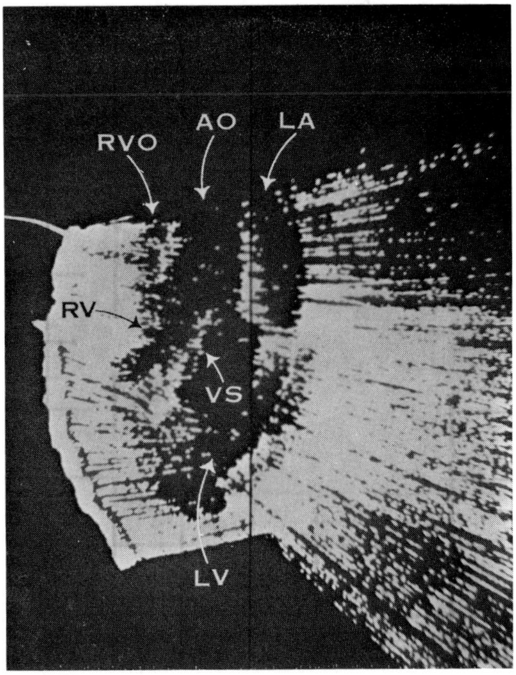

Fig. 9-14. Tetralogy of Fallot. A long axis cross-section is able to demonstrate the features of this congenital anomaly, namely, the enlarged, overriding aorta, a ventricular septal defect, and infundibular stenosis. (From King, D. L., Steeg, C. N., and Ellis, K.: Visualization of ventricular septal defects by cardiac ultrasonagraphy, Circulation **48:**1215-1220, 1973. By permission of The American Heart Association, Inc.)

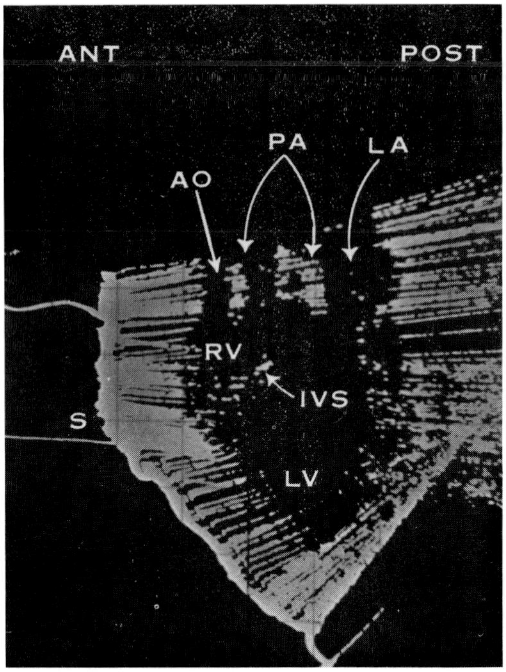

Fig. 9-15. Transposition of the great arteries and double outlet right ventricle. The large posterior pulmonary artery is overriding the ventricular septum. The relationship of the atrioventricular valves to the great arteries is not always apparent from a single cross-section. Note the similarity of appearance to Fig. 9-14.

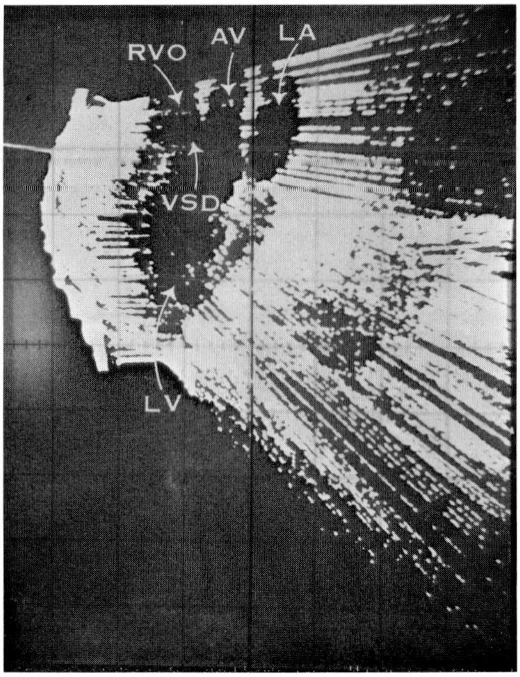

Fig. 9-16. Membranous ventricular septal defect. The aortic valve serves as a landmark for distinguishing high membranous defects and lower muscular defects. (From King, D. L., Steeg, C. N., and Ellis, K.: Visualization of ventricular septal defects by cardiac ultrasonography, Circulation **48:**1215-1220, 1973. By permission of the American Heart Association, Inc.)

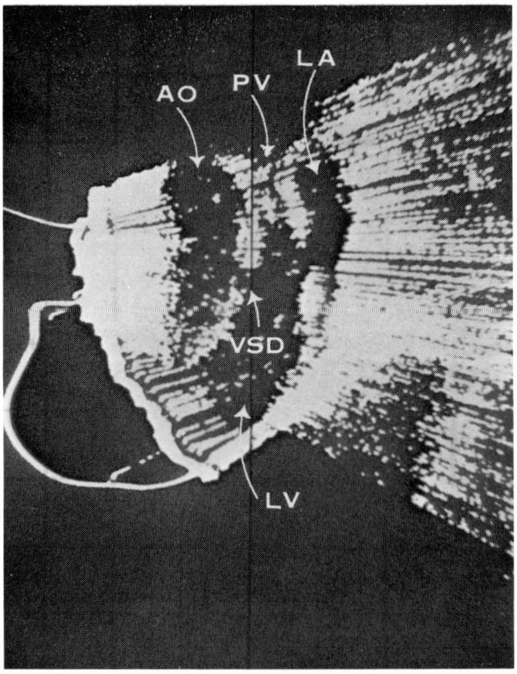

Fig. 9-17. Muscular ventricular septal defect in a patient with transposition of the great arteries. The defect is midway between the aortic valve and the cardiac apex. (From King, D. L., Steeg, C. N., and Ellis, K.: Visualization of ventricular septal defects by cardiac ultrasonography, Circulation **48:**1215-1220, 1973. By permission of The American Heart Association, Inc.)

raphy by recreating cross-sectional images at the rate of sixty per second. As a result not only the anatomic orientation of an echo-producing structure but also its motion are visualized throughout the cardiac cycle. It is suggested that this technique be referred to as sonocardiography. The prefix "sono-" would then distinguish the two-dimensional motion imaging technique from the one-dimensional motion recording technique, echocardiography.

Manual or mechanical scanning of a single-transducer sound beam across the heart cannot be carried out fast enough to view more than a small portion of the heart before significant cardiac motion has occurred. Such motion produces an image blurring or break-up of the image. To obtain a larger field of view and to avoid blurring or image break-up, a faster scanning rate must be used. This is best accomplished by electronic scanning, that is, by shifting the beam position electronically rather than mechanically. Very rapid scanning is often referred to as real-time scanning because the high-speed process permits instantaneous visualization of any change in the structures under observation. At electronic speeds no significant image break-up or blurring is encountered. High-speed real-time electronic scanning[14-16] requires the use of a multielement transducer array (Fig. 9-18). The narrow active surface of the transducer measures 1 × 8 cm. Within it are twenty-four individual piezoelectric crystals. Starting at the top of the transducer, three crystals at a time are used to produce a single sound beam. In sequence, the sound beam position is moved the width of one crystal toward the bottom of the transducer, a step of one-third the beam width. The entire process of sequential shifting of the sound beam from the top to the bottom of the transducer requires approximately 17 msec.

While the sound beam is being scanned across the transducer probe, an image is simultaneously being created on the display television screen. As each scan occurs, the horizontal sweep of the television is made to shift from the top of the screen downward, tracing horizontal lines in the same relative position as each sound beam arising from the transducer. On each "line" the echo signals from the respective sound beams are displayed as intensity-modulated bright dots. Alternate scans are processed together to produce a new image or frame sixty times per second. This

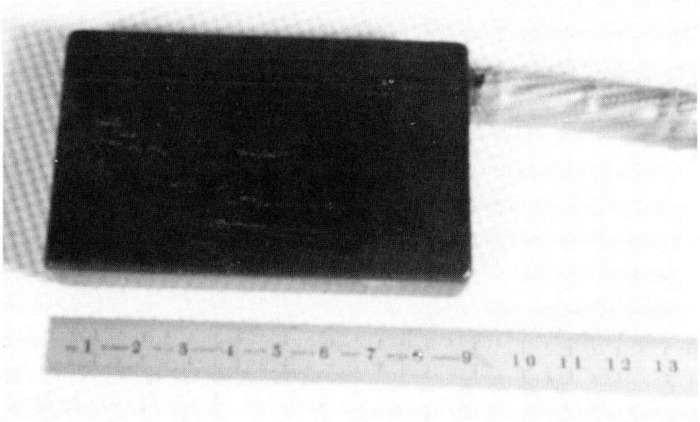

Fig. 9-18. The twenty four–element transducer for dynamic imaging (sonocardiography). The "top" of the transducer, corresponding to the top of the image as it is displayed, is at the left, opposite the cable attachment. (From King, D. L.: J. Clin. Ultrasound **1:**196-200, 1973.)

frame repetition rate is sufficient for instantaneously visualizing the motion of cardiac structures. The frequency of each sound beam is 2 MHz. The lateral and axial resolution, as well as the ultrasound intensity, of each beam is comparable to that produced by a conventional unfocused 1 cm diameter transducer. Smaller, higher frequency transducers for pediatric and neonatal patients are also available.

The transducer is placed directly on the precordium (Fig. 9-19) and its position adjusted by the examiner until the desired cross-section is obtained. The most useful imaging planes are the same as shown for the stop-action technique (Fig. 9-4). Recording of the image may be done by videotape recorder, cinematography, or by an electrocardiogram-triggered Polaroid camera. Fig. 9-20 shows a normal long-axis cross-section of the left ventricle obtained by the multielement transducer. The "top" of the transducer is directed cephalad over the aortic root, while the "bottom" is over the cardiac apex. The cross-section is viewed from the left, anterior and posterior being respectively to the left and right of the image. When the dynamic image is viewed directly or on cine film, the motion of the ventricular walls, septum, and aortic and mitral valves may be observed (Fig. 9-21). This technique permits more accurate study of the complex motion of cardiac structures, such as the ventricular septum, than does one-dimensional echocardiography.

In addition to being especially valuable in the study of cardiac dynamics, sonocardiography is equally useful in the evaluation of the relative size and shape of the heart chambers. Fig. 9-22 shows an example of marked right ventricular enlargement in a child with an atrial septal defect. The enlarged right ventricle has displaced the left ventricular apex away from the chest wall. The ventricular septum lies

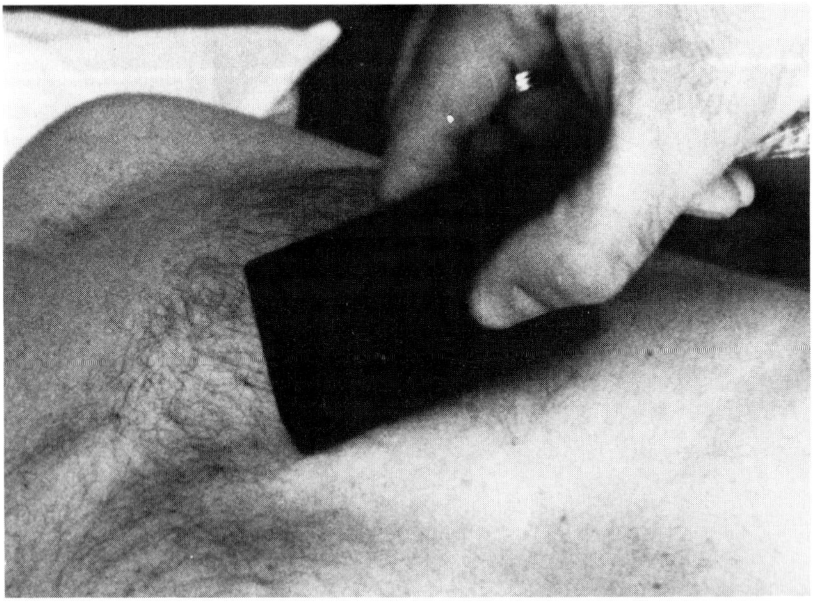

Fig. 9-19. The transducer is positioned on the precordium with the top toward the aortic root and the bottom toward the cardiac apex. The position is adjusted by the examiner while observing the display to obtain the desired cross-sectional image. (From King, D. L.: J. Clin. Ultrasound **1:**196-200, 1973.)

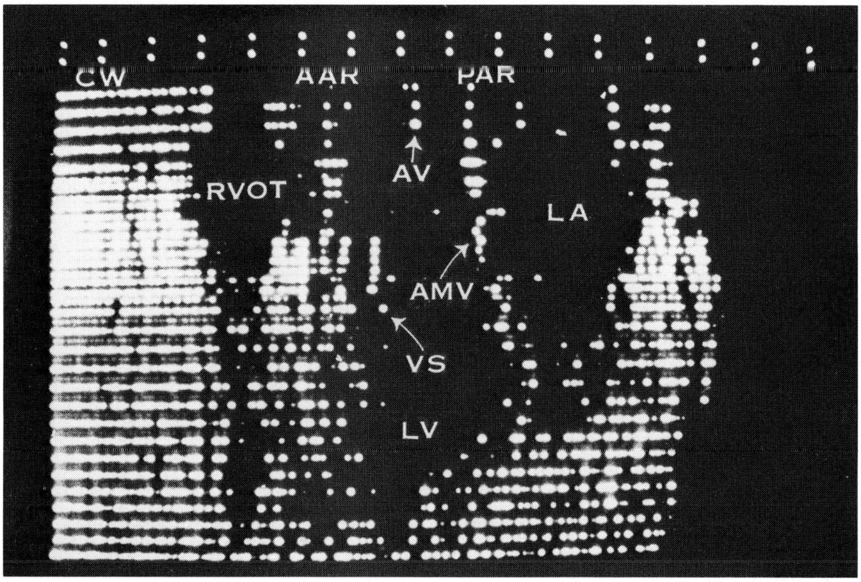

Fig. 9-20. A normal adult long axis cross-section of the left ventricle obtained with the multielement scanner. At a frame repetition rate of sixty per second the motion of structures is readily apparent and aids in their recognition and identification.

A

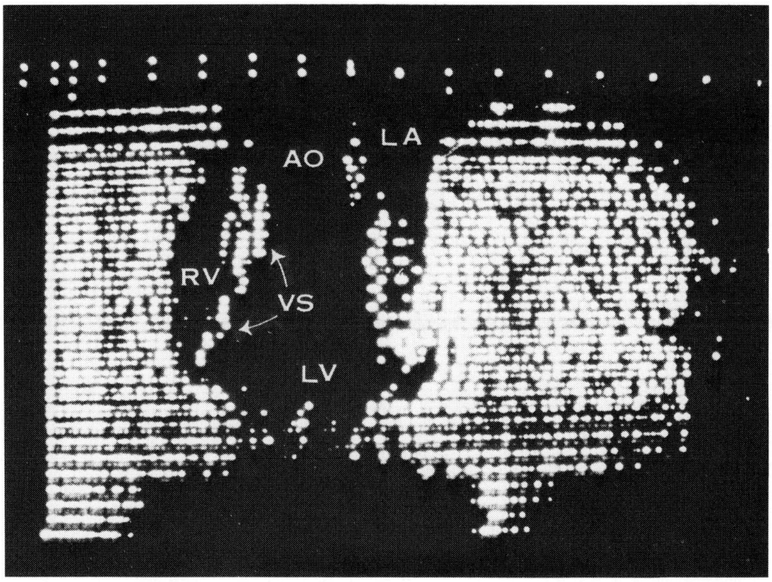

Continued.

Fig. 9-21. Long axis cross-sections of a child with a small ventricular septal defect illustrating the motion of the ventricular septum at different phases of the cardiac cycle. **A,** Diastole; **B,** systole. In cross-section the septum appears to be coiling into an S-shape with systole and uncoiling with diastole.

B

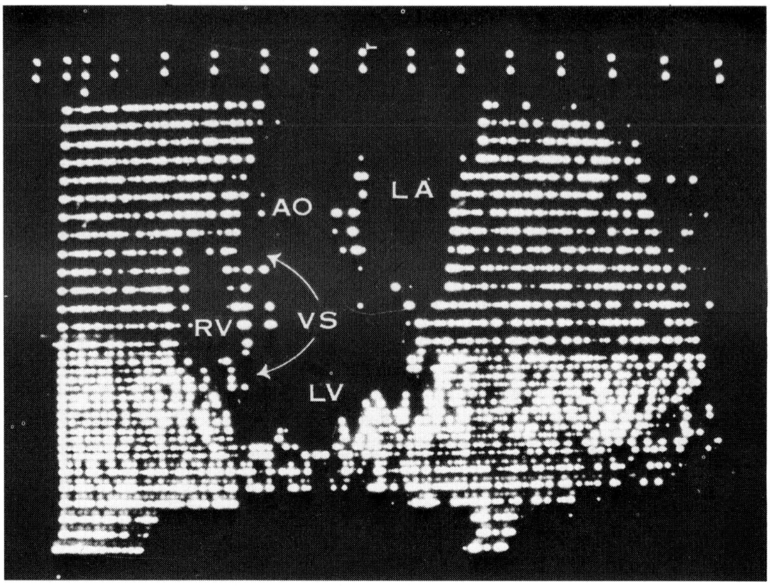

Fig. 9-21, cont'd. For legend see p. 175.

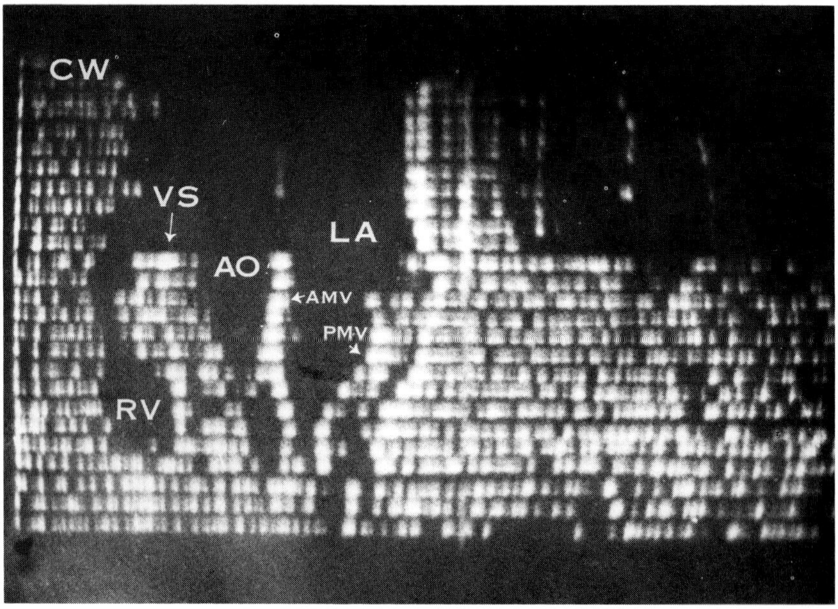

Fig. 9-22. Atrial septal defect. The anterior right ventricle is much larger than normal because of the large left to right shunt in this child. The anterior and posterior mitral leaflets and chordae tendineae were easily visualized.

parallel to the chest wall. Perception of these changes depends partly upon knowing the position and angulation of the transducer on the precordium during the examination. Morphologic abnormalities of the valves, such as thickening and calcification, may also be visualized. Fig. 9-23 compares the appearance of a normal

A

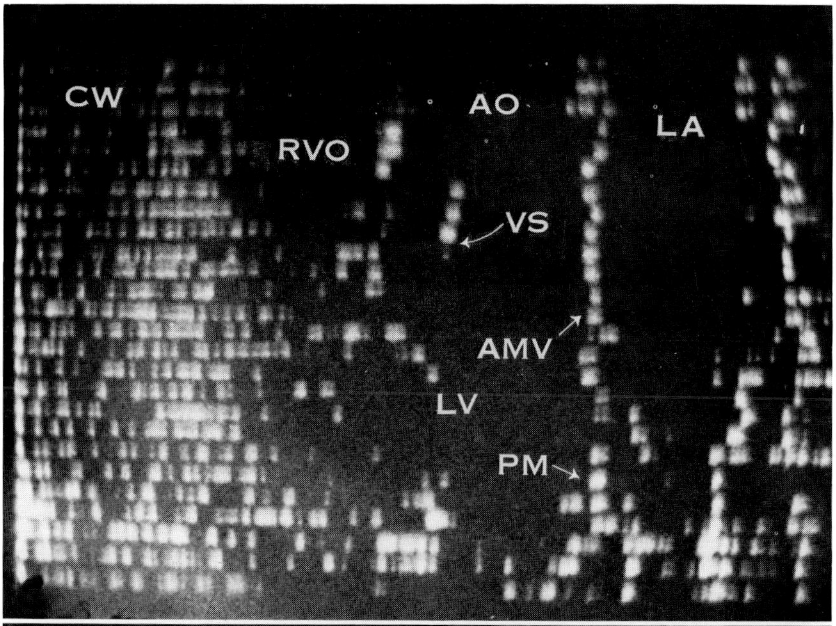

B

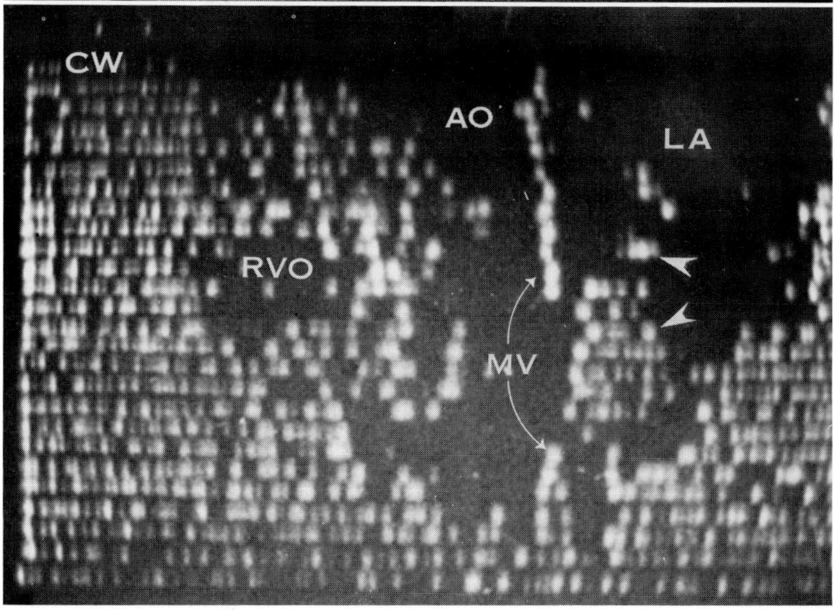

Fig. 9-23. A, Normal anterior mitral valve leaflet. It appears as a thin line of echoes. **B,** Rigid, thickened stenotic mitral valve. The morphologic appearance is readily apparent. The arrows point to a large area of thickening and calcification that moved with the leaflet. (From King, D. L.: J. Clin. Ultrasound **1:**196-200, 1973.)

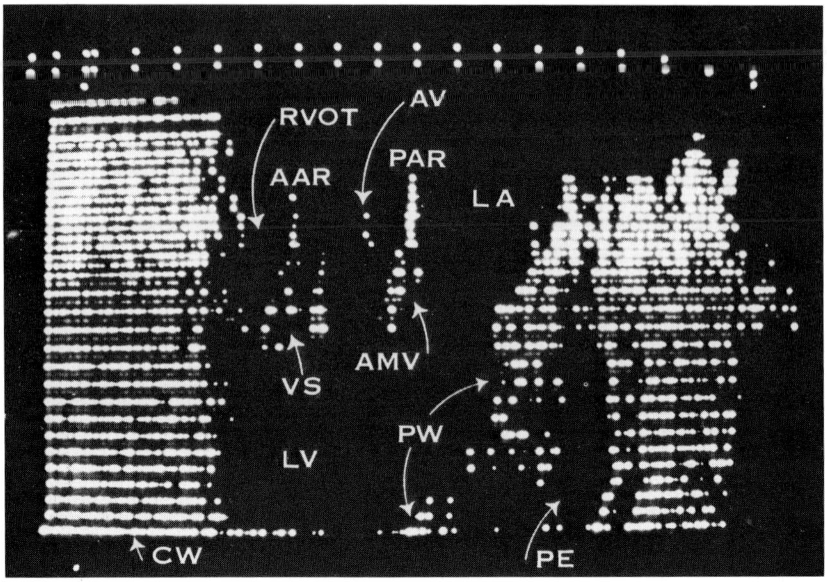

Fig. 9-24. Pericardial effusion. The echo-free space posteriorly between the posterior left ventricular free wall and the left lung represents a large posterior pericardial effusion. The heart was adherent to the chest wall anteriorly in this patient several weeks following open-heart surgery.

anterior mitral valve leaflet in middiastole *(A)* to that of a patient with moderately severe mitral stenosis *(B)*. The *(B)* shows thickening of the valve echo pattern. Many more echoes appear along its posterior aspect than in the normal person. These echoes maintain a constant relationship with the valve leaflet throughout the cardiac cycle. The motion of a stenotic mitral valve is characterized by a diminished amplitude of anteroposterior excursion, a characteristic rapidity of the opening and closing movements, and a sustained anterior deflection of the anterior leaflet in diastole.

Pericardial effusion may be recognized as an abnormal echo-free separation of the posterolateral left ventricular wall from the left lung (Fig. 9-24). The space representing the effusion usually accumulates posteriorly first. With moderate and large effusions an echo-free space will also be seen separating the nonmoving chest wall echoes from the moving anterior heart wall echoes.[17] Whether or not imaging will reveal the presence of the small and minimal effusions detected by echocardiography remains to be determined.

SALINE-CONTRAST SONOCARDIOGRAPHY

Saline-contrast sonocardiography is another promising application for dynamic ultrasonic imaging of the heart. The intracardiac blood-tissue interface acoustically delineates the cardiac chambers and intracardiac structures. The blood itself, however remains echo-free to the imaging sound beam. Its direction and pattern of flow are not apparent without the addition of an acoustic contrast agent to alter the normal acoustic homogeneity of the blood. Saline rapidly injected into the cardiac chambers via a catheter accomplishes this and may serve as a contrast agent.[18]

It appears that the process of injection creates a myriad of microbubbles from dissolved gases in the saline. These microbubbles create an acoustic interface, a gas-blood interface, that is highly reflective of

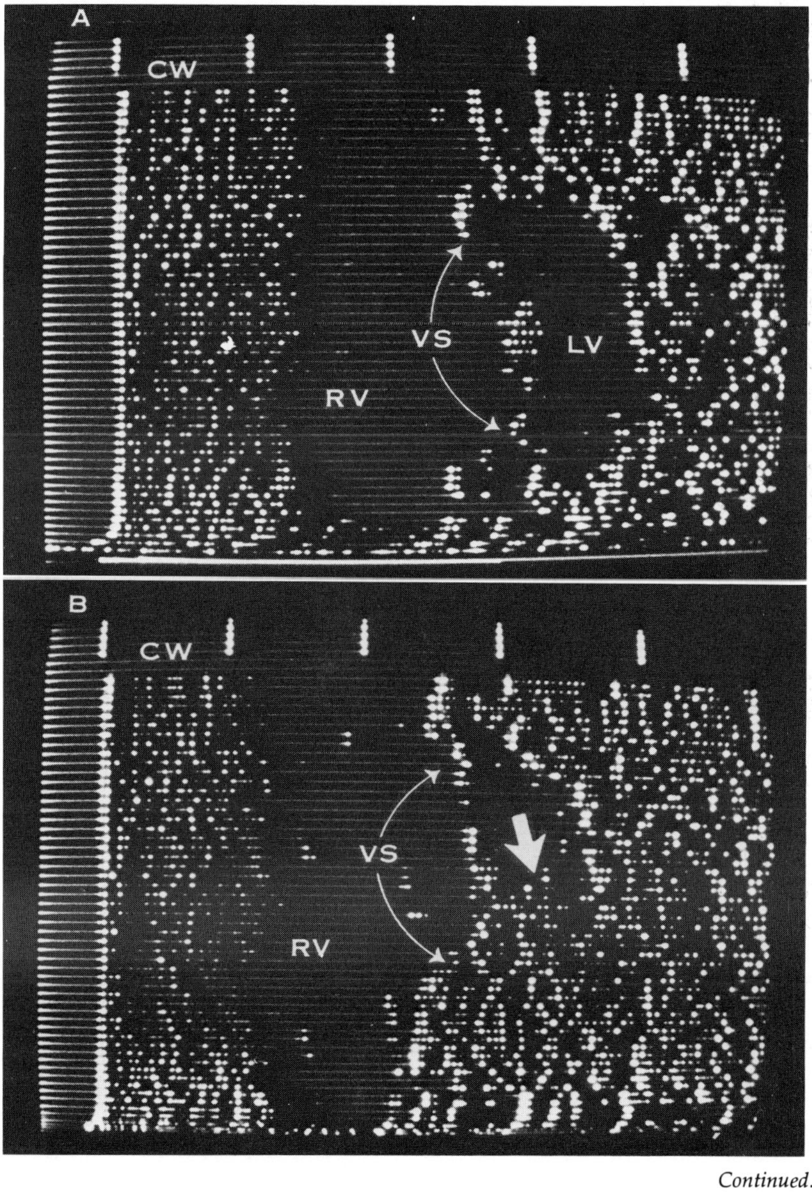

Continued.

Fig. 9-25. Saline-contrast sonocardiogram demonstrating a ventricular septal defect. **A** is a cross-section of the heart prior to injection of saline in the left ventricle via a small catheter. Hand injection of saline produced many highly reflective microbubbles of gas in the blood for a short period of time. **B** shows beginning obliteration of the outline of the apex of the left ventricular chamber by the bubbles (large arrow). **C,** a few milliseconds later than **B,** shows complete obliteration of the outlines of the left ventricle by the cloud of microbubbles with beginning appearance of the cloud in the right ventricular outflow tract (large arrows) via the ventricular septal defect.

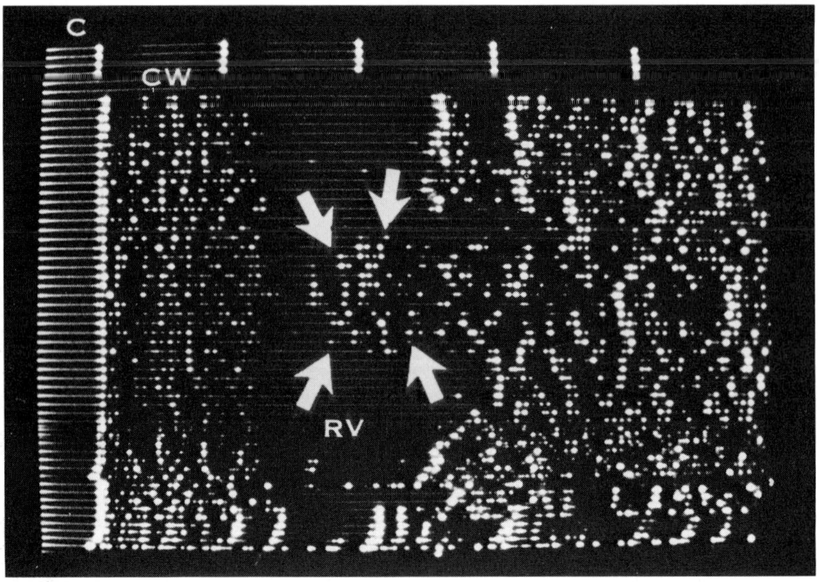

Fig. 9-25, cont'd. For legend see p. 179.

ultrasound. These microbubbles persist for a very short time and are carried along in the bloodstream. The cloud of bubbles in the blood produces a corresponding cloud of echoes filling the injected chamber on the sonocardiogram. Observation of the flow of this transient cloud of echoes may reveal the presence of shunts and valvular regurgitation.

Fig. 9-25 is from a saline-contrast sonocardiogram performed on a 3-month-old infant at the time of cardiac catheterization. The illustrations demonstrate opacification of the left ventricle by the bubble cloud and shunting of the bubbles from left to right through a ventricular septal defect.

Because of its innocuous nature, saline-contrast sonocardiography should prove to be a valuable supplement, if not on some occasions a more desirable alternative, to positive-contrast x-ray angiocardiography. Not infrequently the number of positive-contrast injections used at cardiac catheterization must be less than the number desired. In these instances saline-contrast sonocardiography may help to select the most appropriate and rewarding angiocardiogram injection and to exclude or demonstrate other abnormalities, such as valvular regurgitation, for which an additional angiocardiogram would be unwarranted. Because of these advantages saline contrast sonocardiography may find a role in the evaluation of patients of cardiac catheterization.

DISCUSSION

It is readily apparent that there are no echo data recorded in ultrasonic images of the heart that cannot be recorded by echocardiography. Therefore, what are the justifications and advantages of ultrasonic imaging in comparison to echocardiography? Why is cardiac ultrasonography or sonocardiography needed? What will be its role in comparison to the role of echocardiography? The basic unit of information, the echo signal, is the same for both techniques. The echo signal indicates the presence and depth of an echo source in the path of the sound beam.

The fundamental difference between the techniques is the manner in which that information is manipulated and displayed. In echocardiography the depth of the echo signal, on the vertical axis of a strip chart, is displayed as a function of time, the horizontal axis, yielding a graphic representation of the change in range of any particular echo source with the passage of time. Thus the anteroposterior movement of a heart valve in the sound beam may be observed to describe a characteristic pattern.

In a stop-action image the effects of motion are eliminated and the echo signal is displayed in correct anatomic orientation with respect to many other echo signals from within the heart. As a consequence, the stop-action pictorial image directly resembles the anatomic appearance of the heart while the echocardiogram does not.

Carrying development a step further, the sonocardiogram not only records the anatomic orientation of the echo signals in a pictorial image but also preserves and displays the motion of each echo signal in its correct anatomic orientation. The echocardiogram then yields dynamic information as a function of time while the imaging techniques yield morphologic or anatomic information. For these reasons the echocardiogram is more able to demonstrate functional or physiologic abnormalities while imaging is more able to visualize gross pathologic or structural abnormalities such as congenital cardiac defects. In this sense then the techniques are complementary and mutually supportive in the areas where morphology and function overlap.

In the evaluation of left ventricular function by measurement of the minor axis (to calculate ventricular volume, velocity of circumferential fiber shortening, and percentage wall thickening), sonocardiography should improve the selection of the minor axis. On the sonocardiogram it is possible to select any one of the twenty-four individual sound beams comprising the image for simultaneous display in conventional echocardiographic mode. This will permit selection of the optimum minor axis based on the cross-sectional appearance of the ventricle. Since the one-dimensional volume calculation assumes the perpendicular minor axes to be equal and half of the major axis, the use of imaging should assist recognition of significant deviation of the ventricular shape from the assumed shape. Use of the area-length method should then improve the accuracy of volume estimation. Similarly, ultrasonic imaging should be of great value in recognition of the presence, size, and location of abnormally contracting segments of myocardium in patients with coronary artery disease. It should thus also aid in assessment of the effects of nonuniform ventricular contraction on ventricular function. Clearly, ultrasonic imaging can not only permit rapid visualization of morphologic cardiac abnormalities but can also improve the effectiveness and accuracy of echocardiography for evaluation of physiologic abnormalities.

What will be the relative role of the various cardiac imaging techniques, and what improvements may occur in the future? The single transducer techniques include the conventional, manual B scan, the stop-action technique, including scan converter storage or computer reassembly variations to achieve quasidynamic images, and the motor-driven sector scan for producing real-time images. A conventional long-axis B scan of the left ventricle (Fig. 9-26), when scanned at uniform speed, demonstrates the motion of cardiac structures, particularly the posterior wall, in correct anatomic orientation.[19] This technique requires no specialized equipment other than a scanner and permits a comparatively easy and rapid assessment of the posterior wall for the presence of abnormally contracting segments. It records the same structures as the manual echocardiographic scan but in an accurate anatomic representation. As a consequence it yields a more precise assessment of the relative size and location of an abnormally contracting segment than does echocardiography.

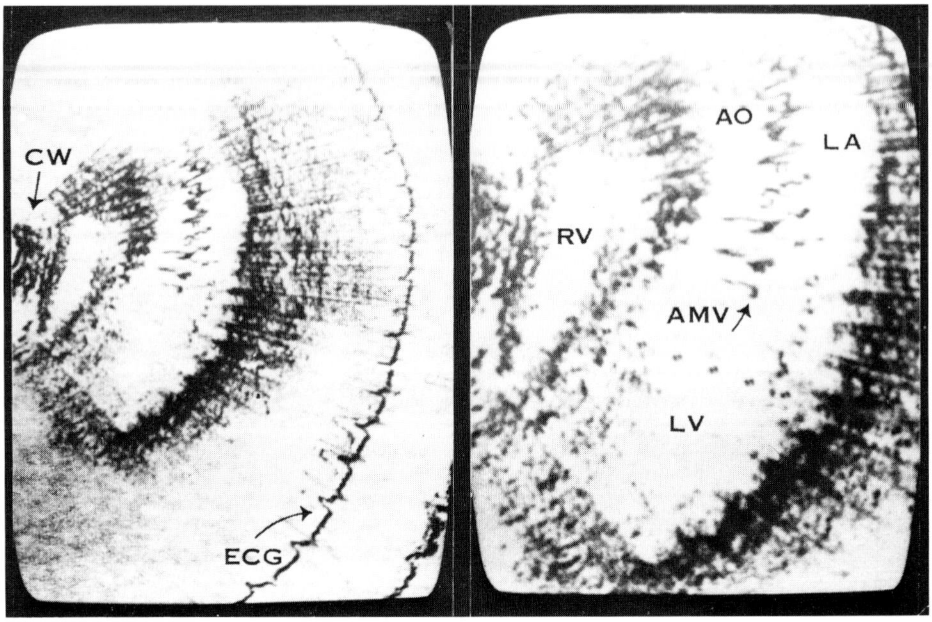

Fig. 9-26. Conventional contact B scan of the left ventricle. The plane of cross-section is anteroposteriorly through the long axis. On the left the electrocardiogram *(ECG)* is simultaneously displayed with the image. On the right is an enlarged view of the cardiac image. The motion of the basilar and apical portions of the posterior left ventricular wall are clearly shown. This technique may be useful in the demonstration of abnormally contracting segments of myocardium caused by coronary artery disease.

A more sophisticated version of single transducer imaging uses the scan converter storage variation of the stop-action techniques. In this technique the long axis scan is made very slowly over a long sequence of cardiac cycles, and a series of images equally spaced throughout the R-R interval is gradually integrated on the storage scan converter[19] in a manner similar to that previously described.[8] These images may then be played out singly or in rapid sequence and recorded on videotape. In rapid sequence the images simulate the heart beating in real-time. It is a pseudo–real-time display, however, because each image is a composite of portions of many sequential heart cycles rather than a series of images of a single heart cycle. A similar pseudo–real-time version of the stop-action technique may be carried out using a computer to perform the positional and temporal reconstruction of the echo data.[20] Motor-driven transducers for producing real-time sector scans have been utilized in both water-path[5-7] and contact[21] scanning systems. The latter system in particular may be practical for clinical use.

The multielement transducer techniques at the present time consist only of rectilinear scanning systems, that is, systems in which the path of the sound beam is perpendicular to the surface of the transducer. These have a comparatively wide field of view but do not have the compound beam motion obtainable with a contact B scanner. The latter permits angling the sound beam so that it may receive echoes from surfaces not parallel to the chest wall. In the future it will be possible to produce angular beam sweeping with multielement transducers electronically by using phased-array scanning techniques. These should greatly improve the image quality obtained by multielement systems.

If multielement imaging systems are available, they most probably will be preferable to single-element systems because of the ease and speed with which they can be used and the comparative lack of skill they require. The real-time scanning systems, whatever their limitations, allow a data acquisition and sampling rate several orders of magnitude greater than the single-transducer conventional or stop-action imaging systems. At these high rates the real-time scanning systems are at a significant advantage and are virtually essential for visualizing complex structural cardiac abnormalities. For evaluation of adult patients for ventricular volume, abnormally contracting segments, and nonuniformity of ventricular contraction, the scan converter storage variation of the stop-action technique may be more desirable, at least until phased-array beam-angling techniques for the multielement systems become available. The scan converter variation of the stop-action technique will also have a cost and availability advantage, being a part of a general purpose ultrasound instrument capable as well of echocardiography and conventional abdominal imaging. Other innovations that may become practical in the future include the use of two-dimensional or area arrays rather than linear arrays and computer processing of image data. It appears doubtful at the present time that transmission holography will become useful for cardiac imaging. The development of a successful reflection holography system might eventually prove superior to pulse echo systems.

REFERENCES

1. Holmes, J. H., Howry, D. H., and Posakony, G. J.: The ultrasonic visualization of soft tissue structures in the body, Trans. Am. Clin. Climatol. Assoc. **66**:208-225, 1954.
2. Hertz, C. H.: Ultrasonic heart investigation, Med. Elec. Bio. Eng. **2**:39-45, 1964.
3. Olofsson, S.: An ultrasonic mirror system, Acustica **13**:361-367, 1963.
4. Asberg, A.: Ultrasonic cinematography of the living heart, Ultrasonics **5**:113-117, 1967.
5. Ebina, T., and others: Ultrasono-tomography for the heart and great vessels in living human subjects by means of the ultrasonic reflection technique, Jap. Heart J. **8**:331-353, 1967.
6. Kikuchi, Y., and Okuyama, D.: Ultrasono-cardiotomography, Jap. Elec. Eng., pp. 53-60, Oct., 1970.
7. Tanaka, M., and others: Ultrasonic evaluation of anatomical abnormalities of heart in congenital and acquired heart disease, Br. Heart J. **33**:686-698, 1971.
8. King, D. L.: Cardiac ultrasonography: a stop-action technique for imaging intra-cardiac anatomy, Radiology **103**:387-392, 1972.
9. Eycleshymer, A. C., and Schoemaker, D. M.: A cross-section anatomy, New York, 1972, Appleton-Century-Crofts.
10. King, D. L., and others: Left ventricular volume determination by cross-sectional cardiac ultrasonography, Radiology **104**:201-202, 1972.
11. King, D. L.: Cardiac ultrasonography: cross-sectional ultrasonic imaging of the heart, Circulation **47**:843-847, 1973.
12. King, D. L., Steeg, C. N., and Ellis, K.: Demonstration of transposition of the great arteries by cardiac ultrasonography, Radiology **107**:181-186, 1973.
13. King, D. L., Steeg, C. N., and Ellis, K.: Visualization of ventricular septal defects by cardiac ultrasonography, Circulation **48**:1215-1220, 1973.
14. King, D. L.: Real-time cross-sectional ultrasonic imaging of the heart using a linear array multi-element transducer, J. Clin. Ultrasound **1**:196-200, 1973.
15. Bom, N., and others: Ultrasonic viewer for cross-sectional analyses of moving cardiac structures, Biomed. Eng. **6**:500-508, 1971.
16. Roelandt, J., and others: Multiscan echocardiography: description of the system and initial results in 100 patients, Heart Bull. **4**:51-56, 1973.
17. Ellis, K., and King, D. L.: Pericarditis and pericardial effusion: radiologic and echocardiographic diagnosis, Radiol. Clin. N. Am. **11**:393-413, 1973.
18. Gramiak, R., Shah, P. M., and Kramer, D. H.: Ultrasound cardiography: contrast studies in anatomy and function, Radiolgy **92**:939, 1969.
19. King, D. L.: Unpublished data.
20. McSherry, D. H.: Digital processing systems for diagnostic ultrasound data. In Second World Congress on Ultrasonics in Medicine, Rotterdam, Netherlands, June 4-8, 1973, International Congress Series, Amsterdam, 1973, Excerpta Medica Foundation.
21. Griffith, J. M., Henry, W. L., and Epstein, S. E.: Real-time two-dimensional echocardiography, Circulation **48**(Suppl. IV):124, 1973.

10 Obstetric ultrasonography

IAN DONALD, M.D.

I propose to approach this subject from the clinician's point of view, as I myself did 18 years ago. By describing the various events that, as the years rolled by, profoundly influenced the way our observations developed, I hope to be able to lead clinical colleagues gradually, and I hope painlessly, into an understanding of what is being done, how it is being done, and why the present methods are used. Fortunately, the technical and engineering aspects have been dealt with by other contributors.

HISTORICAL DEVELOPMENT

There are many reasons for preferring the term "sonar" when describing diagnostic echo sounding. The word stands for sound, navigation, and ranging and is akin to "radar." This at least acknowledges its historic origins in the work originally initiated by Langevin in Paris[1] on behalf of the French and British Admiralties, who formed in 1916 an Anti-Submarine Detection and Investigation Committee (ASDIC) in order to combat the growing German U-boat menace. It may be a very far cry from the science of U-boat detection to studying the fetus in utero, but in certain respects a submarine in the ocean only differs in degree from a fetus in a somewhat limited sea of liquor amnii. The term "sonar" also has the merit of brevity and euphony.

Firestone's work[2,3] in the United States during World War II, which was classified as "secret" at the time, brought miniaturization into the field of engineering in the study of metal structures. Tagging along years later, medicine entered the field of ultrasonics.

In 1954 the late Professor Ian Aird, Hammersmith Hospital, London, where I was then working, introduced me to Wild, who informed me of his hopes of being able to identify malignant ulcers of the stomach with ultrasound. Aird was not sure about whether or not to sponsor a lecture by Wild in the University of London and sought my advice. I was not able to attend the lecture myself, nor do I know of any record of it. At this time I moved to Glasgow and through the literature became, in a distant sort of way, interested in the pioneer work of Wild and Reid.[4,5]

However, it might have ended there were it not for the fact that through a professional contact I became acquainted with the research director of a large engineering firm in Scotland where they were in the habit of testing their welds of atomic boilers by ultrasonic metal flaw detectors. Help was offered and ultrasonic equipment supplied on loan. At that time my major interest was in distinguishing massive ovarian cysts from massive ascites, by no means an easy clinical problem by standard methods of percussion.

A really memorable day was July 21, 1955, when we took to the engineering factory in two cars a selection of very large ovarian cysts and myomata to try out their flaw detection gear on these tumors. All I wanted to know was whether there was a detectable difference between a solid tumor and a cyst. An immediate confirmation that there was convinced me that the matter was worth pursuing.

Through the good offices of Dr. Douglas Gordon and Professor Mayneord in London I had been experimenting with a very primitive flaw detector with such a long paralysis time that I could only operate it through water-filled buckets with plastic bottoms applied directly to the abdominal wall. This provided a situation that had all the ingredients of a shambles and usually resulted in a soaked patient and a wet mattress. From that day I developed a hearty dislike of tanks and came to prefer the engineering technique, with which I am now familiar, of direct contact probe application through a film of olive oil. (I later learned of Kossoff's tank technique[6] but have not pursued it.) My engineering friends in Glasgow also began to lend us more refined apparatus. Then came our greatest stroke of luck. I was invited by a physician colleague to see a patient who was dying of "carcinoma of the stomach," proved radiologically, with hematemesis, progressive loss of weight, and truly massive ascites from portal obstruction and metastases. I fully agreed with the clinical diagnosis and on a purely theoretic basis expected to find with our A-scan probe apparatus numerous vigorous echoes close to the origin of the time base sweep on the left of the cathode ray tube face because of loops of intestine floating up into the center of the abdomen, as one would expect clinically. To my consternation, however, there were no such echoes, only a very wide clear space and, almost at the limit of range of the cathode ray tube, a strong backwall echo implying the presence of a clear fluid-filled cyst. This seemed to invalidate the clinical diagnosis. Fortunately, my physician colleagues encouraged me to undertake laparotomy. I removed a gigantic benign mucinous cystadenoma of the ovary. From that day onward vomiting and hematemesis ceased and the patient, who had previously been given up for lost, made a dramatic recovery. The radiologic diagnosis was now declared an artifact. That was about 17 years ago, and the patient is alive to this day. There could be no turning back now.

We soon began to realize the limitations of unidimensional A-scan probing because of the multiplicity of unpredictable and uninterpretable echoes that could be neither processed nor analyzed. At this time Tom Brown, one of the research engineers of an engineering factory who made the test gear, came on the scene and offered help. His was the real genius behind our future contact scanning apparatus, and our association has continued from that day to the present.[7] Already the case for compound B sector scanning had become apparent to us and was subsequently[8-10] fully described. Although we devised our own apparatus on which our present work is based, it should here be pointed out that the great pioneers of compound scanning were the late Douglass Howry,[11] Bliss,[12] and my friend Dr. Joseph Holmes.[13,14]

For the first few years our work was concentrated upon attempting to depict gynecologic tumor masses. In this we had some success, albeit infrequently. Clinical judgment was seldom altered by our ultrasonic findings, which so far had little more than academic interest. However, with Tom Brown's help and support of loyal colleagues like Dr. John MacVicar, Senior Lecturer in my department, I pressed on. Until 1957 we had not even ventured into a study of pregnancy, mainly because my maternity department was then situated in another hospital at the other side of the city and access was difficult, particularly with complicated cases. In 1957 we still considered it remarkable even to demonstrate fetal echoes in utero by the fourteenth week, but we soon noticed that the fetal head produced very strong echoes on A scan, and we began to use it increasingly for the determination of presentation in doubtful and very obese patients. The need for two-dimensional scanning was so obvious that work on the engineering side was pressed ahead ruthlessly.

Our first publication, perhaps the most important in my whole life, was in *The Lancet* in 1958,[8] and it is interesting in retrospect to see that a number of basic diagnostic criteria that we then enunciated have not had to be reversed since then. Such observations included the ultrasonic clarity or, as one should say, "transonicity" of fluid-containing structures and the readiness with which their distal walls could be visualized. Conversely, the attenuation in solid structures seemed to be related very closely to their density and they could be more easily penetrated by a lower frequency of ultrasound, for example, 1.5 MHz instead of 2.5 MHz. We still insist on checking diagnoses by using different frequencies in the assessment of transonicity. Third, we observed that structures that were of a mushy consistency, as distinct from frankly solid or cystic, occupied a sort of intermediate position between echo-free clarity and a tangle of echoes. This differentiation could be demonstrated by altering the gain setting of the apparatus by somewhere in the range of 10 to 15 dB.

It was in this way that we began our search for the diagnosis of hydatidiform mole, and we asked colleagues throughout the region to give us an opportunity to examine such cases. The response was generous and we were at first successful in diagnosing the presence of fetal echoes and excluding hydatidiform mole, which is after all a relatively uncommon condition, but the theory proved ultimately to be correct and has since become the standard method of diagnosis.[9,15] A disturbing observation, however, was that by turning up the gain setting too high, electronic "grass" could simulate the appearance of a hydatidiform mole.[10,16] This artifact could be provoked by overscanning, usually because of a preconceived expectation of finding such echoes.

For this reason therefore, and at considerable cost, an automatic scanner was built that operated at a constant speed and pressure and sector scanned through a prefixed angular sweep.[7] This effectively stopped further "cheating" and enabled us to work out the optimum scanning technique. However, the method was too expensive and too slow to persist with, but it served a very useful function over the next few critical years. Nowadays, with a little practice, hand scanning can produce perfectly reliable results a great deal more cheaply.

Although compound B sector scanning

was such a dominant feature in our work at this time, we continued to develop the potential of A scanning. This is applicable whenever it is necessary to measure a diameter of a structure whose existence and position are exactly known in advance. As already mentioned, we had observed the strong echoes from the fetal skull. It was evident that, provided a true diameter of the skull and not a chord was struck by an ultrasonic beam at perpendicular incidence, two very large echoes would be produced. If a measurement "off beam" were attempted, the echoes on A scan were not comparable.

Only two true diameters of the fetal head on this basis are to be found, namely, the biparietal and the occipitofrontal. By good fortune the occipitofrontal diameter is not easy to reach because of the position of the head before the onset of labor, and, second, it is a great deal larger and unlikely to be confused with the biparietal.

William Smellie, 200 years ago, was correct in his observation that the fetal head normally enters the pelvis in the occipitotransverse, or lateral, position. This makes the anterior parietal eminence easy to reach unless the head is very deeply engaged. Incidentally, if the biparietal diameter is inaccessible for this reason, it is possible to achieve some disengagement by placing stiff pillows under the patient's buttocks and also by allowing her bladder to fill with urine.

We presented the rationale of this type of measurment to the British Institute of Radiology in 1961[9] and were claiming to get results within an accuracy of about 1 mm. Errors of 2 mm were already considered most unacceptable. The technique of biparietal cephalometry in this manner was very difficult, however, and required great practice involving a search holding the probe by hand until a fleeting glimpse could be obtained of the biparietal diameter. For this reason, for a time we endeavored to overcome the difficulty by using a "coincidence counter" apparatus. This was gated and coupled to a camera shutter trigger so that when the requisite diameter showed up on the cathode ray screen, a simultaneous photograph was taken from which the measurement could be made. This elaborate mechanism, however, was no substitute for a properly acquired skill. The use of graticules and photographic measurements has never been really satisfactory or sufficiently accurate in our view. We now use electronic cursors that take the form of "bright up" dots of light superimposed on the relevant echoes from the parietal bones. The spacing of these cursors is achieved by dials producing an immediate digital read-out in centimeters and millimeters of the distance between them. This eliminates the need for photography or storage pictures and makes it possible to estimate as many as twenty biparietal diameters in an afternoon.

Almost by accident at approximately the same time we hit upon the facility of time-motion scanning while examining an aortic aneurysm.[9] This time-motion facility is now standard in our present apparatus and is used for the early detection of fetal heart movements within the first trimester.

CLINICAL APPLICATION

Fetal cephalometry

In 1962 my colleague, Willocks, began to study the progressive growth of the biparietal diameter throughout pregnancy.[18-20] The technique of biparietal cephalometry was, however, enormously improved by the modifications introduced by another of my colleagues, Stuart Campbell,[21] some years later. Campbell's modification of our technique makes possible readings to within an accuracy of 0.5 mm or less and is carried out as follows.

The head is first identified in longitudinal sectional scanning and by choice of the correct position of scan, the midline echo, believed to be caused by the falx cerebri, is sought. The direction of the beam perpendicular to this is measured in degrees and the point on the patient's abdomen noted. The scanning head is now rotated through a right angle into the transverse scanning position (in our latest apparatus this can be done without the operator moving from his chair) and the scanning frame is also tilted to the angle of head tilt previously discovered. With very minor adjustments, a full transverse view of the fetal skull at the correct angle is quickly obtained with the midline echo, less strong than the parietal bone echoes, showing up midway between them. Cursors are then superimposed over both parietal bones in B scan (Fig. 10-1).* This will bring the measurement to within about 1 mm of the true figure. Further accuracy is now achieved by referring to the second cathode ray tube, which is simultaneously recording in A scan. The fine adjustment of the cursors is now made for the "bright up" dots to superimpose upon the leading left hand edges of the parietal "blips" (Fig. 10-2). With practice great speed of measurement can be obtained. (For a table of biparietal diameter determination of gestational age, see Appendix.)

*Unless otherwise stated, all ultrasonograms taken in longitudinal section are with the patient in the dorsal position, cephalad to the left. In the figures, these abbreviations are used: *B*, bladder; *H*, head; *P*, placenta; *C*, cyst; *U*, uterus; *LS*, longitudinal section; and *TS*, transverse section. All maturities of pregnancy are given as weeks since the onset of the last menstrual period (menstrual age). All ultrasonograms have been taken with the Diasonograph apparatus (Nuclear Enterprises, Ltd.).

Study of early pregnancy

In 1963, I found quite accidentally in an extra nervous patient with a full bladder that I could observe the uterus deeply within the pelvis, though not even enlarged, by using the full bladder as a transmitting tank that also conveniently displaced gas-containing, impenetrable bowel out of the field of view.[22] The real excitement came when a patient presented with a history of four previous abortions and no living children in whom we found a uterus of normal size with a curious white

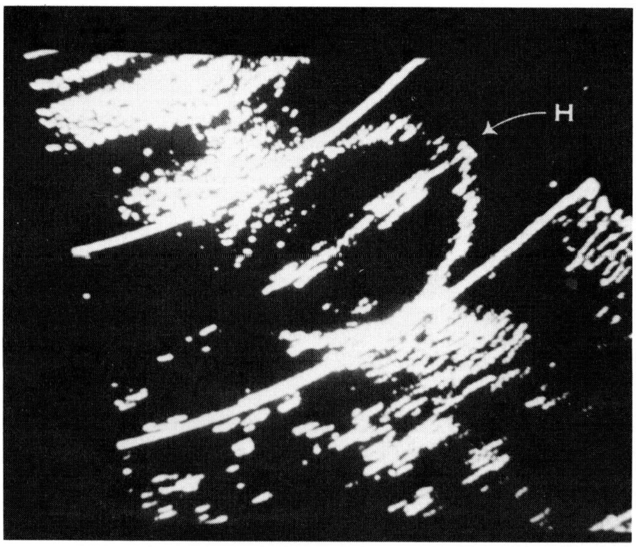

Fig. 10-1. Fetal head taken life size at 13½-weeks' gestation showing electronic cursor marks applied to both parietal bones. Note midline falx.

ring within it. At first it perplexed us until I suddenly realized that I was looking at a very early gestation sac (Fig. 10-3). The patient did not even know she was pregnant. (The patient was delivered on time successfully of a healthy baby.[23])

From now on it was clear that we could study prenatal development from the very earliest weeks, the fifth week of amenorrhea right through to term in all high-risk cases, particularly in patients with a history of recurrent abortion or bleeding in early pregnancy. Subsequently we published a series of landmarks of prenatal development.[24] This work has been fully elaborated in a splendid atlas compiled by Kobayshi and his colleagues,[25] in which illustrations are profusely given of all the commonly and not so commonly encountered abnormalities in obstetrics that lend themselves to investigation by sonar. Our findings throughout are much in common with theirs, although our apparatus is very different.

An intrauterine pregnancy can often be seen after 5 weeks' amenorrhea as a small white ring occupying the upper part of the uterus, if normally nidated. At the sixth week of amenorrhea the intrauterine ring should be clearly visible; in fact, if it cannot be found the diagnosis of pregnancy is suspect. Alternatively, a blighted ovum or, possibly, an ectopic pregnancy may have to be considered (Fig. 10-4). By the seventh week it should be possible to see a "fetal pole" (Fig. 10-5). This appears

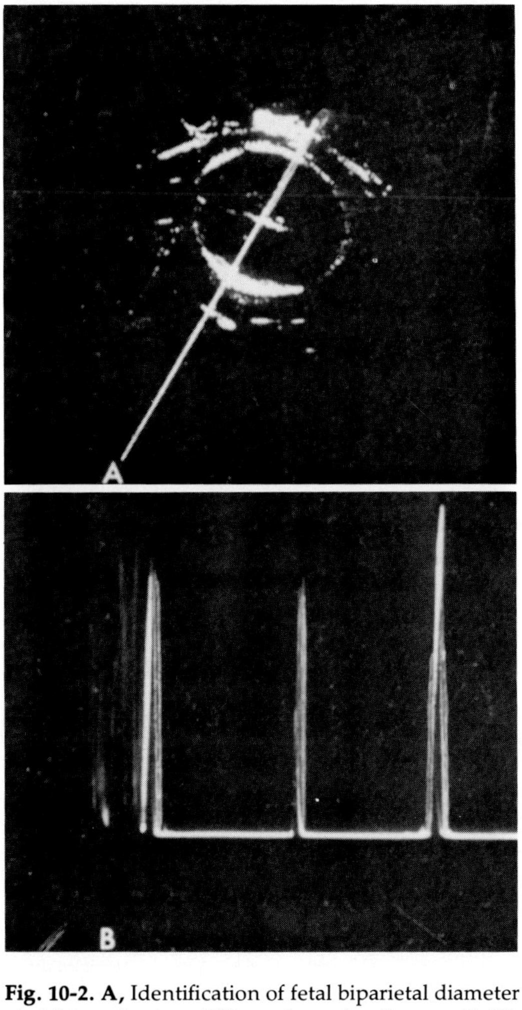

Fig. 10-2. A, Identification of fetal biparietal diameter at right angles to midline echo using B scan. **B,** Biparietal diameter measured on A scan; midline echo is smaller. (Courtesy Dr. Ralph M. Wynn and Meredith Corp.; from Wynn, R., editor: Obstetrics and gynecology annual, New York, 1972, Appleton-Century-Crofts, p. 252.)

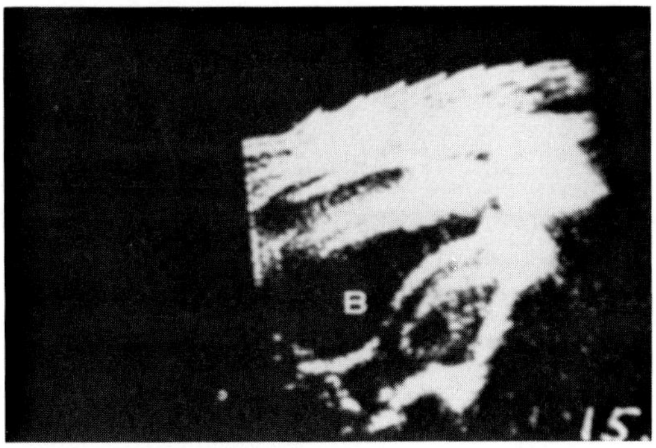

Fig. 10-3. Early gestation sac appears as a white ring-like structure in uterus outlined behind full bladder. LS. Cephalad to right. The last menstrual period was 49 days ago. Urinary Pregnosticon test was negative. Patient had three previous abortions, each at 8 weeks. Pregnosticon test was subsequently positive, with normal delivery at term. (From Donald, I.: Am. J. Obstet. Gynecol. **93:**935-941, 1965.)

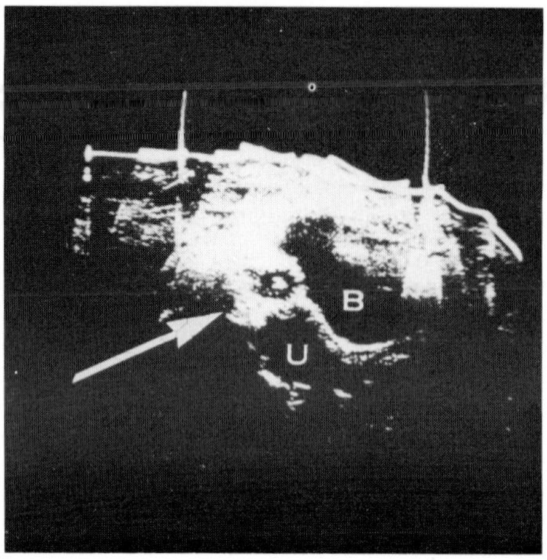

Fig. 10-4. Unruptured tubal pregnancy (right). LS. Symptoms were indefinite but the diagnosis was confirmed by laparoscopy proceeding to laparotomy. Arrow points to ectopic gestational sac above uterine fundus.

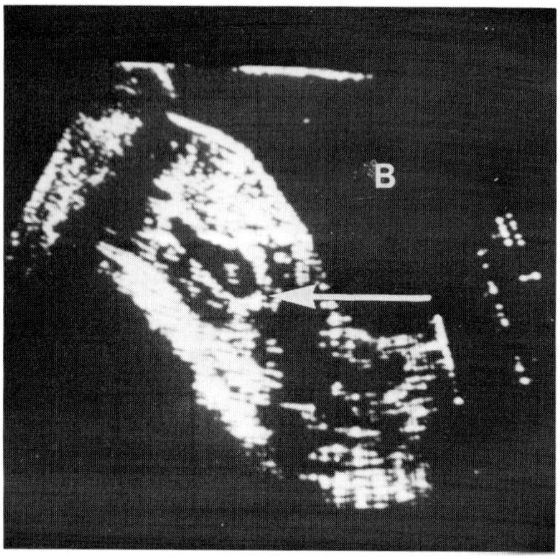

Fig. 10-5. Early gestation sac. LS. Seven weeks and 2 days after last menstrual period onset. Fetal pole can be seen within the sac and fetal heart pulsation demonstrable on time-motion scanning. Arrow points to gestational sac.

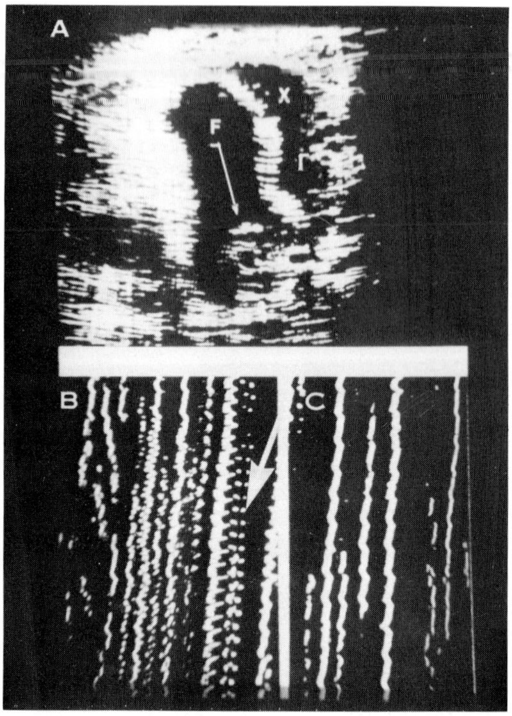

Fig. 10-6. Threatened abortion at 9 to 10 weeks' amenorrhea. **A,** Full-size uterine contents with apparently double twin sac, one containing fetus *(F)* and the other *(X)* apparently empty of fetal echoes are shown. **B,** The time-motion trace shows fetal heart pulsation (arrow) in the left sac. **C,** No fetal heart pulsation is seen in sac to right.

as a little blob within the gestation sac. By carefully positioning the ultrasonic beam through this fetal pole on B scan, fetal heart pulsation is now sought on a simultaneously recording A scan screen. Robinson's method, developed in our department, then employs electronic cursors (as in cephalometry) to identify the pulsating portion of the fetus as it flicks backward and forward from left to right and vice versa on the A scan trace. Then, maintaining watch on the A scan screen, the first screen (originally in B scan) is converted to time-motion scanning and a picture of fetal heart movement, usually between 160 to 180 beats per minute, can be traced and photographed (Fig. 10-6).[26] This is proof absolute of the existence of fetal life. With increasing practice and assurance in the method, one can also find that the ovum is "blighted" and the fetal prognosis hopeless.

About the tenth week the placenta begins to differentiate and can be visible usually on either the anterior or the posterior aspect of the gestation sac.

At 11 weeks of amenorrhea the sac becomes less distinct and begins to break up on ultrasonic appearances, possibly because of the differentiation of chorion frondosum from chorion laeve.[27] The pictures become confused and difficult at about 12 weeks, and it is very hard to see the fetal head with certainty at this time, but by the thirteenth week the fetal head can nearly always be found with assurance. From then on the matter becomes very simple. The head grows extremely rapidly and the placenta is easily seen in its further development. Maturity too can be fixed with great accuracy at this time.

Until about the thirtieth week, the fetal head is practically circular or spheroidal in shape, and cephalometry is relatively simple. Quite often a B scan cursor measurement is all that is necessary (see Fig. 10-1) without invoking the more elaborate Campbell technique. Progressive growth can be studied right through pregnancy. This is particularly useful in dealing with cases of recurrent abortion or alleged threatened abortion where it is clearly worth knowing whether the pregnancy is salvageable or not. In the course of the study of early fetal development by sonar, we naturally came to recognize cases of blighted ovum and the various types of abortion—complete, incomplete, and missed.

Abortion

Sonar is very valuable in cases of abortion. Not only can it indicate whether products of conception are retained (or even that the fetus is still alive in utero), but it can also demonstrate that the abortion process is complete and that the uterus is already empty. Unless a patient is bleeding heavily and requiring urgent transfer to the operating room, it is now our practice to examine by sonar. In this way many patients can be sent home without routine curettage, provided they are not bleeding and the sonar appearances show an empty uterus (Fig. 10-7).[27,28] This practice has materially reduced the number of unnecessary operations. A common finding after a recent abortion is the appearance of a waist of the uterine form on longitudinal scanning. I have not seen this in other conditions.

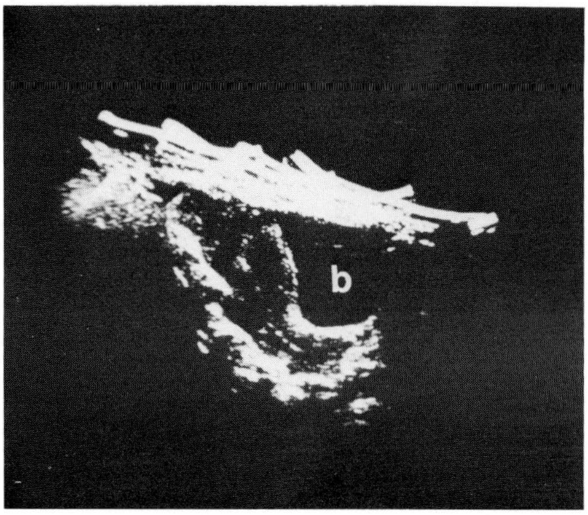

Fig. 10-7. Abortion at 13 weeks occurred a few hours earlier. Uterus is clearly empty, so evacuation is unnecessary.

Missed abortion is altogether more difficult. One has frequently to rely on the absence of a detectable fetal heartbeat by the time-motion scanning method already described or often to wait for a repeat examination in a week's time to make sure there has been no further gestational growth. It is possible that many cases of hydatidiform mole arise from trophoblastic changes in missed abortion.[29] This may confuse ultrasonic diagnosis.[30]

Later on in pregnancy, when the head can be seen, the following signs may indicate intrauterine death.

1. The double line sign described by Kobyashi,[25] which in our experience does not immediately appear (Fig. 10-8)

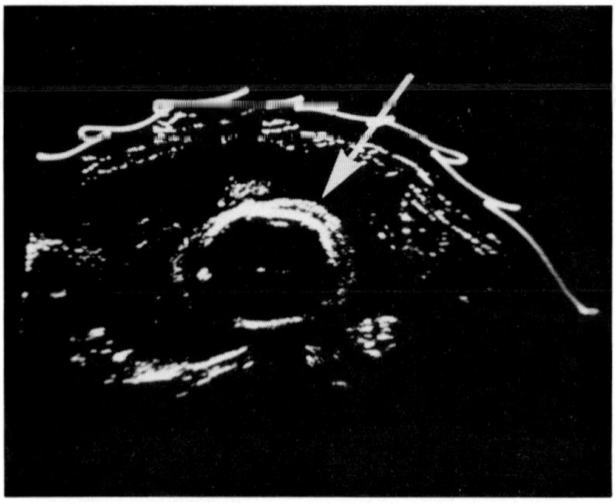

Fig. 10-8. Intrauterine death at 32 weeks. No movements were felt for a fortnight but x-ray reported no evidence of fetal death. Note double line on dead fetal skull (arrow).

2. Some distortion of the fetal head for the same reason
3. Failure of the head to enlarge on biparietal cephalometry

The finding or the absence of fetal heart pulsation, especially on time-motion scanning (even more accurately then by using the Doppler effect), is the method most readily and reliably available in experienced hands.

Blighted ovum

It is almost a quarter of a century since Hertig postulated that the phenomenon of ovum blighting was a common one in early pregnancy.[31]

Blighted ovum can be defined as an impregnated ovum whose development becomes arrested before completion of the first trimester. Clearly the phenomenon is more frequent the earlier in pregnancy it is sought, but even so we are finding that this is every bit as common as Hertig suggested, in fact more so, because many of these patients are unknowingly pregnant and simply declare themselves to have a later menstrual period. Sonar will establish the diagnosis of blighted pregnancy. Furthermore, we have now taken to examining

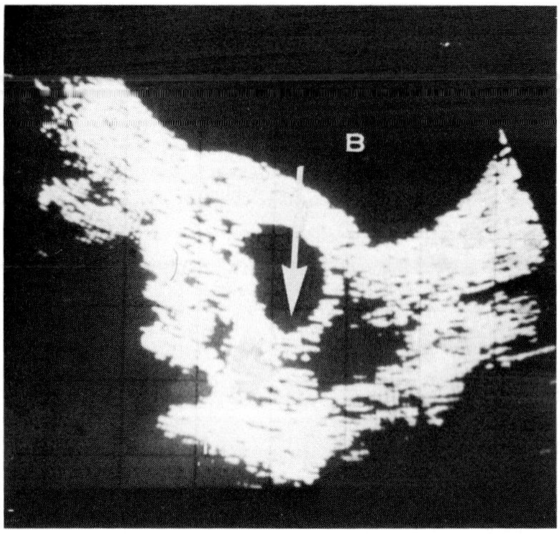

Fig. 10-9. Blighted ovum at 9 weeks (arrow). Although Pregnosticon test was still positive, no fetal echoes could be found within the sac. LS. Patient aborted spontaneously a fortnight later. Small piece of fetal tissue only 2 mm long was recovered too dead for tissue culture and karyotyping.

the tissue passed, if possible by tissue culture and karyotyping, since the incidence of chromsomal abnormality in these cases is high.[32]

The following then are the features of blighted ovum[33]:

1. Poorly defined gestation sac with either fragmentation or C-shaped, incomplete ring
2. Absence of fetal echoes probably by the seventh week and certainly by the eighth week of amenorrhea (Fig. 10-9)
3. An undetectable fetal heart on time-motion scanning after 7 weeks of amenorrhea[26]
4. A gestation sac that is small for date and without further growth over a period of 1 week (the sac may in fact shrink over this period)
5. A discrepancy of 2 weeks in size according to the patient's history
6. A low site of nidation, with the sac sometimes over a partially opened cervix, as seen on ultrasonic scanning

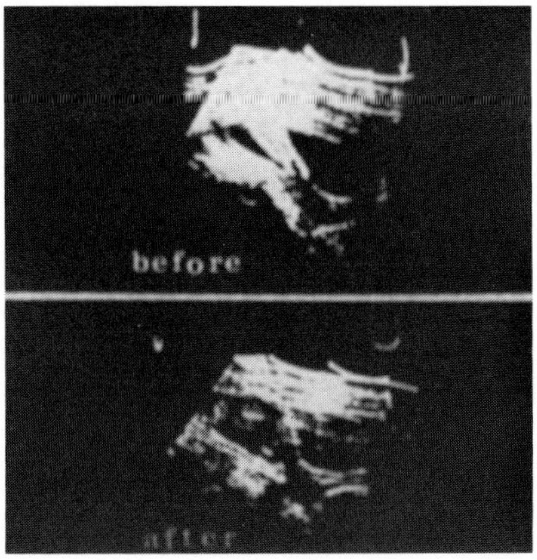

Fig. 10-10. Recurrent abortion. Patient had four previous abortions and no living children. Upper picture at 8 weeks' gestation shows gestation sac elongating toward the lower segment and cervix apparently opening. LS. Lower picture shows same patient a fortnight later following cervical cerclage. Note that the uterus has grown and the cervical canal would appear to be well reconstituted. In spite of cerclage, the patient aborted spontaneously a fresh fetus in conformity with dates at twenty-third week. (From Donald, I.: Proc. R. Soc. Med. **62:**442, 1969.)

behind a full bladder (this may indicate that an abortion actually is in the process of occurring)

These signs may not at once be supported by gonadotropin tests on the urine, and often a diagnosis can be more readily arrived at by sonar.

The method that we use for detecting the fetal heart in very early pregnancy has the advantage of being carried out through the abdominal wall, which causes no disturbance to the patient, which would be undesirable especially if she were bleeding, but it necessitates a full bladder. Jouppila[34] and Kratochwil[35] both had success with vaginal transducers, the former using the Doppler technique, which is serviceable from 8 weeks onward and gives complete accuracy from the tenth week. The latter, using a A scan transducer within the vagina, has picked up the heart at 7 weeks' amenorrhea. We believe, however, that the abdominal approach through the full bladder is quicker and easier, although we have no personal experience with the use of intravaginal transducers.

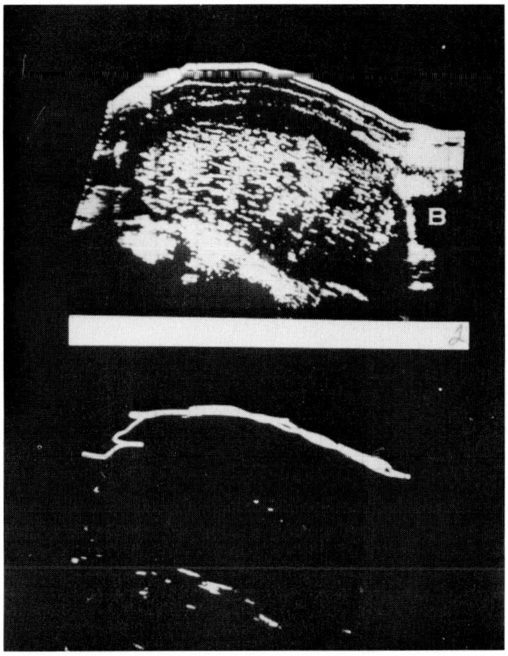

Fig. 10-11. Hydatidiform mole. Upper picture shows speckled mass of the mole (LS). Lower picture shows identical scan but at a gain reduced by 16 dB. The uterus appears empty, but note that its posterior wall can still be seen, indicating high transonicity.

It is now our practice never to undertake cervical cerclage for alleged cervical incompetence in cases of recurrent abortion without first assessing the likely viability of the conceptus by sonar, since many cases of recurrent abortion are in fact cases of recurrent blighted ovum or intrauterine death (Fig. 10-10).

Hydatidiform mole

Not infrequently cases of so-called threatened abortion turn out on ultrasonic examination to be cases of hydatidiform mole. We clarified our criteria for the diagnosis of hydatidiform mole.[15,36,37] The following are the features that must be insisted upon:

1. The appearance of a speckled mass

within the uterus at a given gain sensitivity on the apparatus
2. Its virtual disappearance by reducing the gain by 15 dB
3. The ability even at reduced gain to see the back wall of the uterus; in other words, to establish that the mass of molar tissue is transonic (Fig. 10-11)

Because these appearances can be given by a uterine myoma undergong myxomatous degeneration,[16] we now insist on a fourth criterion, namely;

4. Substantiation of the diagnosis at a very high frequency

We therefore switch from our standard 2.5 MHz probe and amplifier and repeat the investigation at 5 MHz.[38,39] A degenerate myoma is not likely to fulfill these criteria at the higher and less penetrating frequency.

We have not yet had an opportunity of studying a case of choriocarcinoma by sonar.

Placentography

For a surprising length of time placentography eluded us. All along we had believed that the same arguments that made possible the diagnosis of hydatidiform mole could be applied to the identification of the placenta. Up until 1965 and the opening of the new maternity hospital, the Queen Mother's Hospital, in which I could establish full ultrasonic facilities, I had been prevented from investigating cases of antepartum hemorrhage and possible placenta praevia because of the hazards of transporting potentially dangerous cases across the town simply for examination. By 1966 my colleagues in Denver, who were also working along the same lines, had succeeded in placental localization.[40] They clearly had some difficulty in demonstrating a posteriorly situated placenta except by a process of exclusion. We got over this difficulty initially by examining the patient lying on her side. Eventually, by using more penetration and altering our time-varied gain, we were able to get around the difficulty. In our series published in 1967,[41] we included a number of cases of placenta praevia and claimed an overall accuracy of 94% in several hundred cases, a result that compares favorably with other methods. There is also the advantage that placentography by sonar involves the patient in no discomfort or hazard and can be repeated as often as wished. It is interesting to note that a placenta that appears to be situated low over the lower segment or even reaching the internal os at any early stage may alter position as pregnancy advances and the lower uterine segment extends, particularly in the case of anterior placentas.[42]

It is now our practice to examine by sonar placentography:

1. All cases of antepartum hemorrhage in which the diagnosis of placenta praevia has to be confirmed or excluded
2. All cases of unstable lie because of the possibility of a placenta occupying the lower uterine segment
3. Before all cases of amniocentesis at any stage of pregnancy, not only to determine the position and limits of the placenta but also to find a suitable pool of liquor amnii to tap

For the last situation we make a mark on a suitable site for amniocentesis together with notes for the angle of insertion of the exploring needle. Bang and Northeved in Copenhagen use a transducer with a hollow down the center through which they can insert the needle under direct ultrasonic "vision," and they consequently operate with great precision and skill.[43]

The hazards of fetomaternal transfusion and isoimmunization in Rh-negative patients are sufficient to make it likely that in the near future practitioners will expose themselves to lawsuits for failure to localize the placenta by one efficient method or another before running the risk of damaging it at amniocentesis.

One or two points are worth bearing in mind in relation to ultrasonic placentography. The first is that after the fourteenth week the earlier placentography is carried out the more easily the placenta can be seen. Wherever possible, an attempt should be made, by correct positioning of the scanning plane, to identify the fetal surface of the placenta (Fig. 10-12). Its size should be estimated in relation to the whole uterine cavity as well as its ultrasonic density. These last two features appear to us to be more marked in cases of Rh isoimmunization (Fig. 10-13). Certainly a large and opaque placenta is worth an inquiry as to the presence of maternal Rh antibodies. Our work on gray tone scaling is still in a very early stage, but it may help to elucidate more details about placental texture in relation to pregnancy complications.

In the case of the posteriorly situated placenta, an area of shadow may appear behind the fetal trunk and less so behind the fetal head, which is often more transonic. This has to be taken into account in assessing the placental position and dimensions.

In making a diagnosis of placenta praevia, it is worth having the bladder partially filled with urine in order to delimit the lower segment (Fig. 10-14).

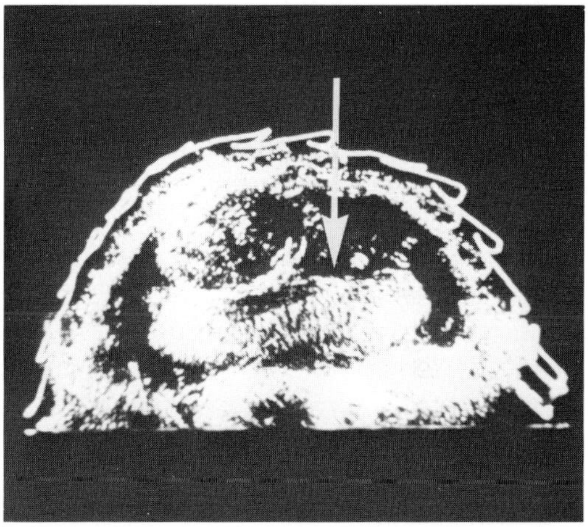

Fig. 10-13. Rh placenta with hydrops fetalis. TS. Placenta is posterior (arrow). Note thickening of placenta and density of placental echoes.

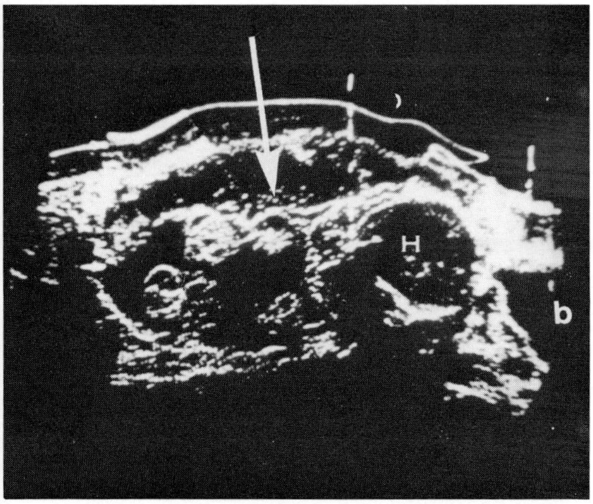

Fig. 10-12. Placentography. Thirty-two weeks' gestation. Upper segment contains anterior placenta. Note line denoting fetal surface of placenta (arrow). There is mild hydramnios and partially filled bladder. Vertex presents. LS.

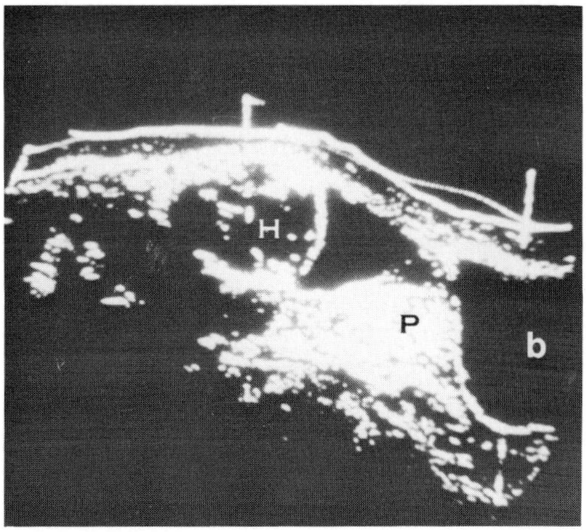

Fig. 10-14. Major degree of posterior placenta praevia. LS. Twenty-nine weeks' gestation. Head is displaced high above the placenta, which fully covers the internal os of cervix. Note partially filled bladder to right.

The correct usage of gain settings will also repay the trouble taken. Our practice is to set the apparatus at sufficient gain just to demonstrate the vertebral column and the area of the sacral promontory and then by time-varied gain to attenuate the more proximal echoes until a clean picture can be obtained. Where the placenta shows up as a speckled mass it will be seen, as in the case of hydatidiform mole, that a reduction of 10, or usually 15, dB in this area will remove the speckles and leave a clearer looking area, but still with the same shape. This helps to distinguish it from artifacts and echoes from within liquor amnii.

The advantages of sonar placentography over other techniques are very obvious, quite apart from its safety and lack of disturbance to the patient. In our department we undertake many hundreds of such examinations in a year, which would be totally impractical by radioactive isotopes or by radioarteriography.

Prolonged examination on the ultrasonic couch, particularly after antepartum bleeding, may occasionally result in nausea, vomiting, or faintness on the part of the patient, owing to the supine hypotensive syndrome. This can also occur in a prolonged examination in a difficult case of cephalometry. The situation is immediately rectified by turning the patient onto her left side as in standard clinic practice. However, this defeats the examination. Another useful measure is to get an assistant to raise the patient's legs straight and hold them up in the air supported by one's shoulders in order to improve venous return to the heart. This often enables the examination to be continued without further untoward incident.

Twins

Diagnosis of twins can be suspected and made with certainty at a very much earlier stage by sonar than by any other technique known. Sometimes it is possible to see two separate gestation sacs at 7 or 8 weeks' amenorrhea[36] (Fig. 10-15). The diagnosis of the Hanson quintuplets in London was made by Campbell with apparatus similar to our own[44] at 9 weeks. This was a dramatic achievement.

As soon as two heads can be separately identified,[17] preferably each in two di-

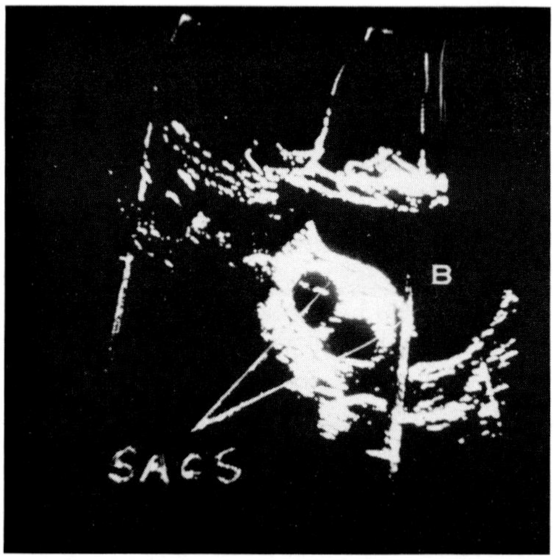

Fig. 10-15. Twin sacs at just under 9 weeks' amenorrhea. LS. There was subsequent spontaneous labor and double breech delivery at 35 weeks. Both babies survived.

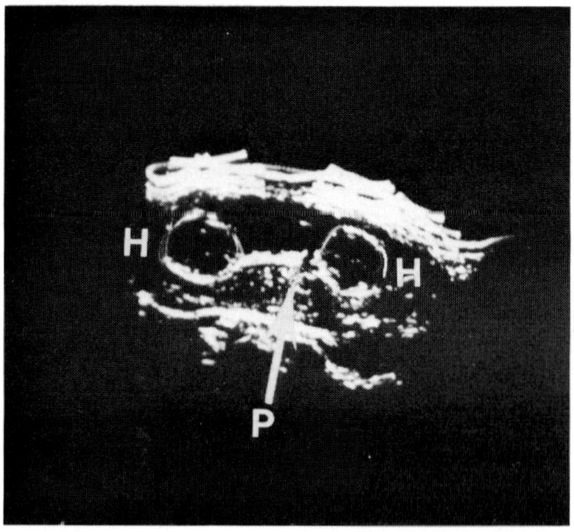

Fig. 10-16. Twins at 17 weeks. Oblique sectional view. There was repeated bleeding during pregnancy. Note twin heads and posterior placenta (arrow).

mensions, the diagnosis becomes certain (Fig. 10-16). To do so may require a certain amount of adjustment of the ultrasonic scanning head. Occasionally one is in doubt about whether a second apparent head is in reality a thorax. This doubt can usually be resolved by taking a further picture in a plane at right angles to the first picture. Even more certain is the method discovered by Mrs. Ida Miller, one of my assistants, that a Doppler apparatus applied in exactly the same area and at the same angle of probe immediately picks up the heartbeat within a thorax, thereby differentiating it from a head. This simple maneuver saves a lot of time in cases of doubt.

The diagnosis of triplets is more difficult, since one is limited to two dimensions at present, and it is this doubt that sooner or later makes one resort to radiography. Nevertheless, many unnecessary radiographs are avoided thanks to sonar.

An important matter is to be able to measure which of twins has the larger head, the first coming or the second. The hazard to the second twin is very much greater, as is well known, if it happens to be the larger of the two.

"Large for dates" problem

This is a very common reason for referring a patient to the ultrasonic department. The possibility of twin pregnancy of course is one and is readily confirmed or excluded by sonar at almost any stage of pregnancy after the second month. Hydramnios is readily identified, but most commonly the case is found to be one of mistaken dates and maturity. The head is practically circular during the first 20 weeks, and clearly precise measurement can be made without going to the trouble of identifying the true transverse axis and the falx, although this is a bonus (Fig. 10-1). At 20 to 30 weeks the job has to be done properly and probably provides the best index of all of fetal maturity.[45]

There is general agreement that biparietal cephalometry provides a better index of maturity than of actual fetal weight, which is far less important. However, the later in pregnancy the measurements are made, the greater must be the care taken in applying the full Campbell technique. Repeated measurements are extremely valuable. By the time that the biparietal diameter has reached 9.8 cm it is unquestionably mature and over 10 cm quite possibly postmature. One hesitates to make a diagnosis of hydrocephalus with biparietal diameters that are not repeatedly over 11 cm.

Another problem is the unexpected coexistence of a pelvic tumor with pregnancy (Figs. 10-17 and 10-18). Even more difficult are cases of hydronephrosis (Fig. 10-19). We have had some notable instances of very gross varieties of this dangerous disorder, dangerous because of the progressive aggravation of the condition as pregnancy advances (Fig. 10-20) and because of the serious risk of superadded infection.

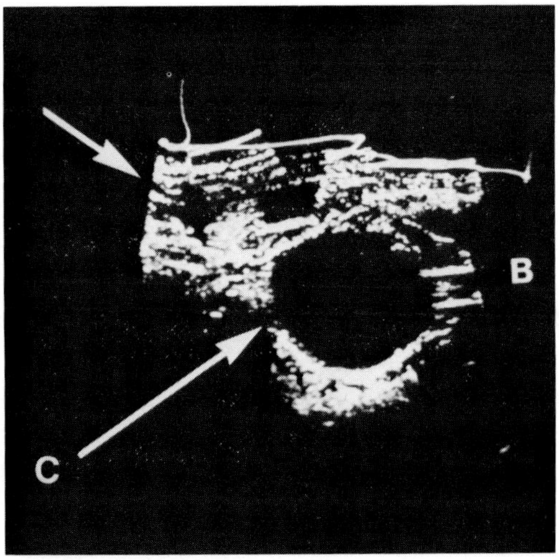

Fig. 10-17. Ovarian cyst complicating early pregnancy. LS. Upper arrow shows displaced gravid uterus; lower arrow shows cyst occupying pelvic cavity. Clinical diagnosis was retroverted gravid uterus. Successful ovarian cystectomy was performed at 13 weeks.

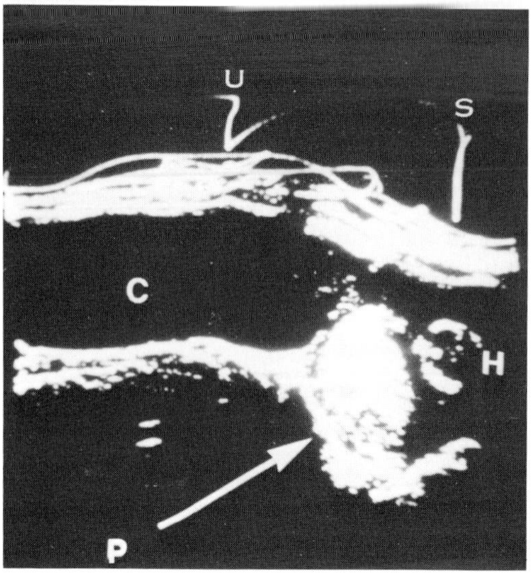

Fig. 10-18. Huge ovarian cyst and 14 weeks' cyesis. The vertical marks on the abdominal wall indicate level of umbilicus *(U)* and symphysis pubis *(S)*, respectively. The upper margin of the cyst cannot be seen because it is out of range. Patient presented clinically as a case "large for dates."

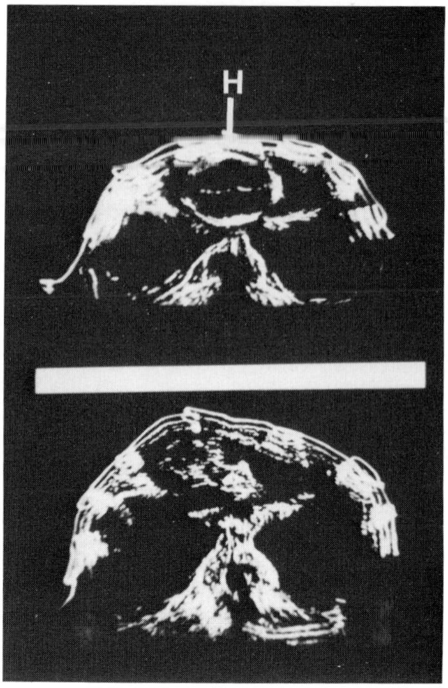

Fig. 10-20. Massive bilateral hydronephrosis and pregnancy. Upper picture (TS) shows vertebral column and huge hydronephrotic sacs on either side. Fetal head, with midline falx, is shown since presentation was by the breech, (30 weeks). The lower picture was taken 6 weeks later after spontaneous cephalic version. Note enormous increase in the size of hydronephrotic kidneys.

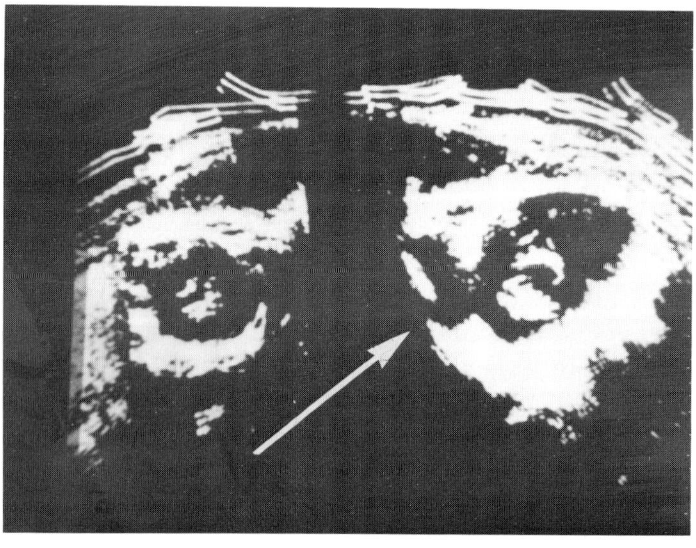

Fig. 10-19. Transverse section of kidneys in a patient who is 20 weeks pregnant and who has recurrent urinary infection. Prone position. Right kidney shows considerable enlargement (arrow) with evidence of hydronephrosis. Antibiotic therapy instituted throughout whole of pregnancy.

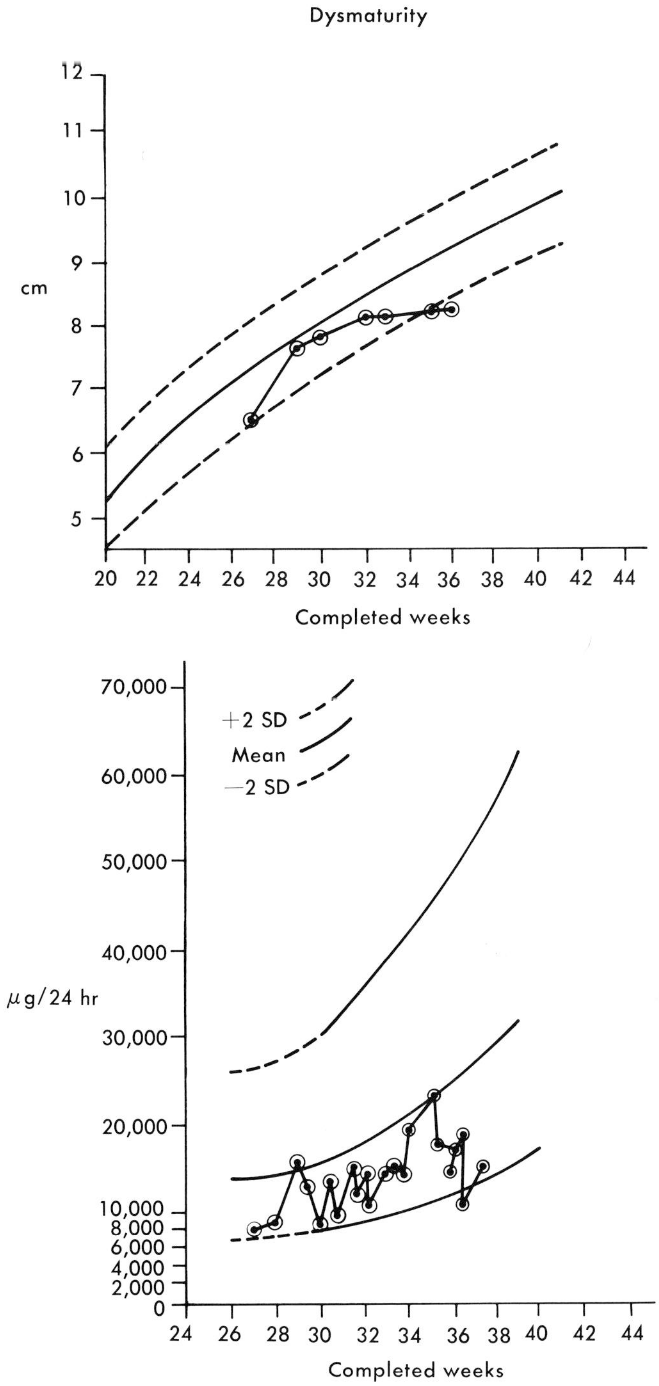

Fig. 10-21. Marked dysmaturity. Patient had a history of two previous dysmature pregnancies. Upper graph shows fall-off in biparietal growth measurement after the twenty-ninth week; lower graph shows failure of estriol excretion curve to rise. There was successful delivery of dysmature baby weighing 1.99 kg at 37 weeks.

Apparent growth retardation

The diagnosis of intrauterine malnutrition resulting in dysmaturity is attracting the attention of the whole obstetric world, and sonar has a large part to play here. It is now standard practice to combine serial biparietal cephalometry with estriol excretion curves based initially on the Mary Coyle curves from Dundee.[46] We now have automated equipment that gives an unlimited number of estimations on 24-hour collections of urine.[47] Although Campbell and Kurjak[48] reckon that cephalometry gives a better index of diagnosing the small-for-date baby than estriol excretion curves, they also admit that there is no difference in predicting the appearance of perinatal asphyxia. It is common practice now to employ both monitoring techniques (Fig. 10-21).

It would be impossible to monitor the growth of every baby in the course of its development and so selection is necessary, usually on the basis of past history of dysmaturity, macerated stillbirth, and all maternal conditions known to interfere with intrauterine development such as hypertensive states, threats to placental integrity from threatened abortion or hemorrhage, diabetes mellitus, and renal disease. A series of measurements must be plotted on a graph to detect abnormal growth. Flamme,[49] in a large series of cases, noted that measurements that were regularly above the ninetieth percentile or below the tenth did not necessarily indicate abnormality. What was significant was a change of course from one interdecile space to another. This may indicate the development of hydrocephalus at one end of the scale or placental insufficiency at the other.

Fetal abnormality

There is a limited usefulness in detecting fetal abnormality mainly because of lack of resolution and limitation to two dimensions. The diagnosis of anencephaly, however, is easily made simply by being unable to identify a fetal head (Fig. 10-22). Likewise, the diagnosis of hydrocephalus is also possible (Fig. 10-23). Unfortunately, lesions of the vertebral column and limbs cannot be detected.

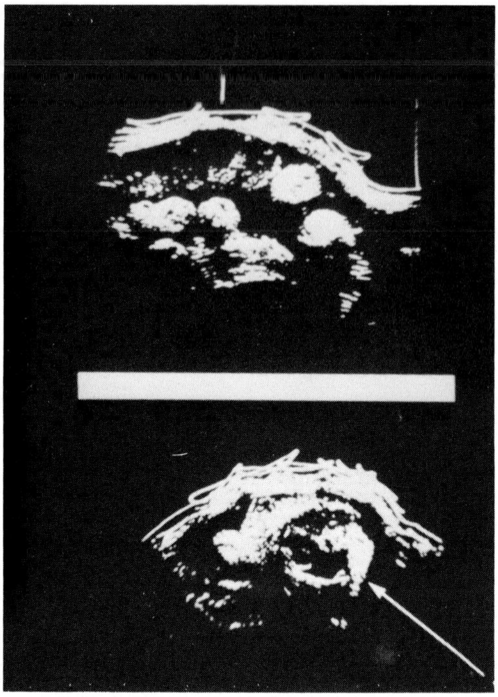

Fig. 10-22. Anencephaly and hydramnios of 35 weeks' duration. Patient presented with hypertension and was "small for dates" with low estriol excretion. Upper picture shows mild hydramnios (LS). No head could be found. Lower picture (TS) shows thorax, (arrow) confirmed by Doppler apparatus. Note fetal heart within the thoracic cage (arrow).

Puerperium

Cases of secondary postpartum hemorrhage are well worth examining by sonar for retained products of conception[50] (Fig. 10-24). Likewise, complications of cesarean section caused by hematoma from the uterine scar behind the bladder can readily be seen and distinguished from puerperal urinary retention[51] (Fig. 10-25).

DOPPLER EFFECT

Although ultrasound is used, Doppler recording is almost a different subject from

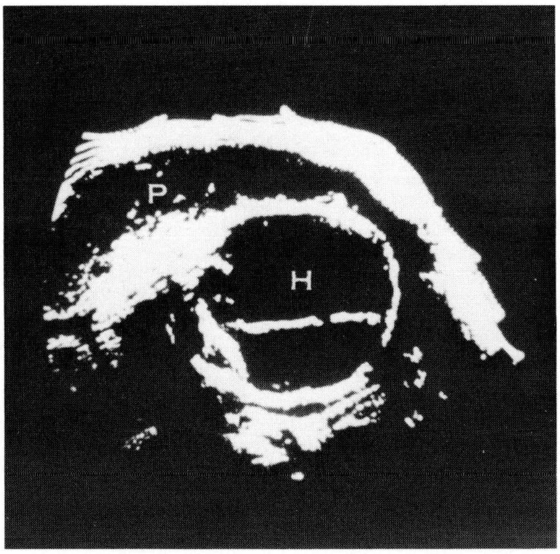

Fig. 10-23. Hydrocephalus, 37 weeks' gestation. Patient had two previous children, first stillborn with abruptio placentae, second anencephalic. She was now small for dates and sonar examination was requested for maturity. TS shows hydrocephalic head (BPD 11.13 cm) with a breech presentation and upper anterior placenta. There was breech extraction, hydrocephalus, and spina bifida stillbirth.

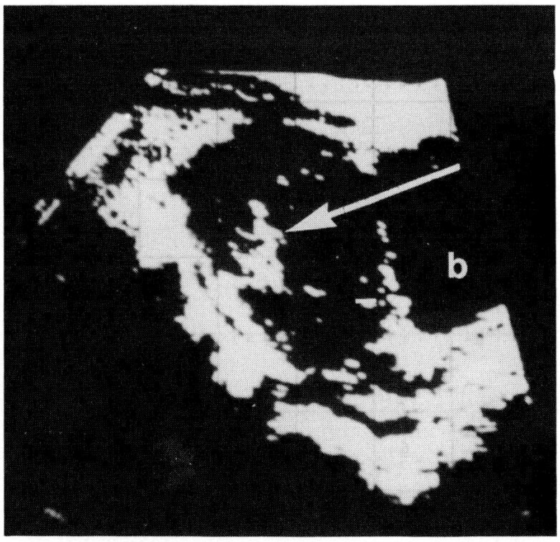

Fig. 10-24. Puerperal retained secundines. Second day of puerperium following manual removal of placenta. Secondary postpartum hemorrhage. Significant quantity of tissue is shown within uterus (arrow). LS. Evacuation of several large pieces of placental tissue was performed same day.

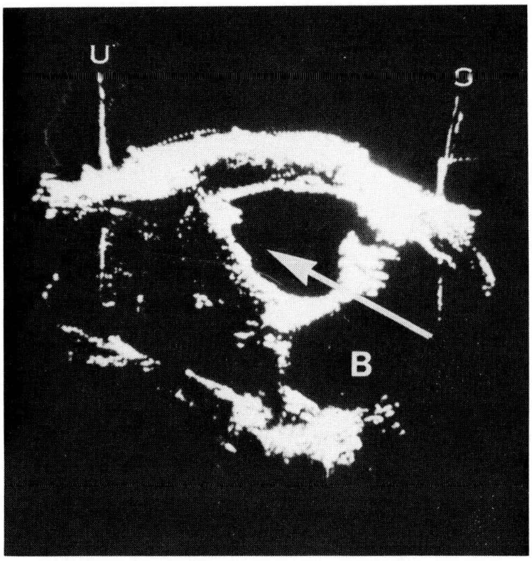

Fig. 10-25. Large hematoma from cesarean section scar of 11 days earlier (LS). The puerperal uterus is to the left, hematoma is marked by the arrow, and the bladder is to the right. The integrity of the uterine scar would appear to be in doubt. (From Donald, I.: Proc. R. Soc. Med. **64:**901-906, 1971.)

the pulsed echo reflection technique with which we have hitherto been dealing. Here a continuous beam of ultrasound is emitted toward a moving structure, such as the fetal heart, and the reflected echoes take more or less time to return to the receiving transducer alongside the transmitter according to the movement of that structure. This produces an apparent alteration in the frequency of the received echo signal. This can be processed and forms an excellent method of fetal heart detection.[52,53]

Many such machines are now on the market, are reasonably cheap, and can reliably establish the fact of fetal life, often from the eleventh week and usually thereafter without any difficulty, although a prolonged search over the uterus is occasionally necessary. As before, some coupling oil or jelly is necessary to secure acoustic coupling. The received signals can be delivered either as sounds simulating the fetal heart or as flashing lights. The most sophisticated technique is applied in studying the blood flow, which

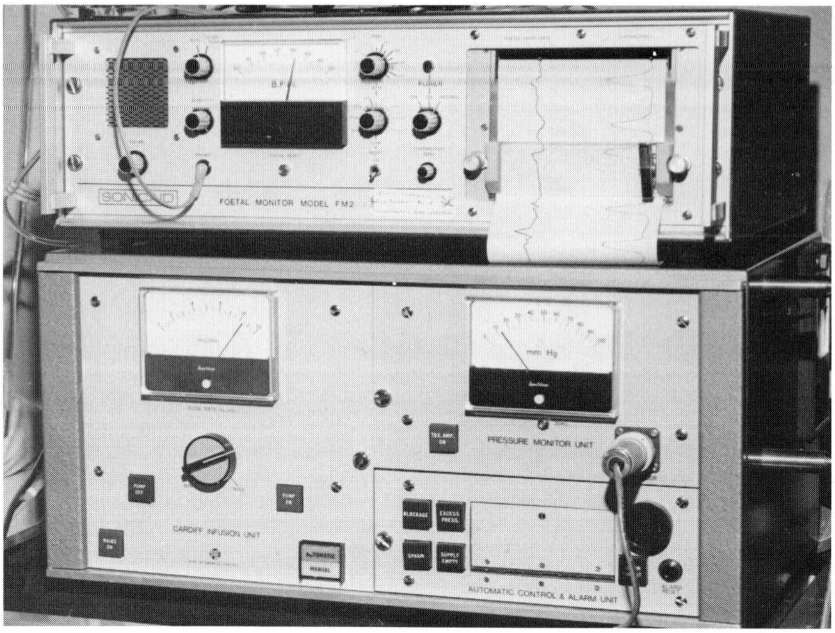

Fig. 10-26. Apparatus used at present for full monitoring of accelerated and controlled labor. Doppler effect is used for monitoring fetal heart rate (left line on trace of upper machine; tocographic trace of the uterine action in the right-hand line). The lower apparatus is the Cardiff Infusion Unit with automatic control and alarm system.

is not yet applicable to obstetric usage.

Fetal heart rate monitoring in labor is possible by the ultrasonic Doppler effect even during the height of a uterine contraction. The information, if properly computed on a beat-to-beat basis, can give early warning of fetal distress often before signs of acidosis appear on fetal blood sampling. The positioning of the transducer over the abdomen is less critical if a diverging beam of ultrasound is transmitted into the abdomen. By using a rosette array of receiving transducers, as in the case of the Sonicaid FM2, returning echoes from the fetal heart can be picked up over a wide area. This apparatus is very useful in stages of labor before the membranes are ruptured and the cervix sufficiently dilated to apply scalp electrodes (Figs. 10-26 and 10-27).

We have often attempted to make a diagnosis of twins by listening for two

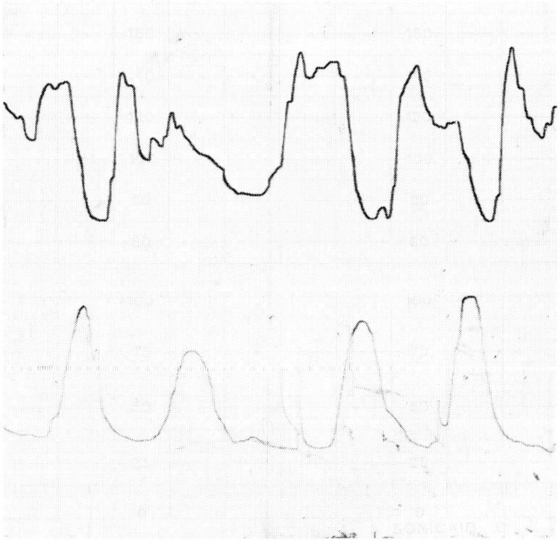

Fig. 10-27. Fetal distress is demonstrated in the first stage of labor by fetal heart monitoring (upper trace) and tocography (lower trace). Patient had a history of four previous pregnancies without a living issue. Subsequent fetal blood sampling showed a pH of 7.19. Delivery was expedited by Ventouse. Recovery was uncomplicated.

fetal hearts beating at different rates, but this requires two separate Doppler machines and simultaneous counting, and we have not found it to be very reliable.

The claim made by some manufacturers that these Doppler instruments can be used for the diagnosis or exclusion of placenta praevia should be treated with the greatest reserve, to put it very mildly. For such an important and dangerous diagnosis the technique is not sufficiently reliable to be acceptable; in fact, there are no cheap shortcuts in a subject like placentography.

SAFETY

Safety is certainly a matter for vigilance and concern, although injury from diagnostic ultrasound has not yet been demonstrated. There is, however, the danger that future machines may become more powerful and exceed the threshold of biologic damage, if one in fact exists.[54] A combined retrospective survey from New York, Glasgow, and Lund[55] for possible teratogenic effects of diagnostic ultrasound yielded negative results. Nevertheless, if any tissue is vulnerable to ultrasonic energy one would, by analogy and comparison with the effects of x-rays, expect embryonic tissues to suffer first. The spectrum of energy is of course totally different, being nonionizing. The possibilities of hazard have been well reviewed by Hill.[56]

An important paper was delivered by Smyth in Pittsburgh[57] in which he showed the absence of teratogenic effects, or effects on fertility, in pregnant rodents subjected to ultrasound and followed through for several generations. Further confirmation came from Guy's Hospital, England.[58]

It is well known that ultrasonic energy, if sufficiently powerful, can produce heat and theoretically cavitation, although the latter has not yet been demonstrated in animal tissue. Most biologic effects hitherto recorded have been associated with appreciable heat production. The energies employed in diagnostic sonar are so small that it has not yet been possible to demonstrate any heat changes even with the most delicate and sensitive apparatus.

A preliminary communication from Cape Town[59] suggested chromosome damage resulting from continuous ultrasonic insonation in the milliwatt range. This work, however, has not been substantiated by other workers.[60-65] The general opinion is that chromosome damage cannot be invoked as an index of ultrasonic biologic effect. Other experiments have been undertaken to see whether placental enzymes could in any way be altered by insonation, again with negative results.[66] Streaming effects may indeed occur on prolonged insonation, but they are difficult to demonstrate. Nevertheless, Dyson has shown temporary aggregation of red cells in blood vessels lying parallel to standing ultrasonic waves applied to a chick embryo placed within a large ultrasonic field[67] The biologic significance of this is not known.

Molecular effects to watch for are the degradation of deoxyribonucleic acid. It may be that electron microscopy, as suggested from Guy's Hospital in England, may show such changes but again with as yet unknown significance.[68]

In the meanwhile the diagnostic benefits of a sonar service are so obvious that they cannot readily be dispensed with. In 1972, at the Queen Mother's Hospital, a total of 4,174 examinations were performed. Of these, 2,542 (61%) were fetal cephalometry, 818 (20%) dealt with pregnancy complications, 578 (14%) were placental localizations, and the remainder (5%) consisted of other indications and types of examinations.

SUMMARY OF PRESENT DAY SONAR USES IN PREGNANCY

In early pregnancy, the indications for use of sonar are: diagnosis of intrauterine pregnancy, early gestation sac, level of nidation, appearance of fetal pole, growth rate, proof of early fetal life, prior to cerclage operation, blighted ovum, maturity, placental differentiation, twins, bleeding in early pregnancy, abortion (threatened, inevitable, complete, incomplete, missed), intrauterine death, recurrent abortion, retention of urine and retroverted gravid uterus, differential diagnosis of large for dates, hydatidiform mole, anencephaly, pelvic tumors with pregnancy, double uterus with pregnancy, renal complications in pregnancy, and ectopic pregnancy.

In late pregnancy the indications are: maturity, fetal growth rate, twins, determination of which twin is larger, presentation, unstable lie, differential diagnosis of large for dates, associated pelvic tumors, hydronephrosis complicating pregnancy, hydramnios, anencephaly, hydrocephalus, disproportion, placental localization, placental development, Rh placental changes, and previous cesarean scar integrity.

Indications for studies in puerperium are: secondary postpartum hemorrhage, puerperal urinary retention, complications of cesarean section, and hematoma and abscess.

The advantages of all the many applications listed are to be weighed against hypothetical dangers whose nature or extent cannot yet be assessed. It would be reckless to deny the possibility of their existence. Only the fullest collaboration between the different centers of the world can determine the extent of risk. In the interval, widespread utilization of this technique of rapidly growing clinical importance is certainly justified.

Acknowledgment

This work is receiving financial support from the Medical Research Council through the University of Glasgow.

REFERENCES

1. Langevin, M. P.: Les ondes ultrasonores, Rev. Gen. Electric. **23:**626-634, 1928.
2. Firestone, F. A.: The supersonic reflectoscope for interior inspection, Metal Progr. **48:**505-512, 1945.
3. Firestone, F. A.: Supersonic reflectoscope, an instrument for inspection of solid parts by means of sound waves, J. Acoust. Soc. Am. **17:**287-299, 1946.
4. Wild, J. J.: The use of ultrasonic pulses for the measurement of biological tissues and the detection of tissue density changes, Surgery **27:**183-188, 1950.
5. Wild, J. J., and Reid, J. M.: Application of echo ranging techniques to the determination of structures of biological tissues, Science **115:**226-230, 1952.
6. Kossoff, G., Garrett, W. J., and Robinson, D. E.: In Kelly, E., editor: Ultrasonic energy. Biological investigations and medical applications, Urbana, 1965, University of Illinois Press, pp. 365-376.
7. Brown, T. G.: Direct contact ultrasonic scanning techniques for the visualization of abdominal masses. In Smyth, C. N., editor: Medical electronics, Proceedings of 2nd International Conference on Medical Electronics, Paris, June 24-27, 1959, London, 1959, Iliffe & Sons Ltd., pp. 358-366.
8. Donald, I., MacVicar, J., and Brown, T. G.: Investigation of abdominal masses by pulsed ultrasound, Lancet **1:**1188-1195, 1958.
9. Donald, I., and Brown, T. G.: Demonstration of tissue interfaces within the body by ultrasonic echo sounding, Br. J. Radiol. **34:**539-546, 1961.
10. Donald, I.: Use of ultrasonic echo sounding in obstetrics and gynaecology, First Charles J. Barone Lecture, Pittsburgh, 1961, University of Pittsburgh.
11. Howry, D. H.: International Radio Engineering Convention Record of 1955, National Convention, Part 9, pp. 75-88.
12. Howry, D. H., and Bliss, W. R.: Ultrasonic visualization of soft tissue structures of the body, J. Lab. Clin. Med. **40:**579-592, 1952.
13. Holmes, J. H., and others: The ultrasonic visualization of soft tissue structures in the human body, Trans. Am. Clin. Climat. Assoc. **66:**208-225, 1954.
14. Holmes, J. H., and Howry, D. H.: Ultrasonic diagnosis of abdominal disease, Am. J. Dig. Dis. **8:**12-32, 1963.
15. MacVicar, J., and Donald, I.: Sonar in the diagnosis of early pregnancy and its complications, J. Obstet. Gynaecol. Br. Commonw. **70:**387-395, 1963.
16. Donald, I.: Diagnostic uses of sonar in obstetrics and gynaecology, J. Obstet. Gynaecol. Br. Commonw. **72:**907-919, 1965.
17. Sunden, B.: On the diagnostic value of ultrasound

in obstetrics and gynaecology, Acta Obstet. Gynaecol. Scand. **43**(Suppl. 6), 1964.
18. Willocks, J.: Fetal cephalometry by ultrasound and its place in clinical obstetrics, M.D. Thesis, University of Glasgow, 1963.
19. Willocks, J. and others: Foetal cephalometry by ultrasound, J. Obstet. Gynaecol. Br. Commonw. **71:**11-20, 1964.
20. Willocks, J. and others: Intrauterine growth assessed by ultrasounic foetal cephalometry, J. Obstet. Gynaecol. Br. Commonw. **74:**639-647, 1967.
21. Campbell, S.: An improved method of fetal cephalometry by ultrasound, J. Obstet. Gynaecol. Br. Commonw. **75:**568-576, 1968.
22. Donald, I.: The use of ultrasonics in the diagnosis of abdominal swellings, Br. Med. J. **2:**1154-1155, 1963.
23. Donald, I.: Utrasonic echo sounding in obstetrical and gynaecological diagnosis, Am. J. Obstet. Gynecol. **93:**935-941, 1965.
24. Donald, I.: Sonar as a method of studying prenatal development, J. Pediatr. **75:**326-332, 1969.
25. Kobayshi, M., Hellman, L. M., and Cromb, E.: Atlas of ultrasonography in obstetrics and gynecology, New York, 1972, Appleton-Century-Crofts.
26. Robinson, H. P.: Detection of fetal heart movement in first trimester of pregnancy using pulsed ultrasound, Br. Med. J. **4:**466-468, 1972.
27. Donald, I., and Abdulla, U.: Ultrasonics in obstetrics and gynaecology, Br. J. Radiol. **40:**601-611, 1967.
28. Robinson, H. P.: Sonar in the management of abortion, J. Obstet. Gynaecol. Br. Commonw. **79:**90-94, 1972.
29. Hertig, A. T., and Edmunds, H. W.: Genesis of hydatidiform mole, Arch. Pathol. **30:**260-291, 1940.
30. Donald, I.: On launching a new diagnostic science, Joseph Price Oration presented at Seventy-Ninth Annual Meeting of the American Association of Obstetricians and Gynaecologists, Hot Springs, Virginia, 1968, Am. J. Obstet. Gynecol. **103:**609-628, 1969.
31. Hertig, A. T., and Rock, I.: Theories of potentially abortive ova recovered from fertile women prior to the first missed menstrual period, Am. J. Obstet. Gynecol. **38:**968-993, 1949.
32. Carr, D. H.: Chromosomal errors and development, Am. J. Obstet. Gynecol. **104:**327-347, 1969.
33. Donald, I., Morley, P., and Barnett, E.: The diagnosis of blighted ovum by sonar, J. Obstet. Gynaecol. Br. Commonw. **79:**304-310, 1972.
34. Jouppila, D.: Ultrasound in the diagnosis of early pregnancy and its complications, Acta Obstet. Gynecol. Scand. **50**(Suppl. 15), 1971.
35. Kratochwil, A., and Eisenhut, L.: Geburtshilfe Frauenheilk **27:**176-180, 1967.
36. Donald, I.: Ultrasonics in obstetrics, Br. Med. Bull. **24:**71-75, 1968.
37. Donald, I.: Diagnostic uses of sonar (ultrasonic echo sounding). In Marcus, S. L., and Marcus, G. C., editors: Advances in obstetrics and gynecology, Baltimore, 1967, The Williams & Wilkins Co., pp. 314-329.
38. Donald, I.: Diagnostic sonar in obstetrics and gynaecology. In Wynn, R. M., editor: Obstetrics and gynecology annual, New York, 1972, Appleton-Century-Crofts, pp. 245-271.
39. Donald, I.: Ultrasonic investigation in obstetrics and gynaecology. In Wells, P.N.T., editor: Ultrasonics in clinical diagnosis, London, 1972, Churchill Livingston Publishing Co., pp. 74-92.
40. Gottesfeld, K. R., and others: Ultrasonic placentography, a new method for placental localization, Am. J. Obstet. Gynecol. **96:**538-547, 1966.
41. Donald, I., and Abdulla, U.: Placentography by sonar, J. Obstet. Gynaecol. Br. Commonw. **75:**993-1006, 1968.
42. King, D. L.: Placental migration demonstrated by ultrasonography: a hypothesis of dynamic placentation, Radiology **109:**167-170, 1973.
43. Bang, J., and Northeved, A.: A new ultrasonic method for transabdominal amniocentesis, Am. J. Obstet. Gynecol. **114:**599-601, 1972.
44. Campbell, S., and Dewhurst, C. J.: Quintuplet pregnancy diagnosed and assessed by ultrasonic compound scanning, Lancet **1:**101-103, 1970.
45. Campbell, S.: The prediciton of fetal maturity by ultrasonic measurement of the biparietal diameter, J. Obstet. Gynaecol. Br. Commonw. **76:**603-609, 1969.
46. Coyle, M. G., Greig, M., and Walker, J.: Blood progesterone and urinary pregnanediol and oestrogen in fetal death from severe preeclampsia, Lancet **2:**275-277, 1962.
47. Barnard, W. P., and Logan R. W.: An automated method for urinary oestriol determination, Clin. Chim. Acta **29:**401-409, 1970.
48. Campbell, S., and Kurjak, A.: Comparison between oestrogen assay and serial ultrasonic cephalometry in assessment of fetal growth retardation, Br. Med. J. **4:**336-340, 1972.
49. Flamme, P.: Ultrasonic fetal cephalometry: percentiles curve, Br. Med. J. **3:**384-385, 1972.
50. Robinson, H. P.: Sonar in the puerperium, a means of diagnosing retained products of conceptation, Scot. Med. J. **17:**364-366, 1972.
51. Donald, I.: Sonar—further scope and prospects, Proc. R. Soc. Med. **64:**901-906, 1971.
52. Johnson, W. L., and others: Detection of life in early pregnancy with an ultrasonic Doppler flowmeter, Obstet. Gynecol. **26:**305-307, 1965.

53. Bishop, E. H.: Obstetric uses of the ultrasonic motion sensor, Am. J. Obstet. Gynecol. **96:**863-867, 1966.
54. Safety of sonar in obstetrics (editorial), Lancet **1:**1158-1160, 1970.
55. Hellman, L. M., and others: Safety of diagnostic ultrasound in obstetrics, Lancet **1:**1133-1135, 1970.
56. Hill, C. R.: The possibility of hazard in medical and industrial applications of ultrasound, Br. J. Radiol. **41:**561-569, 1958.
57. Smyth, M. G.: Animal toxicity studies with ultrasound at diagnostic power levels. In Grossman, C. C., and others, editors: Diagnostic ultrasound, New York, 1966, Plenum Press, Inc., pp. 296-299.
58. Woodward, B., Pond, J. B., and Warwick, R.: How safe is diagnostic sonar? Br. J. Radiol. **43:**719-725, 1970.
59. MacIntosh, I. J. C., and Davey, D. A.: Preliminary communication: chromosome aberrations induced by an ultrasonic fetal pulse detector, Br. Med. J. **4:**92-93, 1970.
60. Abdulla, U., and others: Effect of diagnostic ultrasound on maternal and fetal chromosomes, Lancet **3:**829-831, 1971.
61. Bobrow, M., and others: Absence of any observed effect of ultrasonic irradiation on human chromosomes, J. Obstet. Gynaecol. Br. Commonw. **79:**730-736, 1971.
62. Boyd, E., and others: Chromosome breakage and ultrasound, Br. Med. J. **2:**501-502, 1971.
63. Lucas, M., Mullarkey, M., and Abdulla U.: Study of chromosomes in the newborn after ultrasonic fetal heart monitoring in labour, Br. Med. J. **3:**795-796, 1972.
64. Watts, P. L., Hall, A. J., and Fleming, J. E. E.: Ultrasound and chromosome damage, Br. J. Radiol. **45:**335-339, 1972.
65. Watts, P. L., and Stewart, C. R.: The effect of fetal heart monitoring by ultrasound on maternal and fetal chromosomes, J. Obstet. Gynaecol. Br. Commonw. **79:**715-716, 1972.
66. Robinson, H. P., and others: The effect of pulsed and continuous wave ultrasound on the enzyme histochemistry of placental tissue in vitro., J. Obstet. Gynaecol. Br. Commonw. **79:**821-827, 1972.
67. Dyson, M., Woodward, B., and Pond, J. B.: Flow of red blood cells stopped by ultrasound, Nature **232:**572-573, 1971.
68. Taylor, K. J. W.: Personal communication.

11 Gynecologic ultrasonography

LAJOS I. VON MICSKY, M.D.

Ultrasonic examination of the gynecologic patient presents a greater technical and diagnostic challenge than does examination of obstetric patients. The easy accessibility and well-defined acoustic anatomy of the gravid uterus combine to yield in many instances, on simple morphologic appraisal, pathognomonic information to the obstetrician. Transabdominal scanning of the pelvic organs in the nonpregnant state can, however, be performed only if the intervening, sound-blocking intestinal loops are displaced by pelvic-abdominal masses, by the accumulation of free fluid in the peritoneal cavity, or by what is usually resorted to, the full bladder.[1] The last permits satisfactory visualization of deeper lying structures, but the size of this "sonic window" is considerably influenced by the distensibility, irritability, and intrinsic lesions of this organ and by pathologic alterations of the pelvic anatomy. The complex, variable, and often similar acoustic representation of dissimilar pathologic states of the pelvic organs makes the interpretation of sonogynecograms more difficult and less specific than interpretation for obstetric conditions. Morphologic appraisal often must be supplemented by an analysis of tissue characteristics, a difficult undertaking. Nevertheless, ultrasonographic examination of gynecologic patients may often be of great clinical value by confirming the presence or absence of a palpatory finding, indicating the most likely organ of origin of a mass, and indicating the internal tissue characteristics of the lesion.

An endeavor to upgrade the diagnostic accuracy of gynecologic scans has resulted in the development of novel instrumentation and methodology[2,3] and advanced interpretive criteria.[4] Inspired by Baum's table of "optical characteristics and their acoustic analogues,"[5] a complex set of acoustico-optic tissue characteristics have been identified. Their appraisal, in combination with a detailed assessment of the morphologic properties of normal and pathologic structures, constitutes the ultrasonic analysis. Reevaluation of the latter in the context of the entire clinical picture provides the final sonographic diagnosis.

BIOPHYSICAL ASPECTS OF GYNECOLOGIC SONOGRAPHY

Sonic tomograms are maps of the spatial and amplitude distribution of echoes within cross-sectional planes extending into the scanned body region. Differences in the reflective and absorptive properties of tissues in relation to the sonic beam permit recognition of adjacent antomic structures. The reflected sound waves arise from acoustic impedance discontinuities between juxtaposed histologic structures. The greater the impedance mismatch the higher is the intensity of the reflected beam. The body abounds with such natural contrast media both within normal and pathologic structures. For example, the interface between tissue and fluid or fat and muscle is marked by strong echoes because of the impedance difference. Based on the same principle an almost 100% reflection takes place at tissue-gas interfaces.

Tissues containing structures smaller in dimensions than the wavelength of ultrasound appear sonically homogeneous (acoustically transparent, anechoic, black). Those with components larger than the wavelength are portrayed as heterogeneous (sono-opaque, echo-producing, white). With high frequencies, all tissues appear heterogeneous, thereby providing the normal and often characteristic background pattern.

Sonogynecography enables us not only to outline mass lesions but also to determine their consistency and relationship to and effect upon, surrounding organs and tissue planes. Founded on this consideration, the fluid-distended bladder, the gas-containing portions of the gastrointestinal tract, and the paravesical and ischiorectal fat pads become important landmarks. Distortion, displacement, compression, or obliteration of these structures is of major interpretive significance.

Because of ultrasound's greater sensitivity to tissue density differences, no contrast material is required. Sonogynecography is the method of choice if hysterosalpingography, intravenous pyelography, or pelvic angiography is contraindicated because of known or suspected allergy to contrast media. Acoustic imaging may be the preferred technique or possibly the only modality applicable for the evaluation of very young and very old gynecologic patients when more complex endoscopic or radiologic procedures are unduly hazardous or impractical.

The absence of geometric magnification artifacts found in radiographs permits direct planimetric evaluation of the sonograms. This in turn will considerably facilitate volumetric appraisal of organs and lesions for planning radiation therapy or for monitoring the effects of chemotherapy.[6] An advantage of acoustic imaging is that it enables us to observe tumors while they are functioning in vivo. Studies of spread, persistence, or recurrence will materially supplement other clinicopathologic information.

As a noninvasive technique, transabdominal sonography causes no discomfort to the patient. It is free of any known genetic or toxic effects and thus can be repeated as often as required, thereby allowing meticulous follow-up of disease processes.[6]

METHOD

All the transabdominal sonographic studies were performed with a custom-made Picker Contact Laminograph equipped with a motorized scanning bridge and a twenty-step attenuator calibrated in 2 dB intervals between settings. The execution of precision serial scans and the performance of exacting attenuation studies have been greatly facilitated by the accessory equipment. The 2.25 MHz crystal is slightly focused to compensate for the divergence of the beam. Polaroid films are used to photograph the images on the persistence screen. The graticule on the face of the oscilloscope and electronic magnification circuits permit the accurate determination of the dimensional parameters of physiologic and pathologic structures.

Examination of the pelvic-abdominal organs is carried out primarily in the supine position (anteroposterior or AP). Adequate "sonofluoroscopy" of the entire abdomen performed in both the longitudinal and the transverse directions precedes the actual photographing of the images on the screen. This term denotes a rapid-scan sonographic survey of a particular body region by forming and erasing the cross-sectional images in fast sequence while the scanning bridge is in continuous movement.[7] Subsequently sonograms are taken and photographed at 2-, 1-, or 0.5-cm intervals, depending on the frequency of the transducer used and the dimensions of the structures to be demonstrated. The number of sonograms sufficient for reliable interpretation will depend on the morphologic complexity of the mass and the extent of alteration of topographic relations.

As is apparent from Fig. 11-1, for the transverse (T series) and longitudinal (L series) scans the reference points are the umbilicus and the midline, respectively. Planes above the umbilicus and to the right of the midline are labeled "plus", while those below the umbilicus and to the left of the midline are labeled "minus."[8] The first number in the right upper corner of the sonograms means distance in centimeters measured from the reference point, the second number indicates the attenuator (sensitivity) setting. The key to the other labeling on the AP sonograms is as follows: *S* stands for symphysis, *U* for umbilicus, and *XP* for xiphoid process.

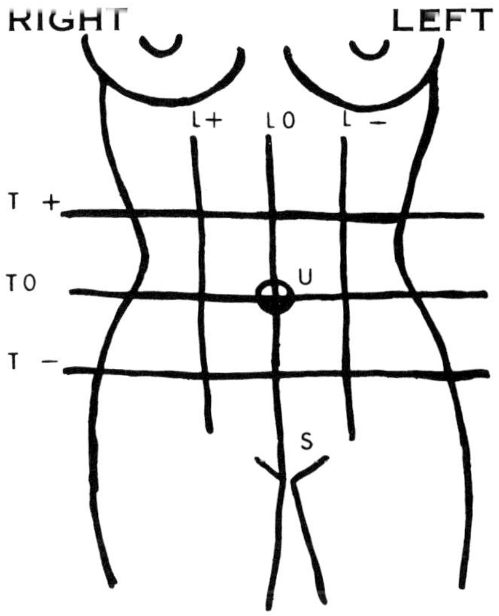

Fig. 11-1. Labeling of transabdominal scanning planes in the supine position (anteroposterior or AP).

Once in a while it is necessary to perform sonographic studies of pelvic-abdominal masses in the prone (posteroanterior or PA) position or in the left or right lateral decubitus positions (LLD and RLD, respectively). The C marking on the transverse and the S marking on the longitudinal sonograms performed in these positions denote the iliac crest and the spine as reference points. Scanning planes above the iliac crest and to the right of the spine are labeled "plus," to the left of the spine "minus."

To provide an optimal scanning path, it is occasionally necessary to tilt the scanning head, as is the case in a markedly protuberant abdomen. Meaningful appraisal of these "tilt scans" is possible only if the precise site of the transducer-skin contact, measured by a tape from the reference point, and the tilt angle are accurately recorded. The tilt is described in degrees of angle enclosed between the sagittal axis of the patient and the longitudinal axis of the transducer. Depending on the orientation of the crystal, it is labeled "cephalad" or "caudad" in transverse scans and "right" or "left" in longitudinal scans.

It is most important to establish a baseline sensitivity (attenuator) setting for each organ system, otherwise false negative and false positive results may occur. Built-in standards, such as the full bladder and the normal liver parenchyma, can be utilized for the daily calibration check of the instrument.

The time-controlled gain (TCG) and suppress controls should also be appropriately adjusted to provide utmost sonographic detail of the organs and pathology being examined.

In the Ultrasonic Division of St. Luke's Hospital Center, mineral oil is used exclusively for acoustic coupling. During the scanning procedure the transducer is not rocked but, in a smooth continuous movement, is positioned as perpendicular as possible to the anticipated orientation of the interface the sonographer wishes to portray. The technique is best described as "contour-following interspersed by one point sectoring at appropriate locations."[7]

The sonographic diagnosis in general is not based on a single sonogram obtained in a particular scanning plane but rather on a three-dimensional image derived through mental integration of the various

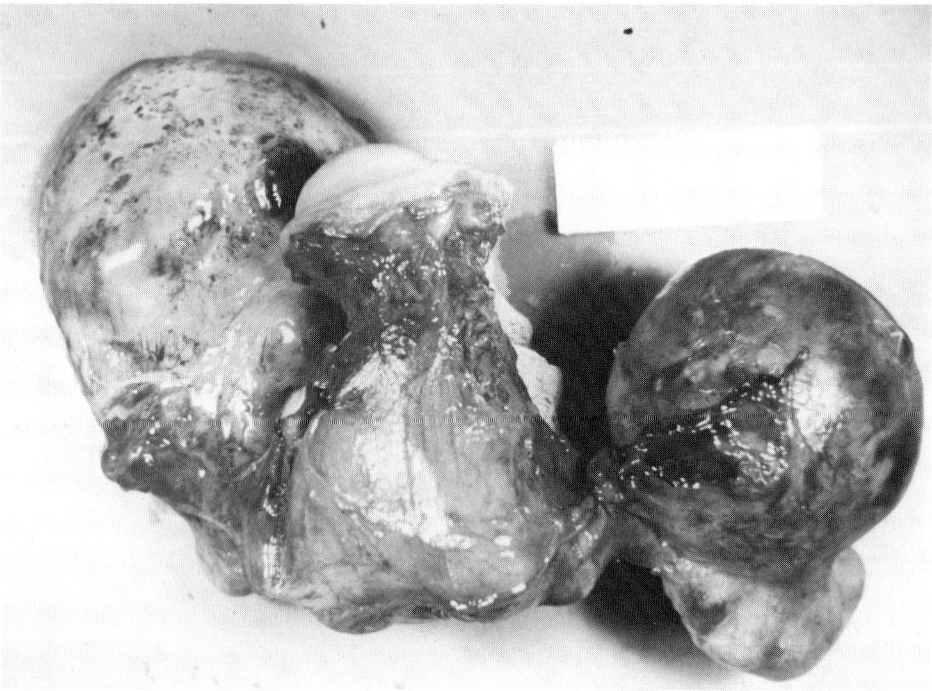

Fig. 11-2. The positioning of the surgical specimen simulates the topography observable at laparotomy when looking into the pelvis from the patient's head. The left tubo-ovarian cyst occupied the cul-de-sac and another tubo-ovarian cyst was fixed to the right pelvic wall. (See Fig. 11-3.)

series or combinations of sonograms (Figs. 11-2 and 11-3).[6]

Sufficient knowledge of topographic anatomy, comprehension of the physical principles of acoustic imaging, and thorough familiarity with the equipment are absolute prerequisites for the production of adequate sonograms and for the reliable interpretation of their data content.

NORMAL ULTRASONIC ANATOMY OF THE INTERNAL REPRODUCTIVE ORGANS AND TOPOGRAPHIC RELATIONS OF THE FEMALE PELVIS

Sonographic recognition of gynecologic pathology is contingent on the establishment of the normal ultrasonic anatomy (acoustic analogue of pelvic topography) of the female pelvis.

Midline longitudinal (L0) sonograms generally demonstrate the distended bladder, the intestines, the vagina, the uterus, and the rectum (Fig. 11-4). The presence or absence, shape, and dimensions of the tomographic sections of these organs will depend on the plane of scan.

The normal distended bladder is a uniformly sonolucent, markedly transonic, smoothly contoured area just distal to the abdominal wall echoes. On the L0 scans the caudal contour of the female bladder is incomplete because of acoustic shadowing by the symphysis. The vagina and the uterus form the dorsal boundaries of the organ, while cranially it is delimited by a zone of intestinal echoes (Fig. 11-4, *A*). The sonographic appearance of the bladder will vary with the degree of its distension and with the size and position

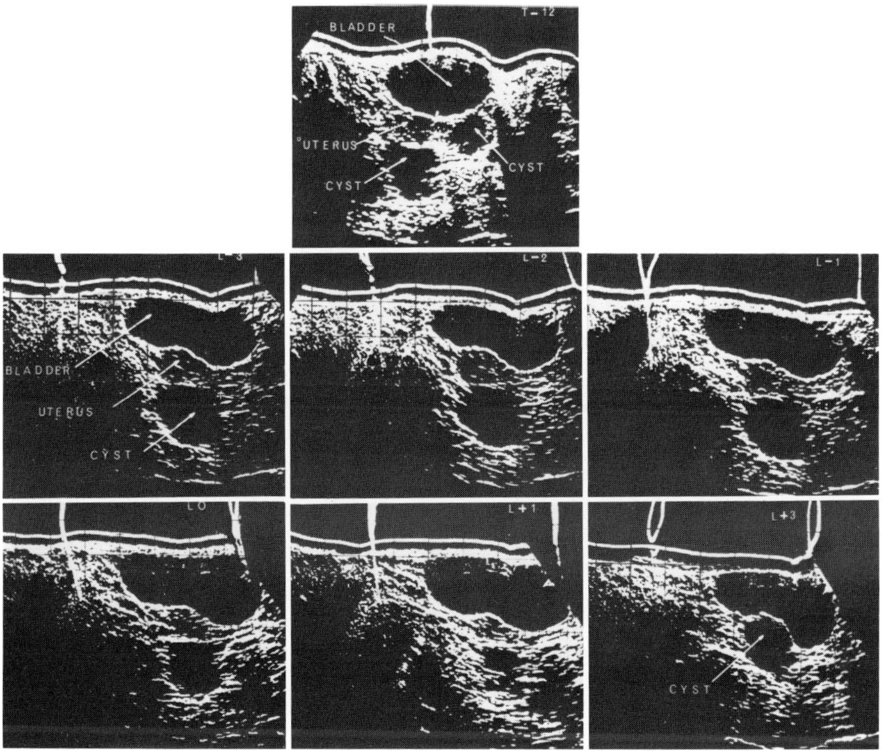

Fig. 11-3. The transverse and longitudinal scans depict the bilateral tubo-ovarian cysts. Note the good morphologic, dimensional, and topographic correspondence with surgical specimen (Fig. 11-2).

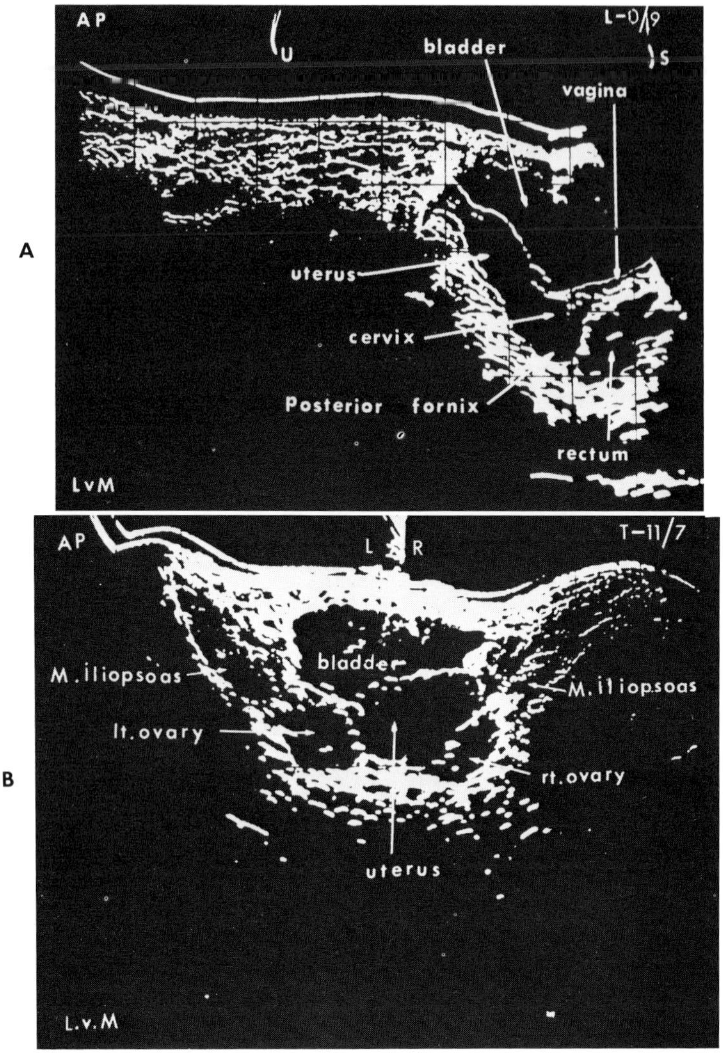

Fig. 11-4. Sonic analogue of the topographic anatomy of the normal female pelvis in **A,** sagittal section (L series) and **B,** transverse section (T series).

of other normal and pathologic pelvic structures. In general, a moderately filled bladder provides the optimal size for sonographic studies: it permits adequate acoustic visualization without causing lateral displacement, rotation, or compression of the pelvic organs.[6,9]

The slightly curvilinear parallel double line located dorsocaudally to the bladder represents the ventral and dorsal walls of the vagina respectively (Figs. 11-4, *A*, 11-8, 11-9, 11-23, and 11-25). They diverge cranially to form the vaginal fornices. The posterior fornix is occupied by the vaginal portion of the uterine cervix (Fig. 11-4, *A*).

At normal sensitivity settings, the uterus is a pear-shaped organ contiguous with the vagina but forming an angle with it (anteversion) (Fig. 11-4, *A*). The nonpregnant endometrial cavity appears as a linear central echo oriented in the craniocaudal axis of the uterus (Fig. 11-9). Since the uterus is a well-perfused organ, its transonicity is moderate to good, thus permitting acoustic visualization of structures located distal to it such as the rectum (Fig. 11-4, *A*) and the hollow of the sacrum (Fig. 11-11). The dimensions and configuration of the "normal" uterus will vary considerably with the age and the obstetric history of the patient.[9] Changes in uterine position (midposition, retroversion) or alterations in the normal relation of the cervix to the corpus (hyperanteflexion, retroflexion) are readily recognizable.

Structures of the broad ligament can frequently be seen lateral to the uterus on both the *L* and *T* series of sonograms (Figs. 11-5, *B*, and 11-21).

The size of the ovaries varies from 2.5 to 5 cm in length, 1.5 to 3 cm in width, and 0.7 to 1.5 cm in thickness. Sonographic demonstration of the normal ovaries can be accomplished only if their size nears the uppermost values of these dimensions. The normal ovaries appear as ellipsoid structures juxtaposed bilaterally to the dorsolateral aspect of the uterus. Their internal texture shows some fine or coarse speckling superimposed on an anechoic background. They are best visualized on the T series of sonograms (Fig. 11-4, *B*).

While in their normal physiologic state, the fallopian tubes cannot be demonstrated by transabdominal sonography.

The gas-containing intestinal loops generally appear as diffusely scattered amorphous echoes confined to a relatively narrow space in the vicinity of the abdominal wall. Occasionally, however, multiple dilated intestinal loops can be distinguished under pathologic conditions (Figs. 11-4, *A*, 11-18, 11-19, *B*, and 11-24). The depth of the intestinal echo zone and the nature of its pattern greatly varies with the fullness and content of bowel.[10] The rectum can usually be identified behind and caudad to the uterus in the sacral hollow and is prominent when distended by fecal material (Fig. 11-4, *A*).

The promontory and hollow of the sacrum are readily visualized in the L series of scans (Figs. 11-11 and 11-20). On the T series of scans the vertebral body appears as an inverted U-shaped structure (Figs. 11-20 and 11-22, *A*). In front of it, the contours of the aorta and vena cava occasionally can be seen (Figs. 11-11, 11-20 and 11-26, *B*). Lateral to the vertebral column, the rounded cross-sections of the right and left psoas muscles are seen (Figs. 11-4, *B*, and 11-20). The para-aortic lymph nodes in front of the vertebral body can be sonographically identified only if enlarged.

In scanning planes corresponding to the lateral gutters, the external iliac artery and vein and the psoas muscle are frequently demonstrable on the L and occasionally in the T series of sonograms (Fig. 11-21).

CLINICAL USES OF ULTRASOUND IN GYNECOLOGY

Contrary to the predictions of published reports by some workers in the field of diagnostic ultrasonics, sonogynecography is no longer merely a research endeavor but a valuable diagnostic modality with an ever-expanding clinical scope.[1,11]

Documentation of presence or absence of suspected pelvic lesions

Since the existence of a pelvic mass is usually known prior to the sonographic study, the role expected from the sonoradiologist is to assist in the differential diagnosis rather than merely document the presence of a pathologic structure.[12] Sonography, however, can be very valuable in the establishment of the presence or absence of a lesion in patients who are difficult to examine clinically (because of obesity, lack of relaxation, or involuntary guarding from pelvic pathology) or where there is a conflict between the pelvic ex-

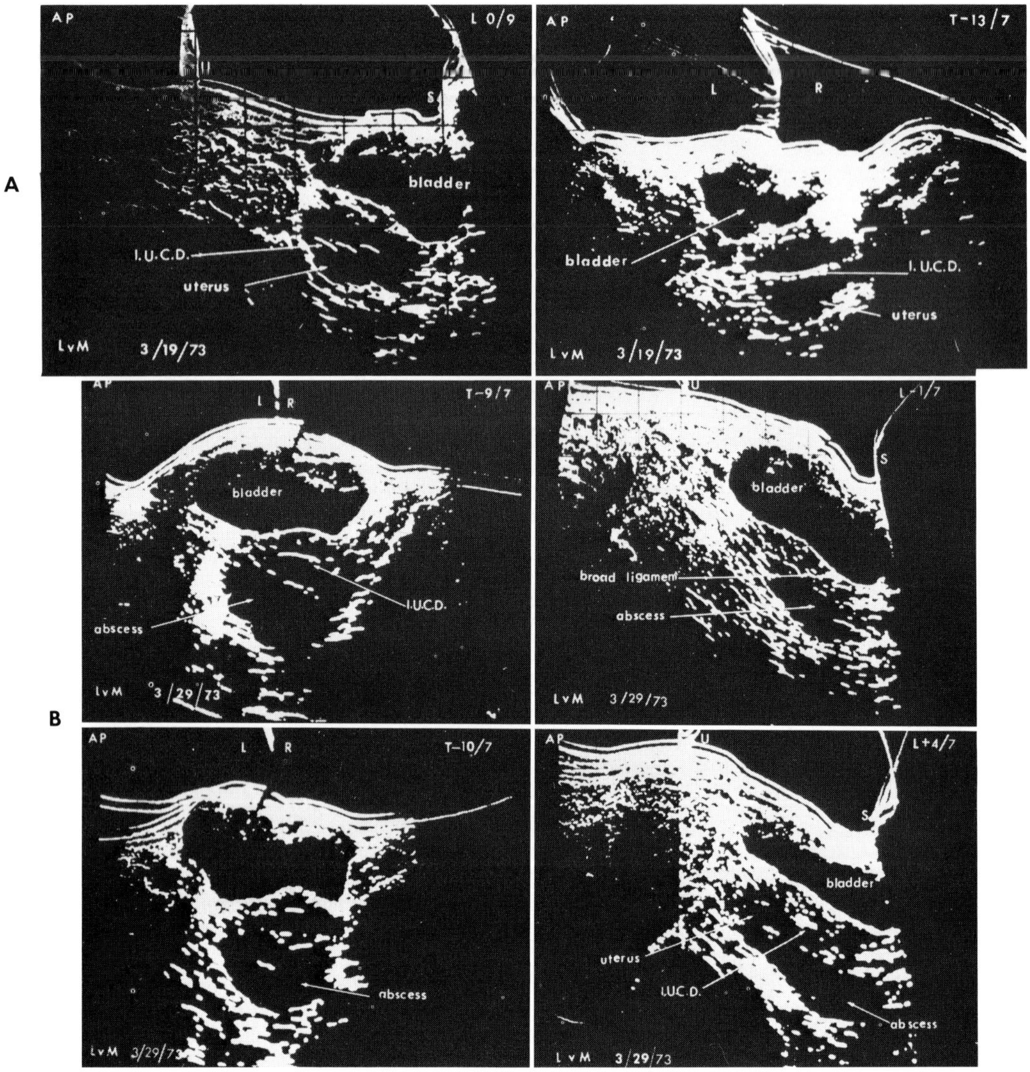

Fig. 11-5. Patient presented with chief complaint of lower abdominal pain and fever. Palpatory findings were difficult because of marked obesity and muscle guarding. **A,** Sonogynecograms show the characteristic echo pattern of an intrauterine contraceptive device within the endometrial cavity. There was no other sonographically discernable pathologic condition. **B,** Repeat scans performed on the same patient 10 days later revealed a massive cul-de-sac abscess.

amination, x-ray, or other diagnostic procedures (Fig. 11-5).

Precise localization and quantitative mapping of pelvic-abdominal masses

Precise localization and quantitative mapping of malignant pelvic-abdominal masses facilitates the staging of disease, the accurate positioning of radiation ports, and the detection of recurrence.[13] Sonographic survey of the pelvis for the "lost IUD syndrome" not only indicates the intra- or extrauterine position of the device but may be of considerable assistance in

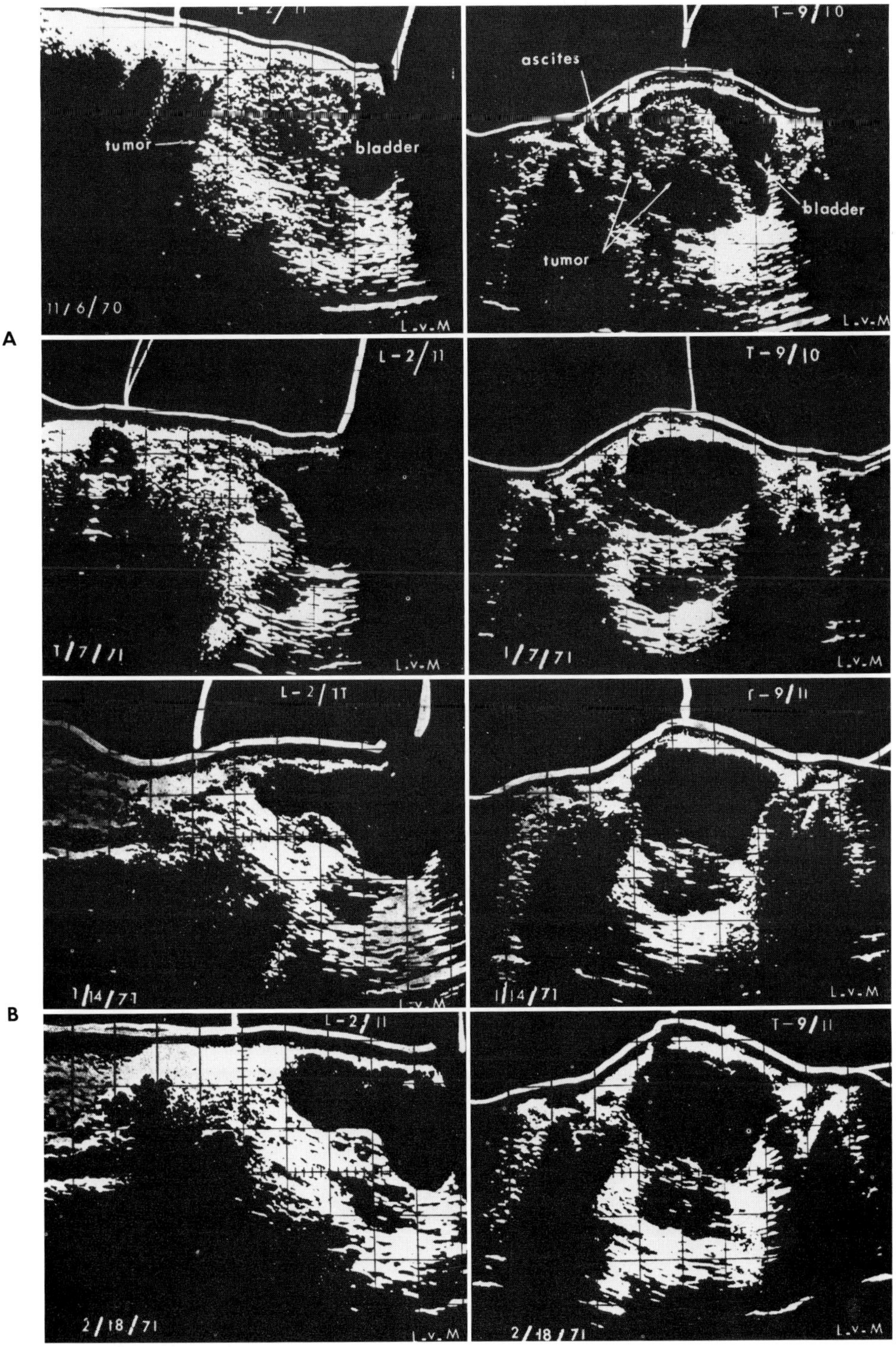

Fig. 11-6. Patient developed primary solid adenocarcinoma of the ovary after total abdominal hysterectomy. Serial sonographic studies objectively document the marked reduction of tumor size under the effect of cytotoxic drugs. Note the areas of necrosis in the neoplasm and the persistence of ascites in the cul-de-sac.

choosing the optimal operative approach for its removal (Fig. 11-5). Serial sonographic studies permit (1) the assessment of tumor growth, (2) the objective appraisal of the effects of hormonal, chemical, or radiation therapy (Fig. 11-6), and (3) the monitoring of the dimensional changes of hematoma, abscesses, ascites, peritoneal fluid, and lymphocysts. Sonographic determination of the size of pelvic inflammatory masses, the delineation of their cystic and solid components, the documentation of the rupture of a hydrosalpinx, and tubo-ovarian cyst or abscess may serve as valuable guidelines for conservative versus surgical management (Fig. 11-5).

Distinguishing between cystic and solid tumors

While differentiation of ovarian cysts from fibroids on pelvic examination can be a vexing problem for the gynecologist, their identification by sonographic means can be successfully accomplished in the majority of cases. Based on observations of other investigators in the field of diagnostic ultrasound and on experience gained in the Bio-acoustical Laboratory of Woman's Hospital, five major criteria have been established for the differential diagnosis of cystic from solid pelvic masses.[9] These are:

1. Topographic relation of the pathologic structure to the uterus
2. Margination of the mass toward surrounding organs and tissue planes
3. Character of the wall-content (cysts) or capsule-substance (solid tumor) interface
4. Nature of internal texture and its alteration with change in sensitivity or frequency
5. Degree of transonicity (range of pene-

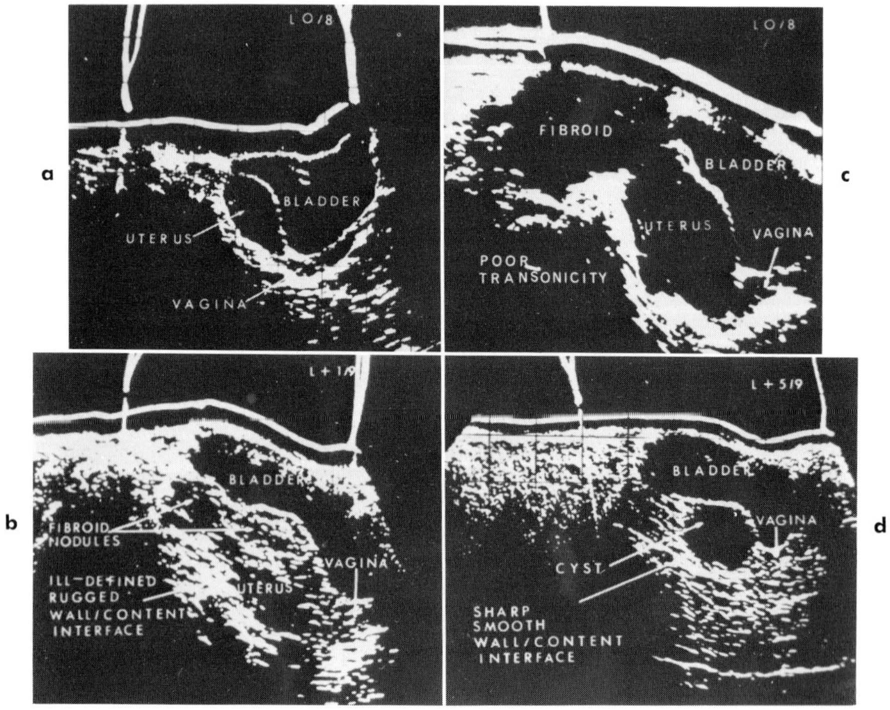

Fig. 11-7. Differential diagnostic criteria 1, 3, and 4 (see text) for distinguishing between cystic and solid tumors.

tration of the incident beam through the mass)

Topographic relation to uterus. The first clue to the nature of the pelvic mass is provided by its topographic relation to the uterus. The sonogynecograms shown on Fig. 11-3 are representative of an extensive study performed on a patient with the clinical diagnosis of bilateral tubo-ovarian cysts subsequent to chronic pelvic inflammatory disease. There is a definite separation of the cyst from the uterus and at no level does the cystic structure appear to be part of the uterus or continuous with the vagina. In contradistinction, the large fundal fibroid on sonogram *c* in Fig. 11-7 is definitely continuous with the uterus and could not be shown separated from it in any of the scanning planes. It has to be emphasized, however, that the separation of the pathologic structures from the uterus should be visualized at multiple scanning planes in order to accept the existence of a true division.[9] Positive identification of the uterus is obviously a prerequisite to fulfill this criterion and, if the organ is distorted or malpositioned, may in itself present a difficult problem.

Margination characteristics. While benign cystic tumors are generally sharply marginated toward the surrounding organs and tissue planes, the interface between solid tumors and surrounding tissues is usually poorly defined. The fibroid tumor shown on sonograms *a* and *b* in Fig. 11-8 is a characteristic example of the poor margination of a solid tumor toward the adjacent tissue planes. The cranial borders of the mass toward the zone of intestinal echoes are ill-defined or nonexistent, and even the bladder-mass interface is poorly delimited and fragmentary. The bladder acts as a contrast organ delineating profile irregularities on the ventral aspect of

a

c

b

d

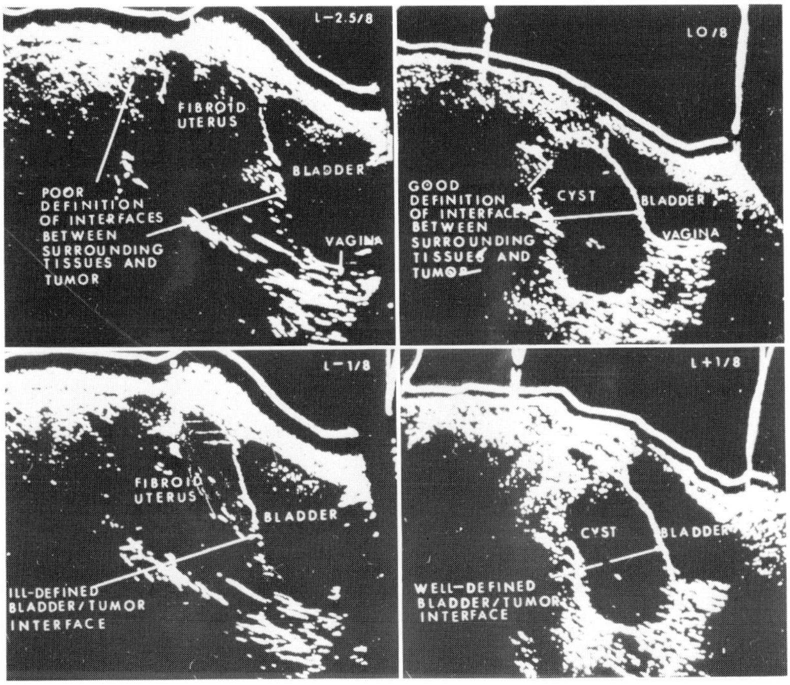

Fig. 11-8. Different margination characteristics of cystic and solid tumors toward the surrounding organs and tissue planes.

the uterus (Fig. 11-7, *B*).[12] Sonograms *c* and *d* in Fig. 11-8 demonstrate the typical margination characteristics of a benign cyst. The bladder-cyst interface is complete, smooth, and even; the junction between the cyst and intestine is also sharply marginated.

Character of the wall-content interface. While the wall-content interface of the solid tumor is generally ill defined and rugged, that of the cyst is usually sharp and smooth. Note on sonograms *c* and *d* in Fig. 11-8 the clear separation of the cyst wall from the anechoic content.

Internal texture. At normal sensitivity settings the internal texture of the solid tumor shows randomly distributed sono-opaque speckling superimposed on an anechoic background in the majority of the cases. With the use of identical acoustic and electronic parameters, the cystic tumor should be uniformly anechoic except for the occasional presence of septae or other solid components. It is also noteworthy that the appearance of the internal texture of the solid mass is dependent on the sensitivity and frequency of the transducer used, whereas that of a cystic tumor is independent. This means that as the sensitivity or the frequency is increased, the solid tumor should become increasingly sono-opaque (with both the density and coarseness of the speckling increasing), whereas the cystic tumor will remain anechoic. While in the majority of ultrasonic departments attenuation studies constitute the keystone for differentiating between cysts and solid tumors, some utilize multiple frequency scanning for the elucidation of the consistency of the mass.[1]

Transonicity. It is a well-known fact that both the incident and the reflected beam are more highly attenuated by a solid medium than a fluid medium. Sonograms *a, b,* and *c* in Fig. 11-9 illustrate the poor penetration of the incident beam through a fibroid tumor: the dorsal wall contours are fragmentary and the acoustic illumination of structures beyond the dorsal limit of the mass is poor or altogether absent. Sonograms *d, e,* and *f* in Fig. 11-9 demonstrate the excellent transonicity of a serous cystoma of the ovary: complete dorsal wall contour and visualization of all the structures out to the skin of the buttocks.

Although in most cases the majority of criteria will favor either cyst or solid tumor, there are certain conditions that may cause diagnostic errors. A homogeneously degenerated fibroid tumor may exhibit a great number of the characteristics of cysts.[1,8,10] If extreme care is taken, however, to show that it is actually part of the uterus, this pitfall can be avoided.[9] Dermoid cysts, lipoid cell tumors and malignant cysts fall into the same category, and their sonographic properties will be discussed under appropriate headings.

Determining the uterine, ovarian, or tubal origin of pelvic neoplasms and forecasting probable malignancy

Uterine masses. The sonographic appearance of fibroids will vary considerably, depending on their size and location and the absence or presence of degenerative processes to which these neoplasms are subject. The major diagnostic features are enlarged uterine size, irregular uterine profile, nodular architecture, poor margination and wall-content interface characteristics, and low degree of transonicity. At normal sensitivity settings their internal texture may be uniformly anechoic, but in the majority of cases it is characterized by fine, discrete, randomly distributed sono-opaque speckling. The coarseness of speckling increases as the size of the histologic components of the fibroid approaches or exceeds the size of the wavelength of ultrasound. This is particularly well seen in cellular leiomyomas and may be the cause of misdiagnosing them as hydatidiform moles.[4,14] The coarse "snowflake" pattern indicates wider separation of the fibrous grid caused by the increased cellular popu-

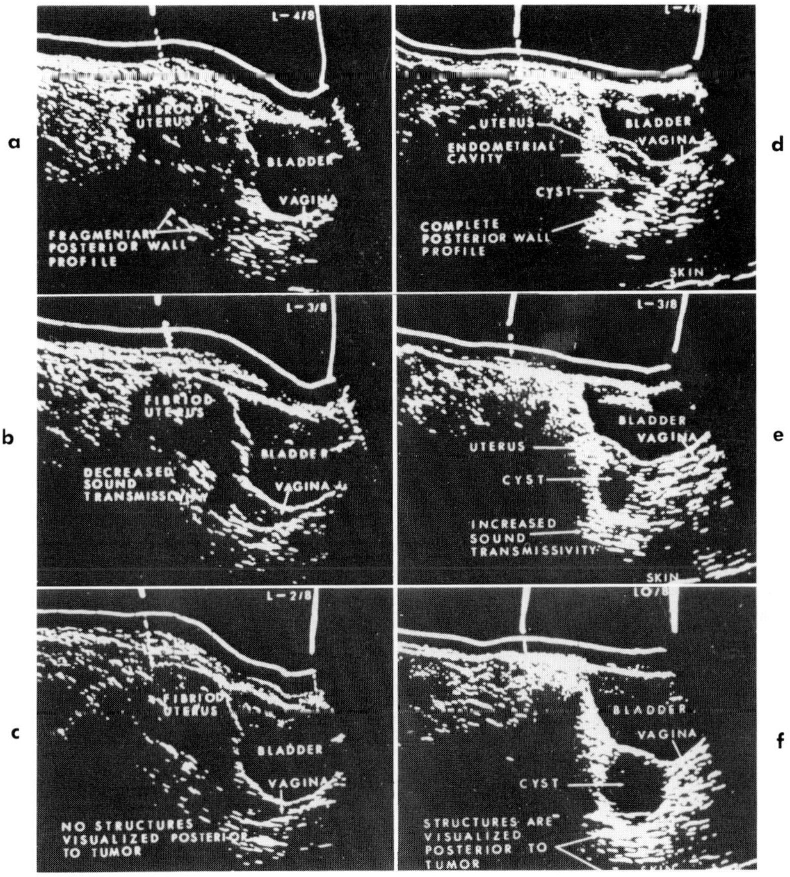

Fig. 11-9. Difference in degree of transonicity between cystic and solid tumors.

lation.[4] On increasing the sensitivity, all fibroids show increase in the coarseness and density of the sono-opaque speckling (Kobayashi's "fill-in" pattern).[4,10,15,16] For unknown reasons, fibroids in the cul-de sac may show a negative fill-in pattern even if they are not completely degenerated, and they frequently have been mistaken for cysts.[10]

Organized echo patterns within the homogeneous internal texture signify various types of degeneration. While the transonicity increases with hyaline and cystic degeneration and in cases of necrobiosis, diffuse calcification causes poor transonicity or outright acoustic shadowing. Myxomatous degeneration with a finely speckled internal texture may lead to the false diagnosis of hydatidiform mole.[1] Small intramural fibroid nodules should be differentiated from adenomyosis. The salient features for differentiation are as follows: adenomyotic foci cause less distortion of the uterine profile; they are generally smaller than fibroid nodules; and they are mostly intramural and located near the endometrial cavity.[7]

Distinguishing subserous fibroid nodules, particularly the pedunculated ones, from solid ovarian tumors is not always feasible at the present stage of development. Even more confusion can arise with large pedunculated fibroid nodules that irritate the peritoneal surface and are

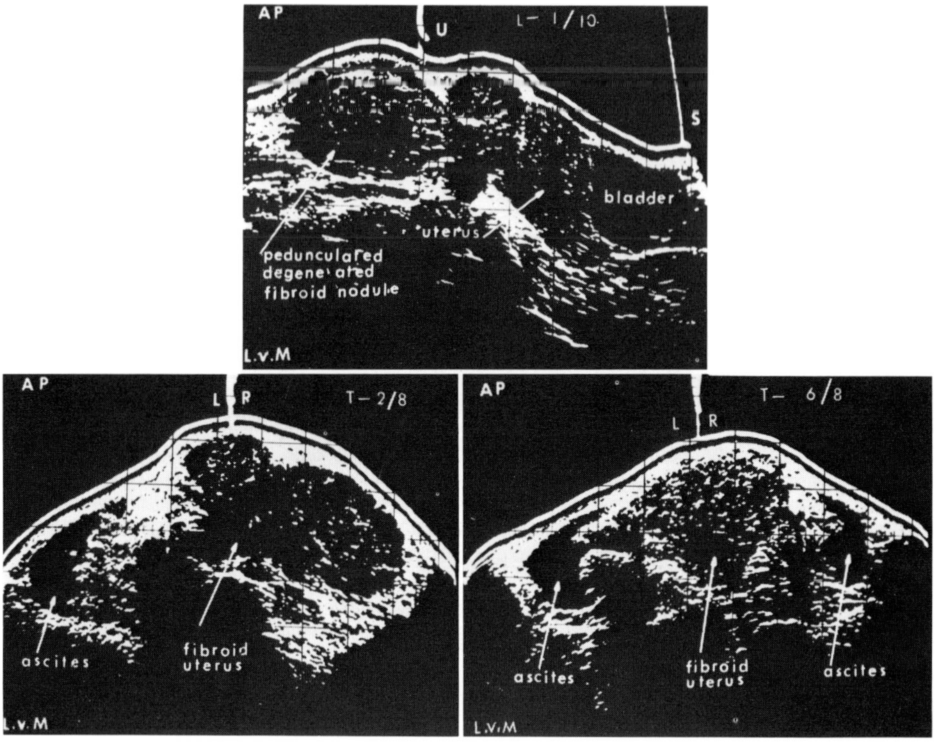

Fig. 11-10. Huge, pedunculated, degenerated, fundal fibroid associated with ascites.

occasionally associated with ascites (Fig. 11-10).

Leiomyosarcoma, carcinosarcoma, and mixed mesodermal tumors show a sonographic appearance similar to fibroids, with the exception that they exhibit large areas of degeneration (because of hemorrhagic necrosis within the mass), bizarre patches of high-intensity echoes (heterogeneous tumor components), and invasive margination characteristics, and they are frequently associated with loculated malignant ascites (Fig. 11-11). While complete or fragmentary contours of nodules are frequently demonstrable around or near the areas of degeneration in fibroids, the internal texture of these tumors does not reveal any nodular structures, and the areas of variable transonicity greatly differ both in configuration and in dimensions.[14,17]

Fig. 11-12 depicts an endometrial carcinoma with metastasis to the anterior abdominal wall. The uterus is irregularly shaped and markedly enlarged. The bizarre aggregates of high-intensity echoes within the endometrial cavity represent polypoid growth of adenocarcinoma. In spite of the presence of serosanguineous fluid in the endometrial cavity, the transonicity of the uterine mass is poor. The greatly reduced penetrability is particularly evident on the T series of scans. Invasion of the myometrium and extension to the parametria and to surrounding organs can also be demonstrated sonographically.[11] In the absence of clinical information, adenomatous hyperplasia, endometrial polyps, unrecognized missed abortion, and retained secundine are some of the conditions that should be considered in the sonographic differential

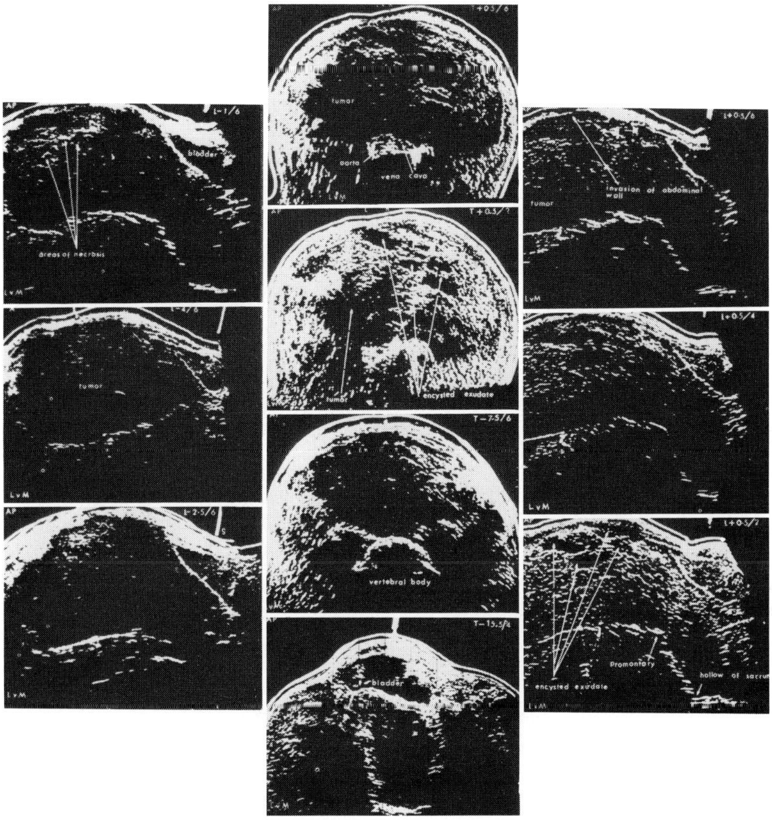

Fig. 11-11. Massive spread of leiomyosarcoma to surrounding organs and abdominal wall. The moderate to good transonicity can be ascribed to the multiple areas of degeneration within the tumor. Note cribriform pattern of encysted malignant ascites.

diagnosis of the cancer of the uterine corpus.

Carcinoma of the cervix can be diagnosed by transabdominal scans only if the parametria are involved and there is a marked extension to the pelvic wall (Stage III or Stage IV). Transvesical pelvic sonography, to be discussed later, can identify Stage I and Stage II carcinomas of the cervix. This procedure is, however, still in an experimental stage and is not performed on a regular clinical basis.

Ovarian masses. The gross morphology, architecture, and consistency of ovarian tumors are subject to great variation. Describing all the distinguishing features of the various pathologic entitites is beyond the scope of this chapter; some differential diagnostic criteria can, however, be stated.

Follicular cysts and serous cystadenomas are generally unilocular, uniformly anechoic, and markedly transonic (Fig. 11-13). Mucinous cystadenomas usually have a multicompartmental architecture and lack the reverberation artifact along their ventral border (negative Staiano's sign).[9] Papillary cystadenomas show multiform conglomerates of fine speckling projecting into the cyst lumen. If the papillation extends outside the cyst wall (reliably recognizable only if ascites is also present), they should be considered potentially malignant.[14,18]

The sonographic diagnosis of ovarian

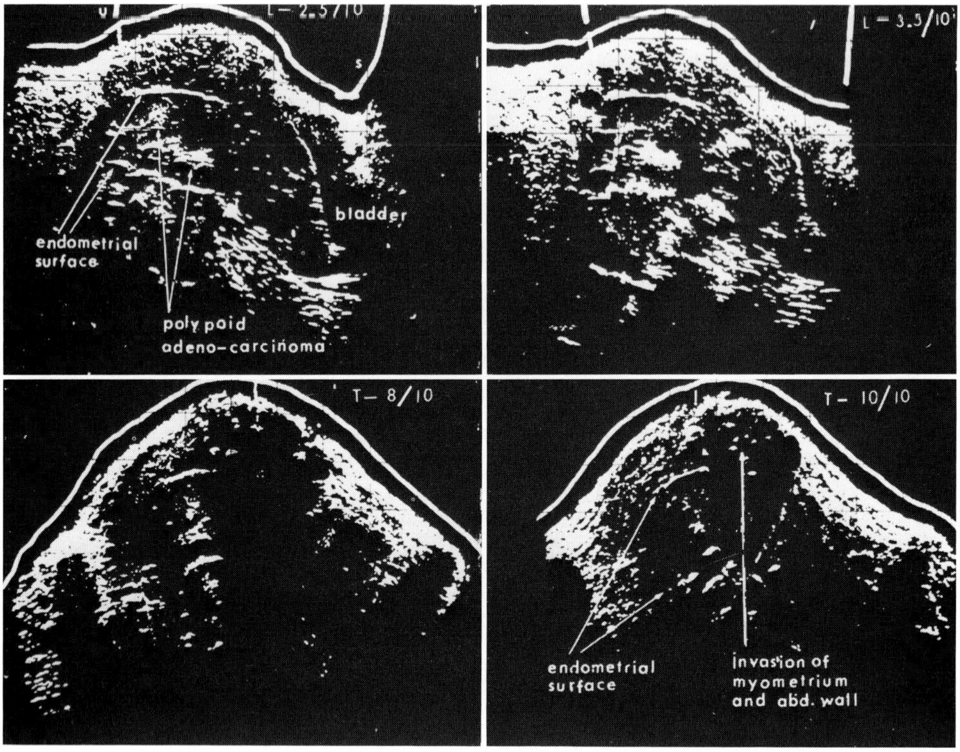

Fig. 11-12. Stage IV endometrial carcinoma.

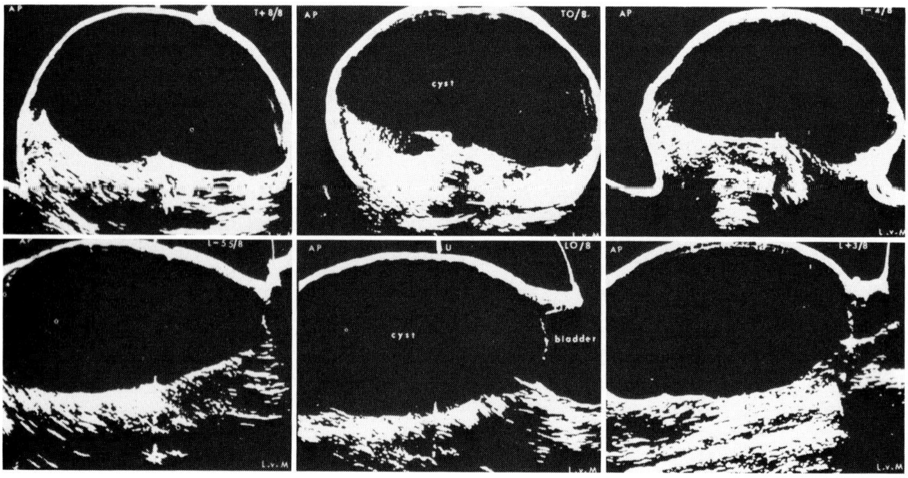

Fig. 11-13. Immense serous cystadenoma in a 15-year-old girl. Note narrow band of reverberation artifact on L + 3 sonogram (Staiano's sign).

malignancy is subject to considerable difficulty. In Sunden's opinion: "It is not possible by means of ultrasound examination to obtain any impression of the histologic structure of a cystic ovarian tumor."[8] Donald states: "As a general rule, the more complex the echo pattern within an ovarian cyst, the greater the suspicion of malignancy, but it is most unwise to attempt an opinion whether a cyst is benign or malignant on ultrasonic findings,"[1] and Kratochwil concludes: "An unequivocal diagnosis of malignancy by ultrasonic examination is not possible at this time. Only the tumor pattern is regarded as suspicious of malignancy."[19] Thompson, while listing several sonographic features suggestive of malignancy, emphasizes that these characteristics relate to the invasiveness of the tumor and have nothing to do with the intrinsic cellular characteristics and architecture of the malignancy.[18]

While it is true that transabdominal scans cannot provide histologic diagnosis and that the detection of small mitotic processes is beyond the modality's present capabilities, advanced malignancy, in our experience, can be identified by sonogynecography in the majority of cases.[7] Kobayashi's and Morley's publications appear to support this view.[10,14] Fig. 11-14 demonstrates the sonic phenotype, and the accompanying legend lists the major morphologic and acoustico-optic characteristics of pseudomucinous cystadenocarcinomas.

The great variability in the macroscopic appearance of teratomas defies any attempt to assign a pattern characterizing the entire group; similar and often dis-

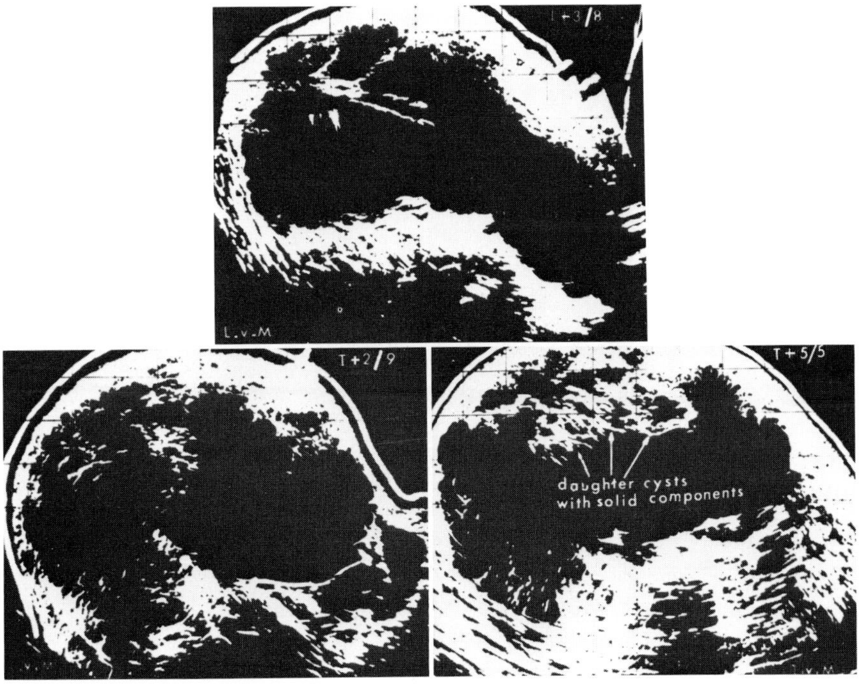

Fig. 11-14. Multilocular pseudomucinous cystadenocarcinoma. Poor margination, invasive wall-content interface, bizarre cluster of daughter cysts, uneven septae interspersed with irregularly spaced solid components, and absence of reverberation artifact (negative Staiano's sign) are the sonographic hallmarks of a pseudomucinous cystadenocarcinoma.

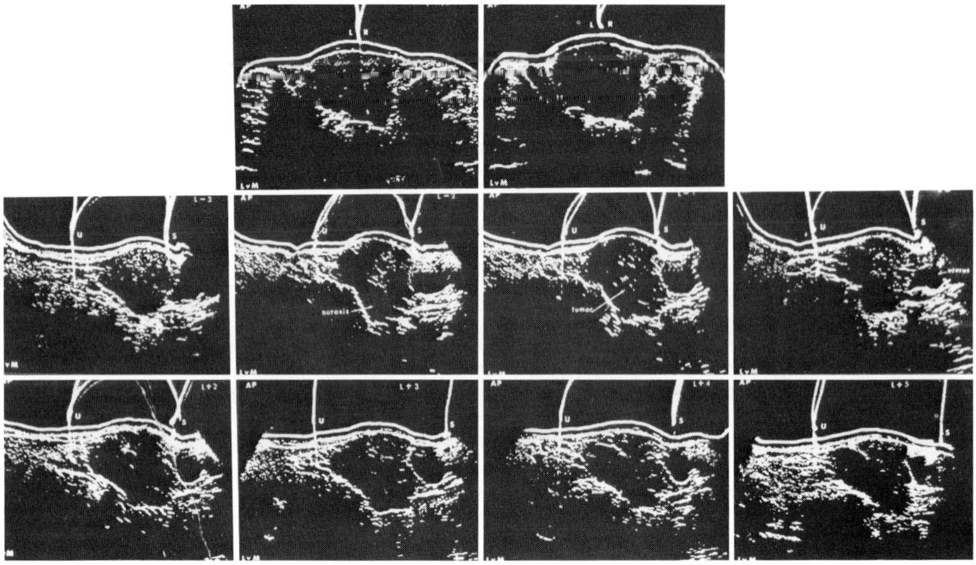

Fig. 11-15. This irregular, solid mass occupying the left adnexal region exhibits a lobular contour and multiple areas of necrosis. Sonographic diagnosis was solid ovarian tumor, ruling out retroperitoneal tumor. Pathologic diagnosis was dysgerminoma.

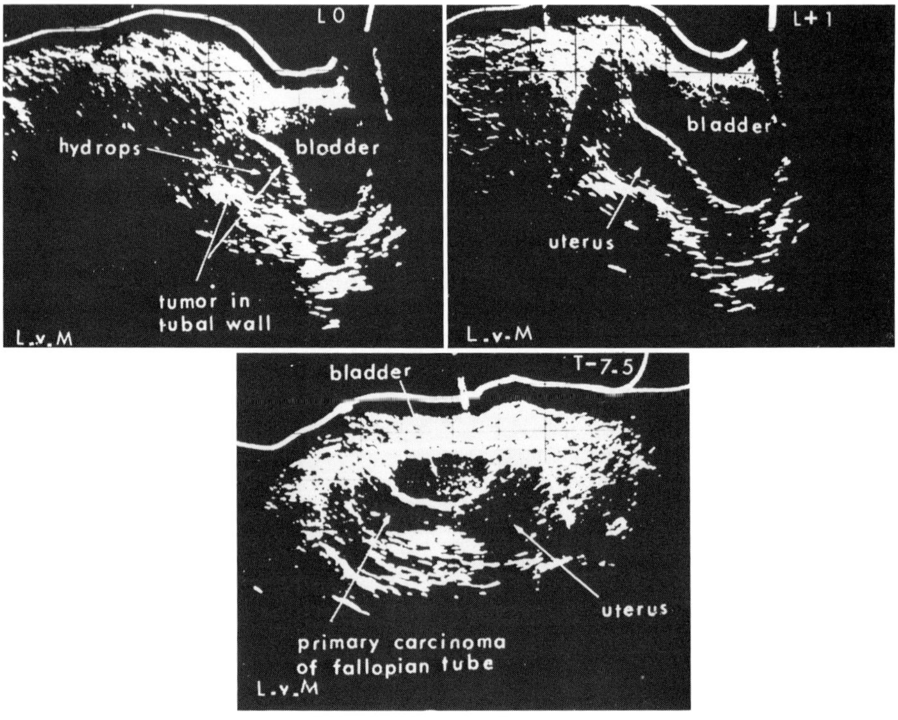

Fig. 11-16. Primary carcinoma of the fallopian tube.

tinctive sonographic properties can, however, be found within the subcategories of these tumors. A benign cystic teratoma, an embryonal carcinoma, and a teratoma associated with pseudomucinous cystadenoma have been described elsewhere.[20-22]

Ovarian fibromas and fibroadenomas cannot be sonographically differentiated from intact or degenerated pedunculated fibroids.[14] Solid malignant tumors of the ovary do not produce a pattern characteristic of malignancy.[18] Granulosa cell tumors frequently show small rounded interlacing necrotic areas or small cystic masses within their internal texture, but their precise identification is not possible.[8] The sonograms shown in Fig. 11-15 depict a dysgerminoma. In the absence of a meticulous attempt to identify the uterus as a separate structure, this lobulated solid mass can be easily confused with a nodular uterine fibroid.

The least common malignancy of the female reproductive organs is the primary carcinoma of the fallopian tube. The characteristic features include a unilateral sausage-shaped adnexal mass, markedly thickened and irregular bladder-mass interface, thick tumor-infiltrated wall, and fluid-filled lumen. History of hydrops tubae profluens in a geriatric patient associated with the preceding sonographic findings confirms the diagnosis (Fig. 11-16). In the absence of this, salpingitis isthmica nodosa, old tubal pregnancy, and tubal tuberculosis should enter into the differential diagnostic considerations.[7]

Differentiation of adnexal tumors from other pelvic conditions simulating ovarian or tubal neoplasms

Cystic masses not associated with pregnancy. Paraovarian cysts make up approximately 10% of all adnexal growths in the 30- to 40-year age group. Expanding between the leaves of the broad ligament, they are always located lateral to the uterus. At first they cause a contralateral displacement and rotation and later a marked elevation of this organ. The nonspheroid unilocular cystic mass is closely juxtaposed to the uterus and appears to have a continuous contour with it. The bladder-cyst and wall-content interfaces are sharp and smooth. The serous cyst content is manifested by the anechoic internal texture, Staiano's artifact, and marked transonicity (Fig. 11-17).[7,8]

Because of their bizarre sonic phenotype, endometrial cysts of the ovary may closely mimic cystadenocarcinomas. Although their frequent coexistence with external endometriosis and adenomyosis may provide some clues, their exact identity cannot be deduced from ultrasonic examination (Fig. 11-18).[7,8]

The inflammatory lesions of the tubes and ovaries show great morphologic variety, depending on the nature of the causative organism and on the acute or chronic stage of the disease. In cases of gonococcal infections occlusion of the distal extremity of the tube is the rule with the resultant pyosalpinx or hydrosalpinx. The usually bilateral tubular masses originating from the cornual region generally occupy the adnexal regions or the cul-de-sac in the beginning, but then because of secondary infections, they become large and may extend to the middle or upper abdomen. The sausage- or retort-shaped masses of pyosalpinx or hydrosalpinx are usually unilocular but may appear multicompartmental as the scanning path transects several convolutions in the same plane. The thickness, smoothness, or ruggedness of the bladder-mass interface, the anechoic or speckled internal texture, and the degree of transonicity provide additional data for discriminating between the acute and chronic stages of the disease.[3,7,10] Unequivocal sonographic differentiation between pyosalpinx and tubo-ovarian abscess or between hydrosalpinx and tubo-ovarian cysts is not yet feasible (Figs. 11-3, 11-19, and 11-20).

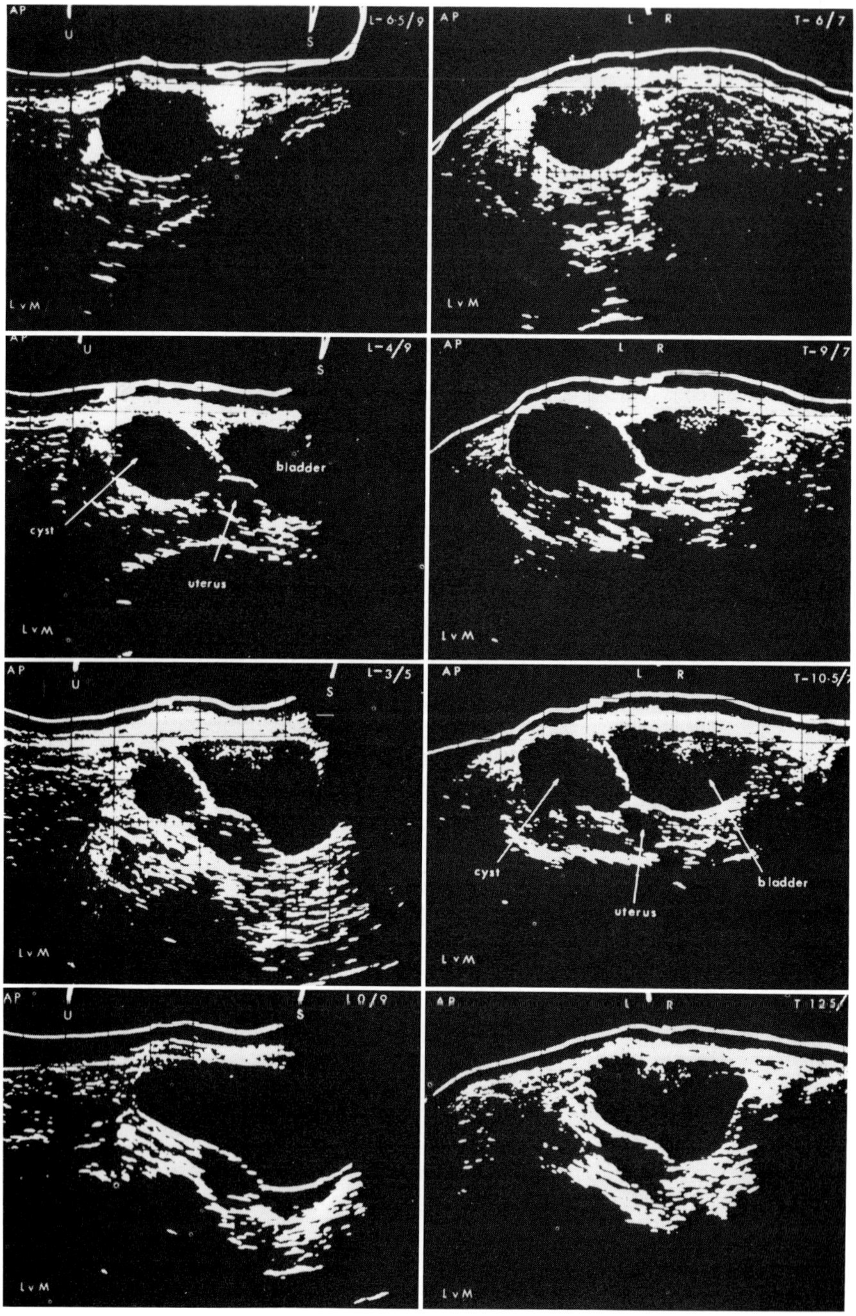

Fig. 11-17. Paraovarian cyst.

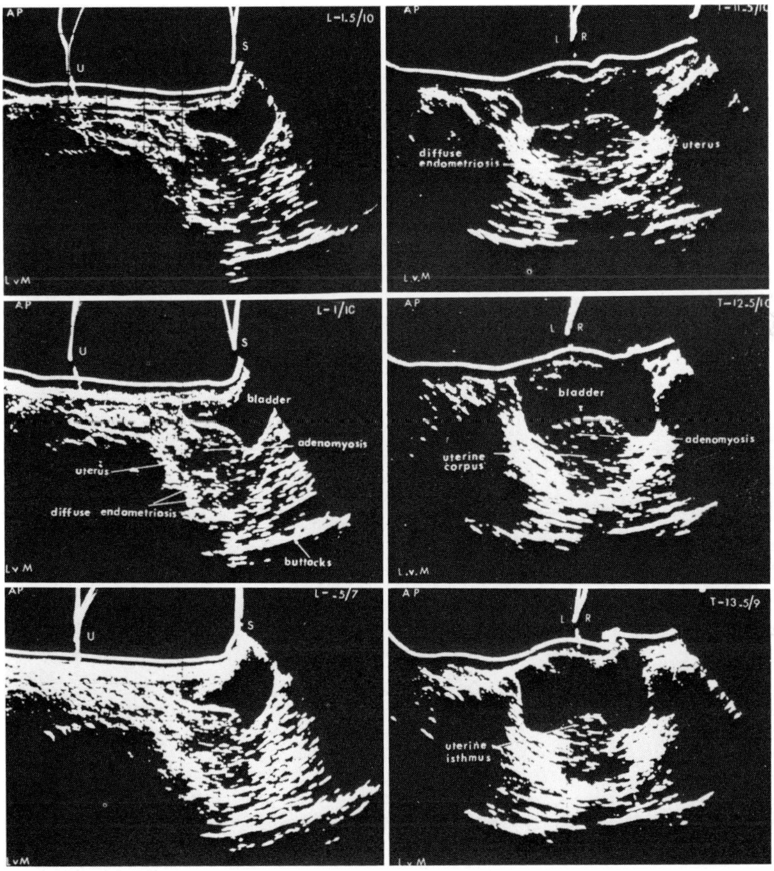

Fig. 11-18. Pelvic endometriosis and adenomyosis. These sonograms represent a classic example of the sonographic phenotype of both conditions.

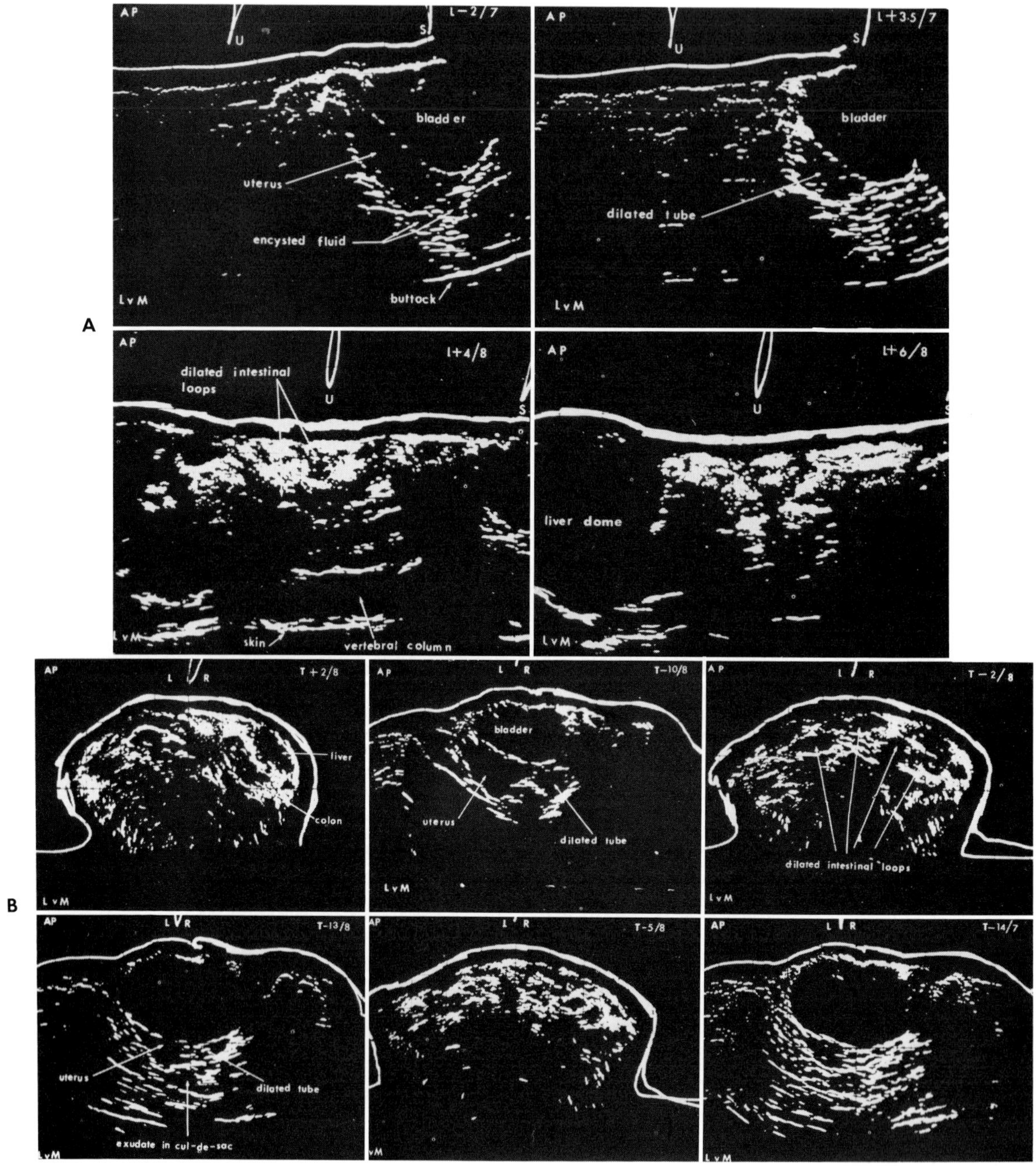

Fig. 11-19. The right-sided sausage-shaped mass with speckled internal texture and thickened wall is a pyosalpinx. The dilated intestinal loops and marked transonicity noted throughout the abdominal cavity are indicative of a paralytic ileus secondary to pelveoperitonitis.

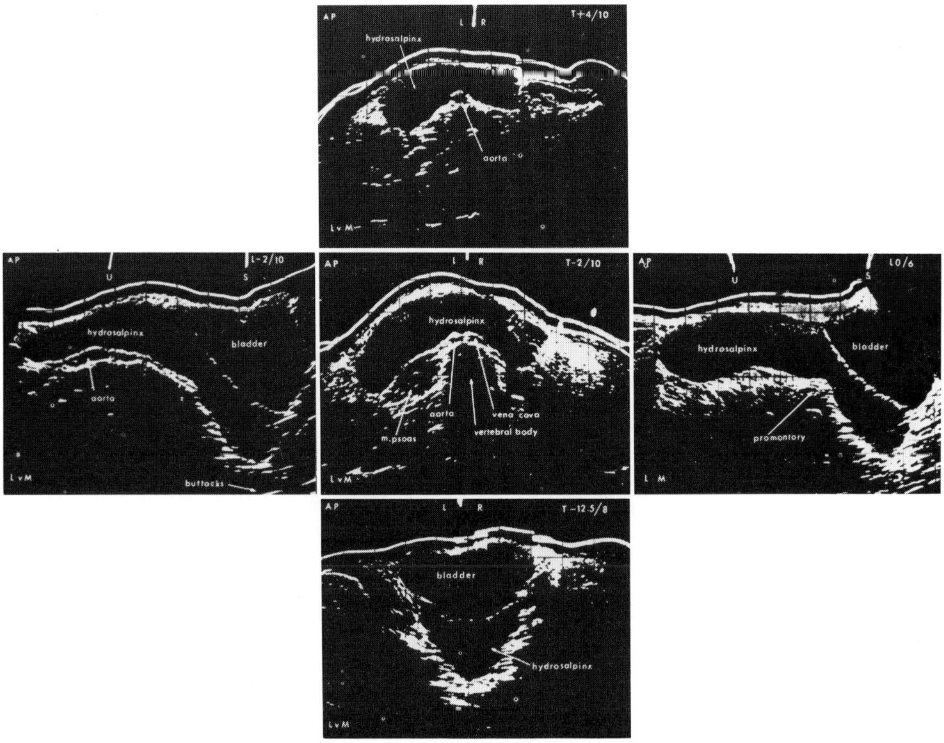

Fig. 11-20. Immense hydrosalpinx following total abdominal hysterectomy. The narrow band of fine speckling along the ventral border of the cystic mass is reverberation artifact indicating serous content (Staiano's sign). The indentation of the mass by the bladder on both the T and L sonograms suggests low internal pressure and a practically impalpable flaccid mass.

Cul-de-sac and other pelvic abscesses not contained within a preformed space have distinctly discernible morphologic and sonographic characteristics (Fig. 11-5, *B*).[7,10] Other conditions that should be borne in mind include hematometra (vaginal atresia or absence of vagina), pyometra (conglutination of the cervical os, endometrial carcinoma), hematocele secondary to bleeding follicle (Fig. 11-21), peritoneal cysts, lymphocysts, carcinomatosis peritonei (Fig. 11-22), mesenteric cysts, pancreatic pseudocysts, and oversized hydronephrosis.[6,10] On many occasions an overdistended bladder (neurogenic, acute retention in a 3-degree retroverted and fixed pregnant uterus) has been mistaken for cyst. When in doubt, the patient should be catheterized and the scan repeated.

Cystic masses associated with pregnancy. Unruptured ampullary pregnancy or ruptured tubal pregnancy with hematocele between the leaves of the broad ligament can closely mimic neoplastic or inflammatory lesions of the ovaries and tubes (Fig. 11-23). Interstitial pregnancy may simulate an adherent adnexal mass.[23] The pregnant cornu of a bicornuate uterus might be misdiagnosed during the first trimester as a semisolid ovarian mass or degenerated fibroid.[23]

Lutein cysts associated with hydatidiform mole may become another source of erroneous diagnosis of neoplastic ovarian disease if the amount of molar tissue is minimal.[7,23,24]

Solid masses. The following conditions have been misdiagnosed by ultrasonog-

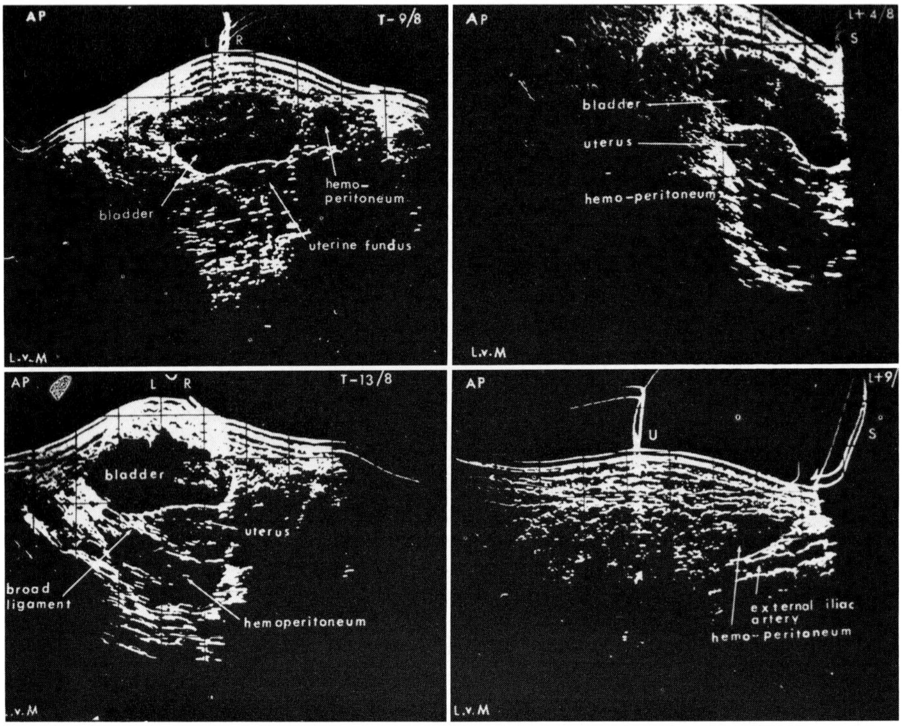

Fig. 11-21. Hemoperitoneum secondary to bleeding follicle. The triangular-shaped anechoic area anterior to the large vessels and psoas muscle in the lateral gutter exhibiting sharp ventral and dorsocaudal but ill-defined cranial margins (von Micsky's sign[23]) suggests intraperitoneal fluid accumulation in excess of 200 to 300 ml.

A

B

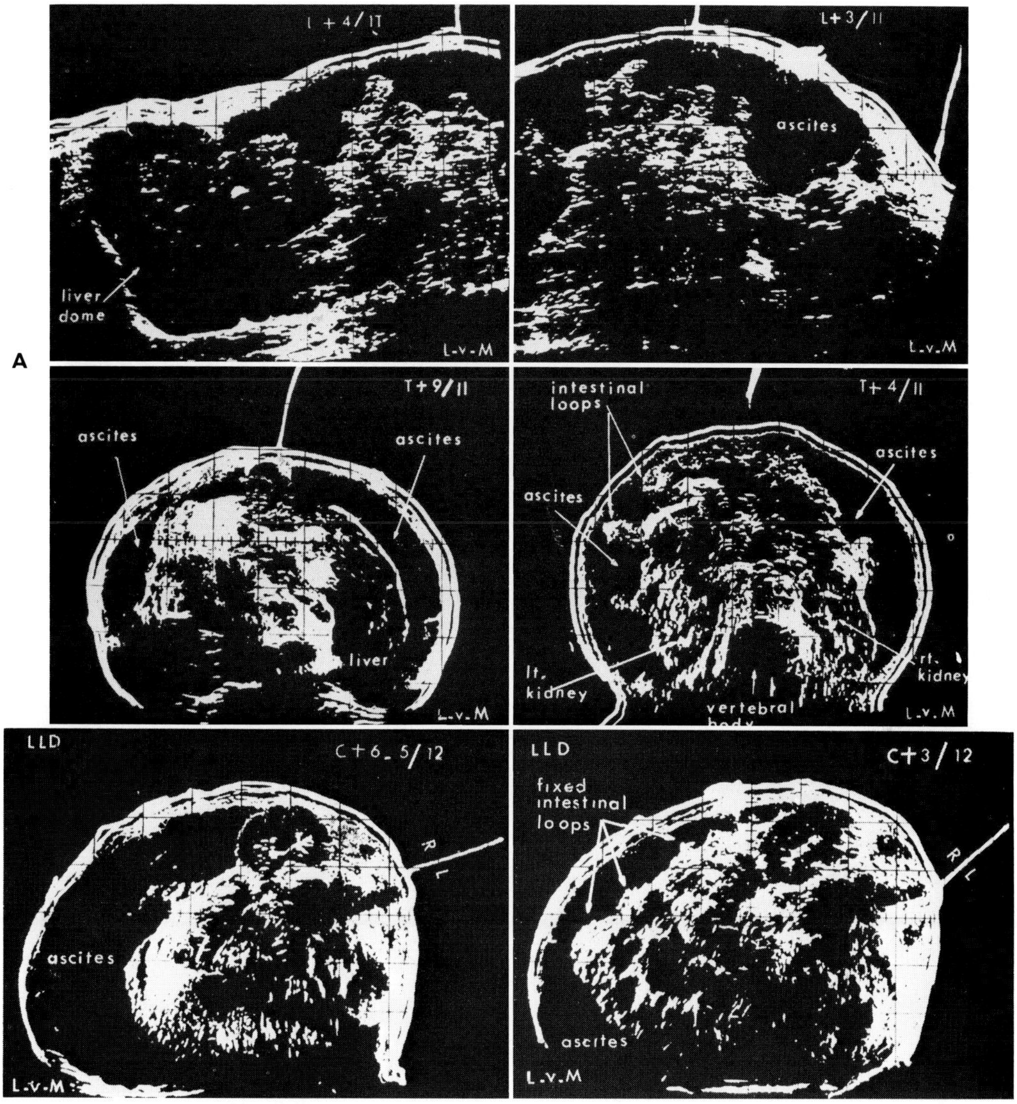

Fig. 11-22. Carcinomatosis peritonei. **A,** The vast expanses of anechoic areas located ventrally to the bowel and the bizarre contour of the intestinal loops highlighted by the ascitic fluid suggest malignant ascites. The discrete aggregates of high-intensity echoes within the liver parenchyma suggest intrinsic lesion, most probably metastasis. **B,** The anechoic areas in the flank and the apparent floating up of all the intestines toward the midline noted on sonogram T + 4 on **A,** cast some doubt as to the malignant nature of the ascites. The original assumption that the intestines are adherent to the dorsal abdominal wall is confirmed by the fact that there is no change in the intestinal echo pattern on the LLD echograms.

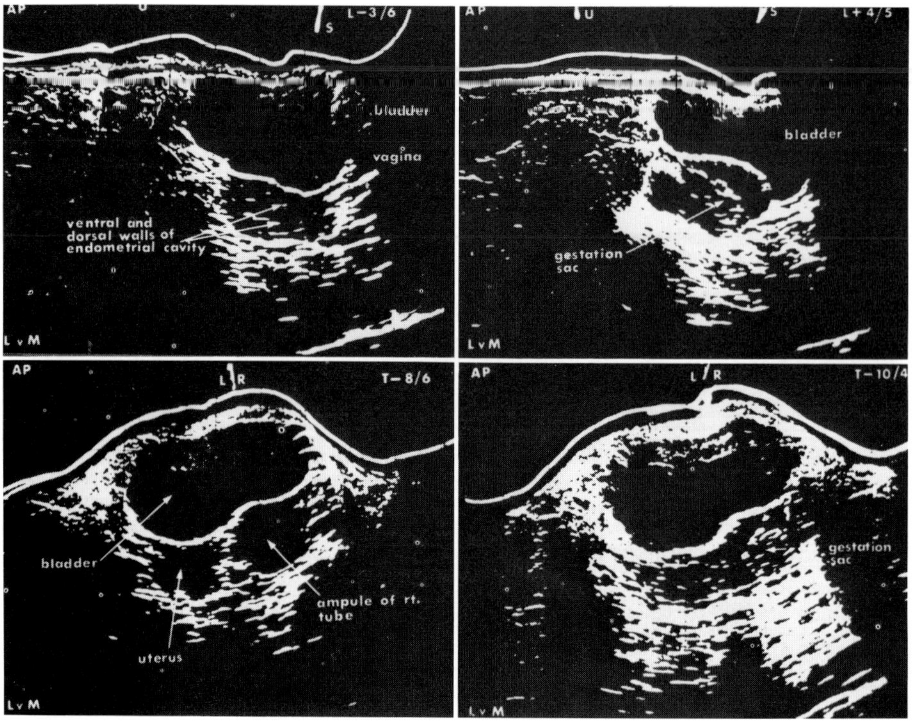

Fig. 11-23. Unruptured tubal pregnancy. Occupying the right adnexal region is an irregularly shaped sonolucent mass in which the fragmentary contours of the gestation sac are visualized. Note the marked burst of transonicity dorsal to the ampullary portion of the right tube. The separated decidual cast within the endometrial cavity may give the false impression of intrauterine pregnancy.

raphy for ovarian neoplasms: impacted feces, adherent bowel and omentum secondary to previous surgery (Fig. 11-24), low-lying cecum, redundant sigmoid colon, and carcinoma of the cecum or sigmoid. On the other hand, based on meticulous multiplane, multisensitivity scannings, malignant retroperitoneal tumors and pelvic kidneys were readily differentiated from ovarian neoplasms (Fig. 11-25).

Documentation of bladder, rectum, liver, lung, and brain metastases of pelvic tumors

Metastatic neoplastic masses within the sonolucent liver are seen as irregularly shaped, bizarre aggregates of coarse high-intensity echoes. Uniform replacement of liver substance by tumor tissue is a more difficult diagnostic problem. Sonohepatography should always be performed in cases of pelvic carcinomatosis since radiotherapy is generally witheld if the liver is grossly involved.[1]

Fig. 11-26 depicts the primary lesion and a massive pleural effusion caused by lung metastasis. Sonograms of brain metastasis secondary to squamous carcinoma of the cervix have been published elsewhere.[2]

Transabdominal sonograms can reveal only very advanced metastatic lesions of the bladder and rectum. Endoscanning methods offer the hope of detecting infiltrations of the vesicouterine ligaments and rectovaginal septum at a considerably earlier stage.[3,19,25]

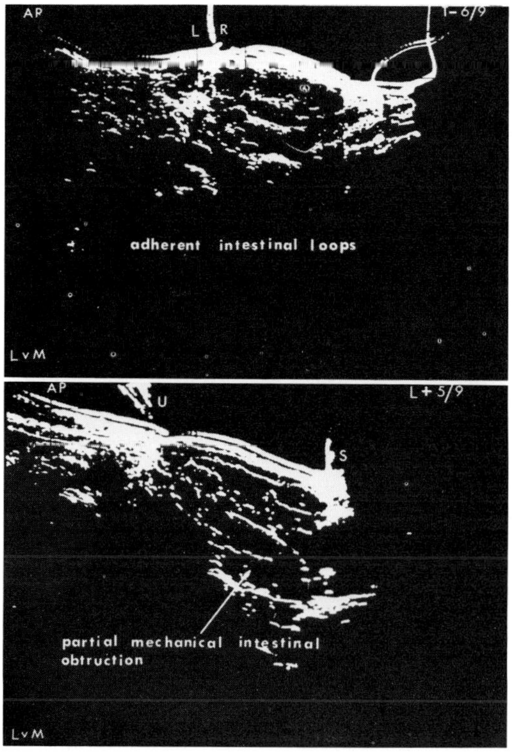

Fig. 11-24. Adherent intestinal loops and omentum may present on palpation as an irregular matted mass and give the impression of a pelvic tumor.

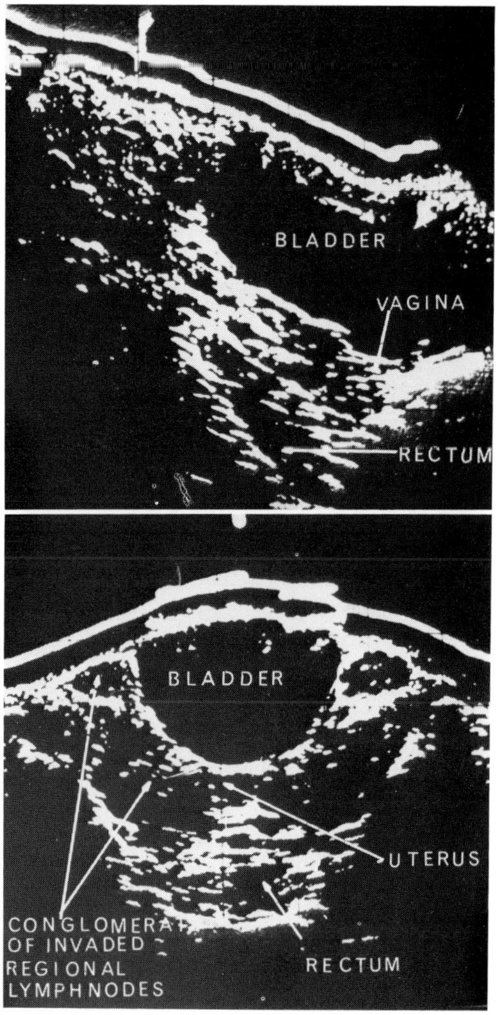

Fig. 11-25. Patient with known chronic lymphatic leukemia developed bilateral hydronephrosis and frozen pelvis, suggesting the possibility of secondary primary lesion in the pelvis. Sonogram showed large conglomerates of invaded regional lymph nodes; biopsy revealed reticulum-cell sarcoma.

DISCUSSION

Rapid progress over the past few years in ultrasonic instrumentation has advanced the production of an interpretable sonogram from a research experience to a routine clinical procedure. The main difficulty now lies in identifying, cataloging, and differentiating the sonographic characteristics of various pathologic entities.

The sonic image is the compound effect of many simultaneously operating physical phenomena evoked by the acoustic properties of the tissues. Although it appears to be of paramount importance for intelligent interpretation, relatively little is known of the physical mechanism of high-frequency acoustic wave propagation in biologic matter. Awareness of this fact is motivating a great deal of investigative effort for the elucidation of the tissues' structural characteristics responsible for the echo pattern. While in light and electron microscopy and in radiology the differentiation of tumors is founded on the electromagnetic characteristics of their structural components, in sonography it is based on acoustic optics. It has been generally observed that tumor tissues return more energy than normal tissues. The exact mechanism of this effect is unknown. Although the higher concentration of nucleic acids and the increased nuclear/cytoplasmic ratio may represent considerable alteration in density, and thus in acoustic impedance, it is assumed that the factor most responsible for the reflected beam's energy content is the heterogeneity of malignant tissues. The multiformity of neoplastic cell clusters, the general orientation of these minute reflectors to the propagating beam, their size and thickness, and their peak to valley surface roughness in relation to the wavelength are major contributory factors in generating the reflected beam radiation pattern (nonspecular reflection).[4]

It has been postulated and partially supported by laboratory evidence that the fibrous matrix of the tissues, over which the cellular population is supported, provides an acoustic grid. This, by effecting diffraction and interference phenomena, may play a major role in determining the configuration and parameters of the reflected ultrasonic field. Since it is further hypothesized that these physical processes are influenced by the dimensions of the structural components of this interstitial network as well as by the pattern and width of the interstices separating them,

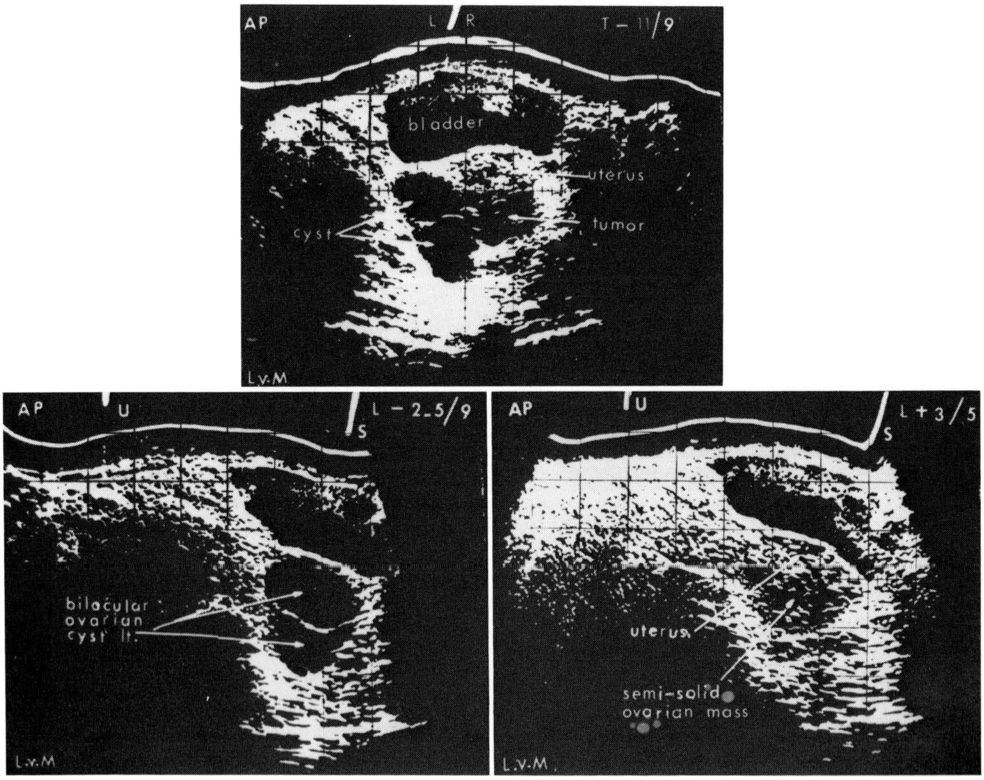

A

Fig. 11-26. There is no substitute for a meticulous multiple-plane scanning to arrive at the correct diagnosis. The bilocular cul-de-sac structure on the left had all the characteristics of a benign cyst. The solid portion of the tumor on the right, however, heralds a potential malignancy. Radiographic examination suggested pleural effusion, and pathohistologic examination of the sediment button obtained by thoracocentesis confirmed lung metastasis.

it can be theorized that the particular desmoplastic properties of tumors might prove to be a major factor in the sonographic identification of neoplasms. Since the dimensions of the grid are in the submillimeter range, achieving resolution of equal magnitude is a prerequisite for the establishment of the sonic phenotype of various physiologic and pathologic tissue entities.[4]

As sound absorption increases with increasing frequency, the data content of the sonograms obtained by external scanning must by necessity be a compromise between resolution and penetration. Consequently, reduction of the penetration requirements is the only feasible means for attaining good sonographic resolution of deep-seated organs; that is, only by bringing the transducer closer to the area of interest can one provide acoustic discrimination of the magnitude required by the nature of information sought. This rationale led to the concept of internal scanning and the development of an entire new family of scanners.[3,19,25,27]

The vagina, cervix, uterus, bladder, and rectum are conveniently accessible organs for direct study. By the utilization of miniaturized scanning equipment, sonography can be carried out in the vicinity of pelvic organs without traversing the numerous interfaces of the abdominal wall. This reduction of penetration requirements (the probe is either in direct contact with the internal genital organs or separated from them only by the thin bladder or rectal walls) permits the use of 10- to 15-MHz transducers with a practical resolution capability of 300 to 500 μ. The information

B

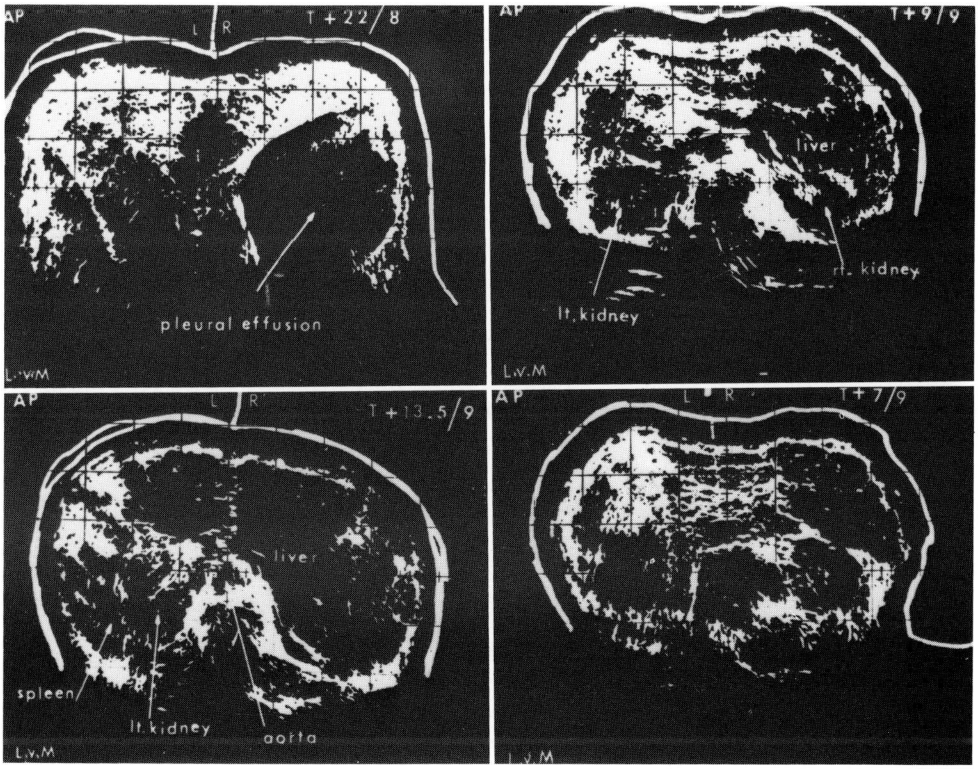

Fig. 11-26, cont'd. For legend see opposite page.

thus obtained is quasihistologic, not in terms of cellular but of submacroscopic histology (that is, observable at 20× to 30× light magnification).

Murooka, Ishihara, and Uchida published A mode echograms of gynecologic conditions as early as 1964.[27] Mizuno and his co-workers utilized specially constructed fingertip transducers to diagnose and differentiate solid and cystic pelvic tumors.[26] While A-mode studies of the eye (an organ of simple acoustic architecture) can be very informative, time-amplitude echograms of the pelvic organs with their literally thousands of interfaces are much too complex for reliable interpretation.[28]

The transvesical scanner designed by von Micsky and built by Hoffrel Instruments Corporation represents the first imaging endoscopic ultrasonic probe. Fig. 11-27, *a*, illustrates the concept of transvesical pelvic sonography. The fluid-distended bladder, utilized as a built-in water delay tank, provides the optimal scanning path through the thin bladder wall to the juxtaposed pelvic organs. The linear transvesical scanner depicted in Fig. 11-27, *b*, consists of a small ultrasonic transducer combined with a cystoscope and a precision scanning bridge. The instrument is mounted on a manipulator (Fig. 11-27, *c*), also of original design. This apparatus, in the form of a movable stand, is counterbalanced in such a manner that the scanning unit appears weightless and is capable of moving with all degrees of freedom. A pantograph type arrangement of the arms allows the cystoscope probe to move on a level in and out of the bladder. Once the desired location is obtained the operator can release the foot switch, which simultaneously locks the magnetic brakes of all joints, fixing the mechanism in the required position.

The prototype instrument has been ex-

a

b

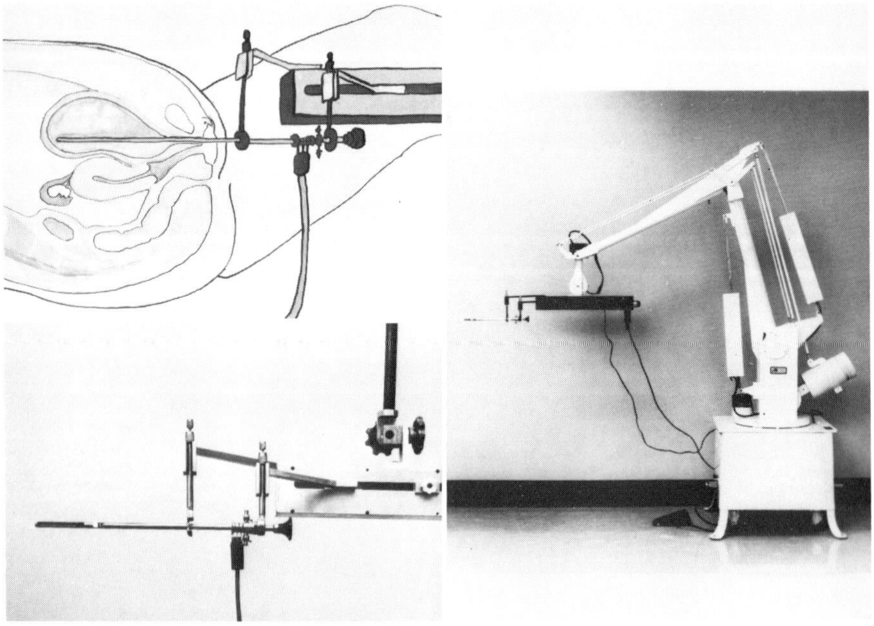

c

Fig. 11-27. Transvesical pelveosonography. *a*, Methodology; *b*, cystoscope probe and scanning bridge; and *c*, manipulator.

tensively used in a research project aimed at (1) forecasting the histologic nature of pelvic lesions, (2) staging the advancement of cervical cancer, and (3) studying the spread, persistence, and recurrence of pelvic tumors (Fig. 11-28). On one occasion it was also utilized to map the extent of transitional cell carcinoma in the bladder wall of a patient with total procidentia. Guided by the sonograms, a partial transvaginal cystectomy was performed at the time of vaginal hysterectomy.

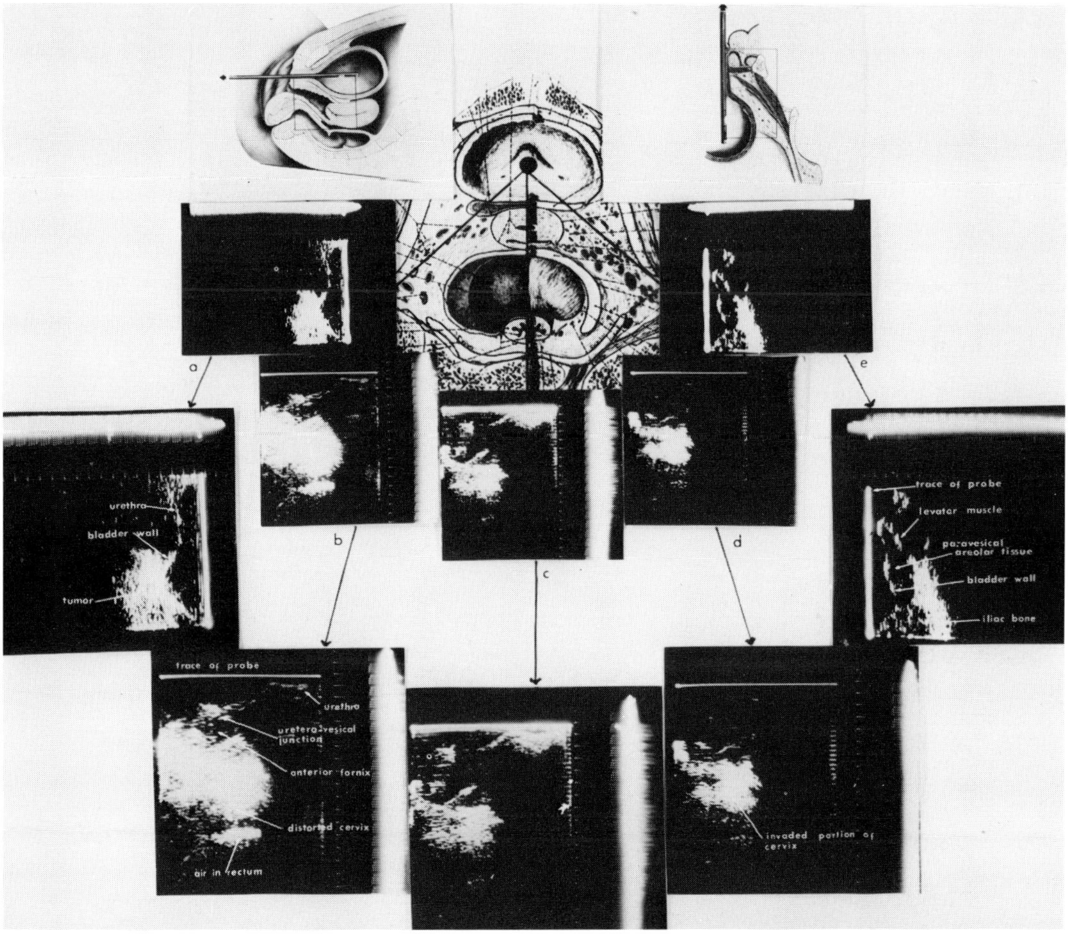

Fig. 11-28. Sonographic staging of cervical cancer. Sonograms *b, c,* and *d* taken in the sagittal plane at progressively reduced sensitivity show a large exophytic cervical lesion. The 20 dB difference in electronic attenuation between sonograms *b* and *d* clearly demonstrates that decreasing the sensitivity will reduce the intensity of echoes returning from normal tissues but not those reflected by cancerous infiltration. While the *contours of normal anatomic structures disappear, echoes from the invaded portion of the cervix still persist—the cancer "lights up."* Sonogram *e,* taken at 45 degrees to the right of the sagittal plane, shows the normal ultrasonic anatomy of the paravesical region. Sonogram *a,* taken at 45 degrees to the left of the sagittal plane, reveals a massive conglomerate of high-intensity echoes replacing the areolar tissue adjacent to the bladder. These indicate parametrial extension of the mitotic process. Its location and dimensions were in good agreement with those of a nodular lesion palpable over the lateral fornix.

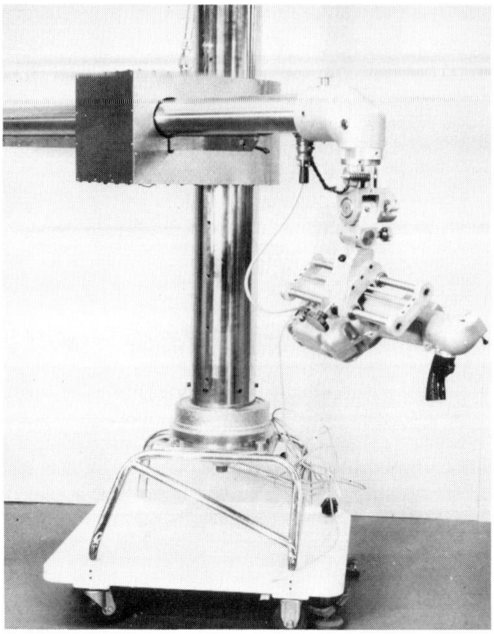

Fig. 11-29. Scanning bridge and manipulator of the new Son-Endoscope. (Courtesy Rohe Scientific Corp.)

As of now, the patient has survived for over 6 years.

The Son-Endoscope, a new endoscanner, conceived by von Micsky and developed in cooperation with Rohe Scientific Corporation, is provided with cystoscope, vaginoscope, hysteroscope, and sigmoidoscope probes (Fig. 11-29). While the first three are designed for sector, linear, or programmed sector scan, the larger lumen of the sigmoidoscope accommodates a miniaturized compound scanning system (sector scan superimposed over a linear main scanning path) (Fig. 11-30). The instrument has various auxiliary and safety devices to permit introduction of the probes and docking of the scanning bridge with them without discomfort or injury to the patient. The instrument is expected to be extremely useful in both gynecology and urology (Fig. 11-31). Besides the already proved applica-

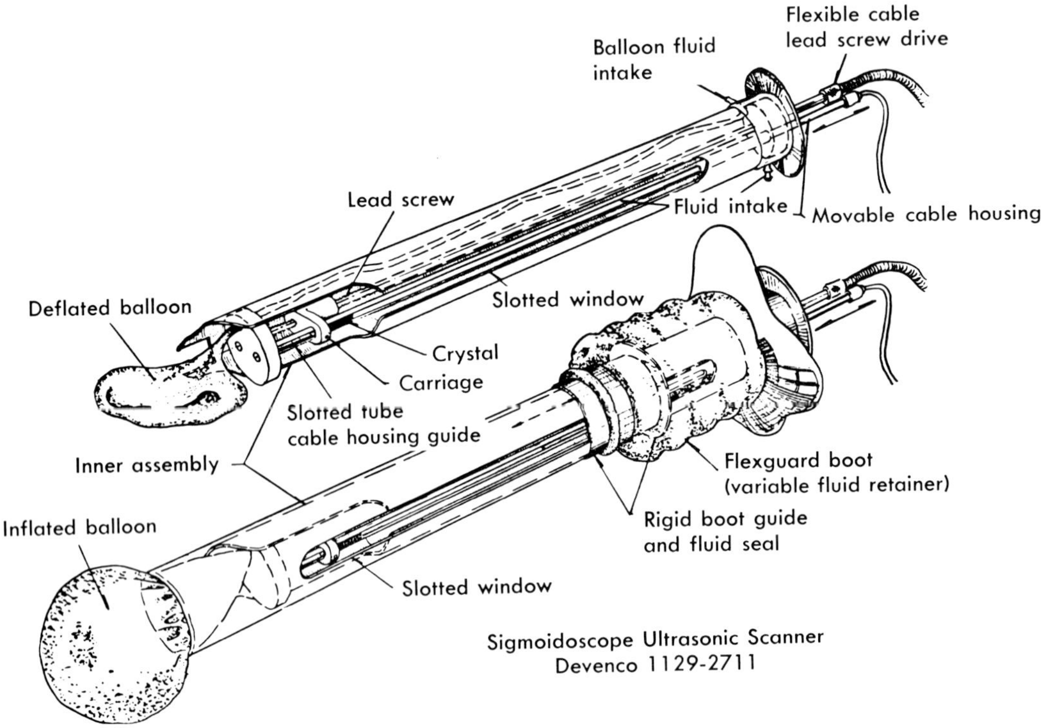

Fig. 11-30. Artist's representation of the transrectal scanner.

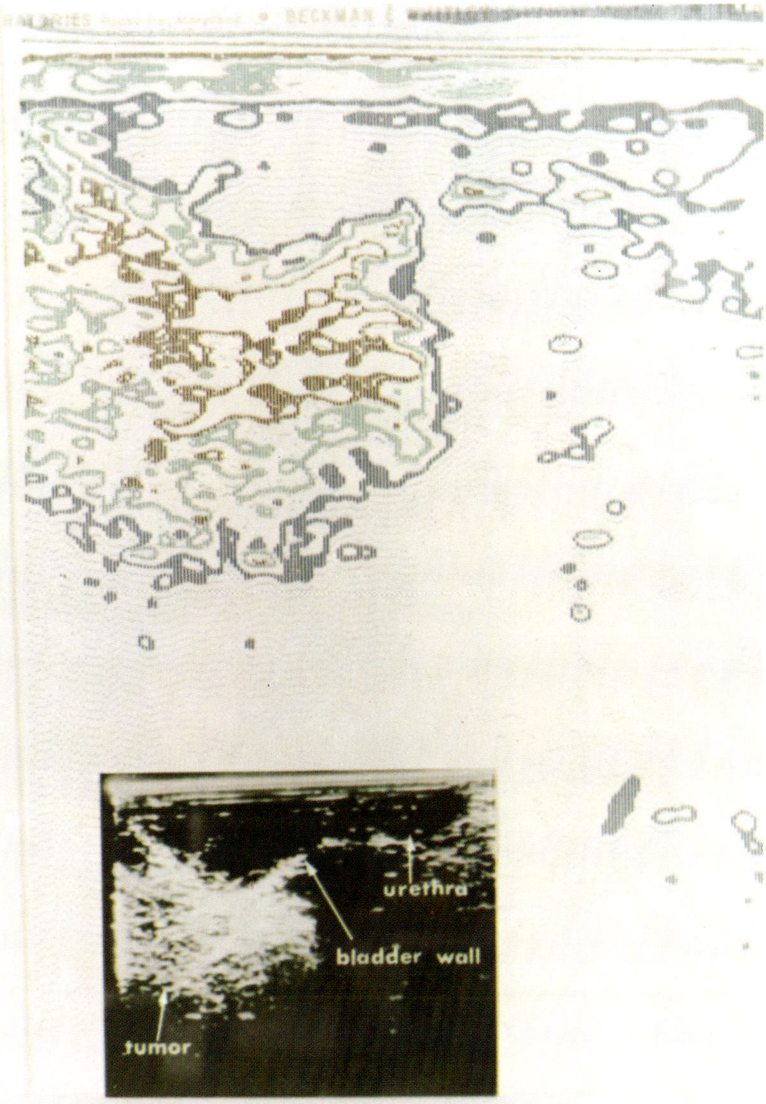

Plate 1. Color isodensitracing. Because of the acoustic shadowing caused by scattering in the tumor tissue, the pelvic wall is not visualized on sonogram *a* of Fig. 11-28, thus it cannot be determined whether we are dealing with a Stage II or Stage III lesion. The area shown in reddish brown on the color isodensitracing marked the extent of the cancerous spread, thus assigning to it a Stage IIA classification. The clinical and ultrasonic staging was verified at surgery and by pathohistologic findings.

tions, the gynecologist may be able to detect early ovarian cancer by screening ovarian masses larger than 6 cm or those persisting longer than 90 days. By being able to map the extent of the tumor in the bladder wall, the urologist can plan his surgical approach more adequately but more sparingly; that is, instead of performing total cystectomy, he may be able to choose a partial one and leave a residual functioning organ. The primary target organ for transrectal pelvic sonography is the prostate, but it is hoped that it will make many other pelvic lesions accessible to investigative sonic survey.

A thorough perusal of the ultrasonic literature makes it apparent that in evaluating the sonograms published, the distribution of the light and dark areas is used only qualitatively as an aid to what might be called the photogrammetric analysis of the sizes and shapes of picture components comprising the sonogram. Thus most of the vast amount of information present in these photographs remains untapped. To further complicate the prob-

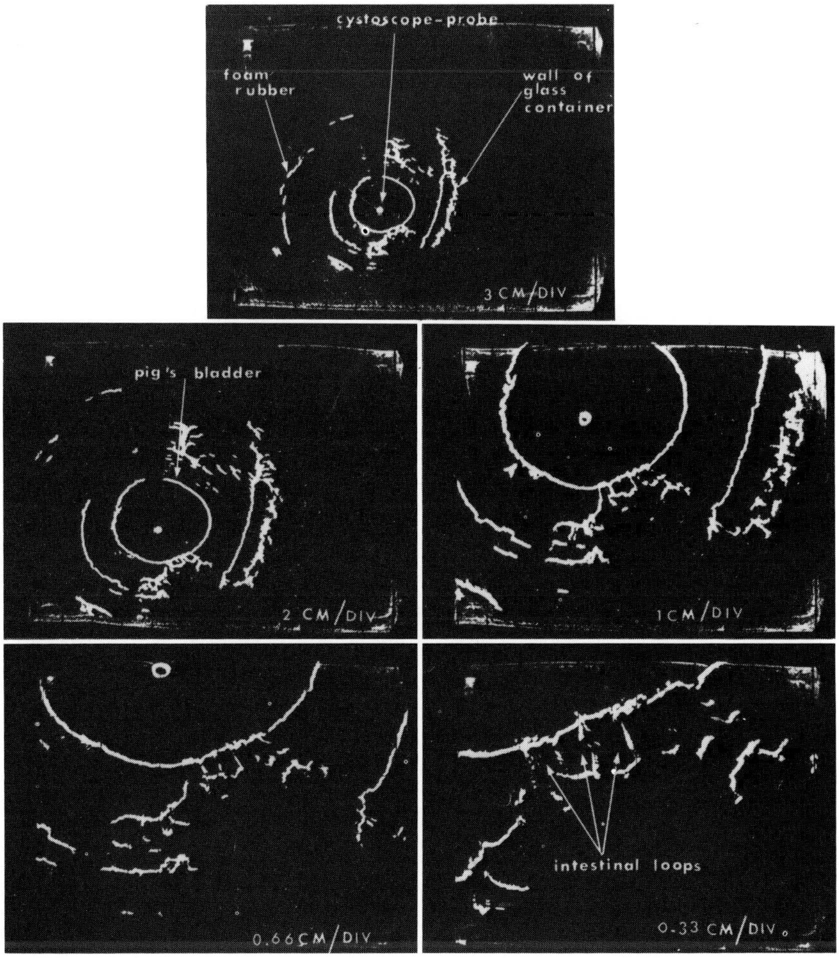

Fig. 11-31. This in vitro experiment with the new Son-Endoscope illustrates the combined effects of high-frequency and electronic magnification on resolution.

lem, the process of appraising the acoustic images is one of subjective interpretation. Thus to further improve diagnostic accuracy, various methods have been tried for the extraction of all the photometric data stored in the photographic emulsion of the gray-scale sonograms (produced and photographed on a nonstorage scope of 40-dB dynamic range). In all attempts at semiquantification, best results were obtained by evaluating the sonograms with an isodensitracer. This is a high-speed, direct recording isophotometer that automatically scans and measures the optic density on the Polaroid pictures or transparencies and plots the quantized density values in a coded (dot, line, blank, with change of the code at each density gradient) two-dimensional isodensitracing of the scanned area. An improved version, the color translating isodensitracer, can be programmed in such a fashion that preselected portions of the density spectrum are printed in particular colors, as is seen in Plate 1.[3]

Since in both linear and sector scan modes each target is acoustically illuminated only from one direction, quantitative evaluation of sonograms obtained by these techniques can readily be performed by isodensitracings. Compound scanning characterized by acoustic illumination of each target from a multiplicity of angles introduces artifacts (overlap images) that invalidate direct extraction of quantitative data by isodensitracings. The linear-sector scan employed in the sigmoidoscope attachment of the Son-Endoscope provides a predictable density distribution of the overlap images, thus facilitating compensation and quantitative evaluation. A simple but only semiaccurate method of compensation involves an add-on correction circuit for the isodensitracer. The complex but precise solution is to utilize a digital computer both for compensation and for the quantitative analysis of the sonographic data so as to obtain morphologic and structural characteristics, which will ultimately lead to automatic pattern recognition, though this is not as yet in sight.

It is confidently expected that the multiplex approach to improved diagnostic accuracy outlined will extend our capabilities to the detection of ever smaller lesions and that, in accordance with medicine's latest aspirations, it will update sonogynecography's role from a primarily documentary or differential one to a preventive one.

Acknowledgments

I wish to express my grateful thanks to Drs. Nathanial Finby and Harold M. M. Tovell for their unwavering support, advice, and encouragement since the inception of the Radiology Department's Ultrasonic Division at St. Luke's Hospital Center. Thanks are also due to Dr. Joshua Becker for his permission to include among the illustrations some of the sonograms I had the privilege to evaluate as a consultant to the Ultrasonic Department at Downstate Medical Center. My sincere appreciation is offered to medical sonographers Shirley Staiano, Mary Bright Noyes, and Ellen Cromb Campos. The acoustic images here reproduced should be considered a tribute not just to their pervasive knowledge and superior technical skill but, beyond those, to an assiduous, inspiring devotion to the cause of diagnostic ultrasonics. Special thanks are extended to research fellows Drs. Elsa Brea and Hyon-u Lee for their assistance and to my secretary, Mrs. Margaret Alt, for typing the numerous drafts.

REFERENCES

1. Donald, I.: Sonar in obstetrics and gynecology. In Greenhill, J. P., editor: Year book of obstetrics and gynecology, Chicago, 1967, Year Book Medical Publishers, Inc., pp. 242-266.
2. von Micsky, L. I.: Ultrasonic tomography in obstetrics and gynecology. In Grossman, C. C., and others, editors: Diagnostic ultrasound, New York, 1966, Plenum Press, Inc., pp. 348-368.
3. von Micsky, L. I.: Transvesical pelveo-sonography: a new theoretical and experimental approach to the investigation of gynecological cancer, Obstet. Gynecol. **27**:597, 1966.
4. von Micsky, L. I.: Experimental investigation into the origin of tissue echoes with particular

reference to signals arising in pelvic neoplasms, Obstet. Gynecol. **31:**584, 1968.
5. Baum, G.: Ophthalmic ultrasonography. In Gordon, D., editor: Ultrasound as a diagnostic tool, London, 1964, E. & S. Livingstone, Ltd., pp. 181-184.
6. von Micsky, L. I.: Clinical sonography in urology, Urology **1:**506-522, 1973.
7. von Micsky, L. I.: Clinical sonography in obstetrics and gynecology. In Ayromlooi, I., and Mukherjee, T., editors: Advanced concepts in obstetrics and gynecology. In press.
8. Sunden, B.: On the diagnostic value of ultrasound in obstetrics and gynecology, Acta Obstet. Gynecol. Scand. **43**(Suppl. 6):1964.
9. Staiano, S. J.: Sonographic differentiation of cystic from solid pelvic tumors, unpublished paper presented at the Fifteenth Annual Meeting of the American Institute of Ultrasound in Medicine, Cleveland, Ohio, Oct. 13, 1970.
10. Kobayashi, M., Hellman, L. M., and Cromb, E.: Atlas of ultrasonography in obstetrics and gynecology, ed. 7, New York, 1972, Appleton-Century-Crofts.
11. Damascelli, B., and others: B scan ultrasound exploration of neoplastic disease, Am. J. Roentgenol. Radium Ther. Nucl. Med. **105:**428-437, 1969.
12. Asher, W. M. Sonographic diagnosis of pelvic malignancy, personal communication.
13. Brascho, D. J.: Clinical applications of diagnostic ultrasound in abdominal malignancy, Southern Med. J. **65:**1331-1339, 1972.
14. Morley, P., and Barnett, E.: The use of ultrasound in the diagnosis of pelvic mass, Br. J. Radiol. **34:**602-16, 1970.
15. von Micsky, L. I.: Ultrasonics in obstetrics and gynecology, Obstet. Gynecol. **24:**420, 1965.
16. von Micsky, L. I.: Ultrasonics in obstetrics and gynecology, Hosp. Topics **43:**104, 1965.
17. Gottesfeld, K. R.: The practical application of ultrasound in obstetrics and gynecology. In Grossman, C. C., and others, editors: Diagnostic ultrasound, New York, 1966, Plenum Press, Inc., pp. 428-449.
18. Thompson, H. E.: Ultrasound techniques in pelvic cancer, Clin. Obstet. Gynecol. **12:**354-371, 1969.
19. Kratochwil, A.: Ultrasonic diagnosis in pelvic malignancy, Clin. Obstet. Gynecol. **3:**898-909, 1970.
20. Finby, N., and Begg, C. F.: Enlarging abdomen in teenage girl, N. Y. State J. Med. **72:**1615-1619, 1972.
21. Hyman, R. A., von Micsky, L. I., and Finby, N.: Ovarian teratoma in childhood, Am. J. Roentgenol. Radium Ther. Nucl. Med. **116:**673-676, 1972.
22. Finby, N., and Begg, C. F.: Embryonal teratoma of ovary, N. Y State J. Med. **70:**2570-2573, 1970.
23. von Micsky, L. I.: Clinical sonography in early pregnancy. In The Alliance for Engineering in Medicine and Biology: Proceedings of 25th Annual Conference of Engineering and Medical Biology, Vol. 14, Washington, D. C., 1972, p. 134.
24. von Micsky, L. I., Heelan, R. T. and Finby, N.: Sonographic differentiation of gestational corpus luteum cysts from ovarian neoplasms complicating pregnancy. In press.
25. von Micsky, L. I.: Transvesical pelveo-sonography, unpublished paper presented at the third International Symposium on Ultrasonic Diagnostics in World Congress, Vienna, Austria, June 5, 1969.
26. Mizuno, S., and others: Diagnostic application of ultrasound in obstetrics and gynecology. In Grossman, C. C., and others, editors: Diagnostic ultrasound, New York, 1966, Plenum Press, Inc., pp. 452-64.
27. Murooka, H., Ishihara, M., and Uchida, R.: Ultrasonic wave diagnosis of pelvic tumors, Aust. N. Z. J. Obstet. Gynaecol. **4:**139-142, 1964.
28. Kratochwil, A.: Ultraschall Diagnostik in Geburtshilfe und Gynekologie, Stuttgart, 1968, Georg Thieme Verlag.

12 Urologic ultrasonography

JOSEPH H. HOLMES, M.D.

Ultrasound can contribute additional information to expand current diagnostic capabilities for demonstrating pathology of the kidney and genitourinary tract. Ultrasound has certain characteristics that make it particularly valuable for study of the kidney and genitourinary tract.[1] Its cross-sectional display provides an additional dimension in looking at the kidney. Its unique capability of visualizing fluid is particularly valuable in demonstrating cysts, hydronephrosis, and bladder pathology. The examination technique is simple and thus readily accepted by patients, which makes it valuable for use in early detection programs for polycystic kidney disease and bladder tumor. Further, ultrasonic examination does not require use of contrast media and thus provides diagnostic information in uremic patients in whom contrast or isotope uptakes are insufficient to provide adequate studies. Since repeat studies are feasible as often as every hour, ultrasound is particularly valuable for following patients with acute renal injury or those with suspected complications after transplantation or after needle biopsy. This chapter presents some of the diagnostic applications of ultrasound related to the genitourinary tract that have proved of greatest value in our unit. I will also discuss briefly some of the future developments of ultrasound that promise to make this technique even more valuable for the diagnosis of renal disease.

Although this presentation will focus on the direct diagnostic application of ultra-

Supported in part by a grant from the U. S. Public Health Service HEO2115; the General Clinical Research Center Program, Division of Research Resources, National Institutes of Health, RR51; and a General Research Support Grant RR-05357.

sound to the kidney and genitourinary tract, there are several other applications of ultrasound that have contributed significantly to the care of patients with kidney disease. For example, some 20% to 25% of the patients on hemodialysis have hypertension and cardiac complications. In these patients echocardiography has proved helpful in assessing their cardiac status. One specific application has been the determination of the reason for cardiac enlargement—that is, pericardial effusion, ventricular wall hypertrophy, or left ventricular chamber dilation. In addition, ultrasound has been used to evaluate the presence of ascites, which is a not uncommon complication in renal and dialysis patients, and for assessing the fluid distribution during peritoneal dialysis. It is useful in the chest to locate pleural effusion and other pulmonary complications. Undoubtedly, ultrasound will have additional applications in the management of patients with renal disease because of its very effective demonstration of fluid and internal hemorrhage.

EXAMINATION TECHNIQUES

The types of ultrasonic equipment required for diagnostic B scan studies are adequately described in other sections of this book and in previous publications.[1-3] In the work described here, we utilized either a Unirad Sonograph II or a Picker Model 102 scanner.

For examination of the kidney, the patient is placed in the prone position and mineral oil applied to his back to provide sonic contact between the skin surface and the transducer face. A series of horizontal scans is made at approximately 2-cm intervals to include the entire kidney region. Each scan takes 30 to 40 seconds. Several vertical scans are made to visualize the longitudinal axis of the kidney, usually several centimeters to each side of the midline. Then the patient is placed on each side and lateral views of the kidney area are obtained. The total time required for the examination is approximately 30 minutes.

The technique for examining the bladder is essentially the same except that the patient lies in the supine position and scans are made horizontally across the lower abdomen extending from the symphysis pubis up to about the umbilicus. Vertical scans are also made to either side of the midline. If the bladder is not sufficiently filled for good visualization, the patient is required to drink additional water and the examination is rescheduled. Repeat scans are always made after voiding and the urine volume recorded.

A technique of considerable value in renal studies is the calculation of volume of either bladder urine or the volume of the transplanted kidney. The outline of the kidney or bladder is traced with a planimeter to obtain the area of that segment. Then, by repeating the scans at 1-cm intervals, one can add the separate volumes to obtain total volume. In the case of the urine-filled bladder, the accuracy checks to within ±10% of the catheterized or voided volume.[4]

Normal kidney

The normal kidney, when scanned from the back, has a very characteristic ultrasonic pattern, as shown in the upper part of Fig. 12-1. Two parallel white lines representing echoes reflected from the spine are placed to either side of a black area because of lack of penetration of the ultrasound through bone. To either side of the spinal echoes are two ovoid sonolucent areas 5 × 6 cm in diameter, representing the kidneys well outlined by echoes from their surface. Within each kidney is a discrete echo nest representing reflections from calyceal-pelvic structures and called by us the calyceal-pelvic "echo blob." These normally occupy no more than 15% of the total area of the kidney. Usually there are no definitive echo patterns be-

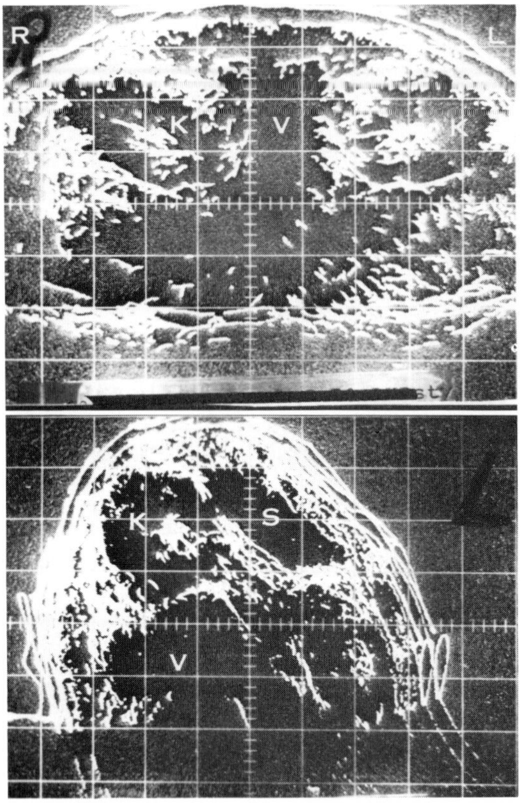

Fig. 12-1. Upper scan made across the back of a healthy 18-year-old female shows the kidney region with a well-outlined sonolucent area to either side of the dense spinal echo band that contains a discrete calyceal pelvic "echo blob." This is the characteristic configuration of a normal kidney. The lower picture is a left lateral scan showing the same kidney echo pattern and a sonolucent area to the right representing the spleen. *K*, Kidney; *V*, vertebra; *R*, right; *L*, left; *S*, spleen.

yond the kidney, but occasionally one sees laterally a sonolucent area representing liver or spleen.

In the lower part of Fig. 12-1 is a left lateral scan with the kidney outline shown to the top and left. The skin surface to the left is the back and to the right the anterior abdominal wall. The sonolucent area just to the right of the kidney represents the spleen. A similar pattern is seen for the right kidney except that the anterior sonolucent area represents liver. Both posterior and lateral scans are essential for a good kidney study.

The list below gives some of the most useful applications of ultrasound in the diagnosis of renal disease.

1. Determination of renal size and position
2. Evaluation of polycystic kidney disease
3. Differentiation of renal masses between cyst and tumor
4. Assessment of size changes in transplanted kidney
5. Positioning for renal biopsy and detecting postbiopsy complications
6. Detection of hydronephrosis and renal calculi
7. Demonstration of aortic lesions that may impinge on renal circulation
8. Detection of acute renal injury, perirenal abscess, retroperitoneal hemorrhage

Renal size and position

In many instances, when a patient is admitted with severe uremia, knowledge of renal size may contribute significantly in the differential diagnosis. Since it is sometimes difficult to get good sonograms of the poles of the normal kidney, we have chosen to express kidney size based on the two maximum diameters observed. We have not used the expression of maximum renal circumference. We have compared the diameter with the corresponding width of the kidney as shown by x-ray. With proper corrections applied to each measurement, we have found approximately 90% of comparable measurements to be within 5 mm. In our series, most normal kidneys have measured 5 × 6 cm, large kidneys up to 6 × 7 cm, and small kidneys 4 × 5 cm. Perhaps some standardized technique for ultrasonic expression of renal size should be developed.

Because of its cross-sectional presenta-

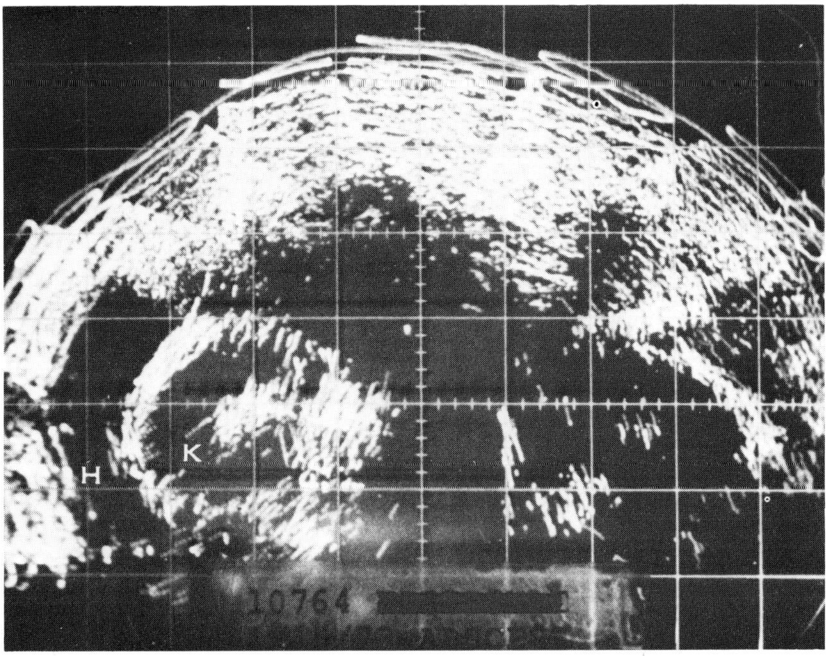

Fig. 12-2. Left lateral scan of the kidney region in a dialysis patient who had just had surgical repair of the aorta. The kidney is pushed forward and the echo outline of the kidney is quite discrete and dense, a distinct difference from the normal kidney. Posteriorly is a sonolucent area, presumably representing retroperitioneal hemorrhage. *H,* Hemorrhage.

tion, ultrasound has proved useful in a number of instances in demonstrating displacement of the kidney from its usual position in relation to the spine and other organs. One example of this is shown in Fig. 12-2. This is an anterior abdominal scan of a 73-year-old chronic dialysis patient who had retroperitoneal hemorrhage following aortic surgery. The kidney outline is accentuated and there is a black area behind and lateral to the kidney suggestive of retroperitoneal hemorrhage. Similar displays might be seen when retroperitoneal hemorrhage occurs after acute renal injury, after renal biopsy, and in patients with hemophilia. By outlining the area of hemorrhage on tracing paper and comparing successive scans, one can detect continued bleeding. A similar pattern may be seen in association with retroperitoneal abscess or tumor.

Polycystic kidney disease

The ultrasonic pattern in advanced polycystic kidney disease is quite characteristic.[5] In early polycystic kidney disease there will often be changes in the ultrasonic pattern before the "routine" intravenous pyelogram shows definitive changes. In addition, ultrasound can demonstrate cysts in the liver, and thus both organs can be checked at the same examination.[6]

Fig. 12-3 (upper part) shows an ultrasonic scan of the right kidney area made by moving the transducer across the back. It demonstrates an echo pattern of interlacing echo lines surrounding black areas of irregular size and shape distributed in an indiscriminate pattern. Each black area represents a fluid-filled cyst. In the lower part is a single large cyst located at the lower pole of the same kidney.

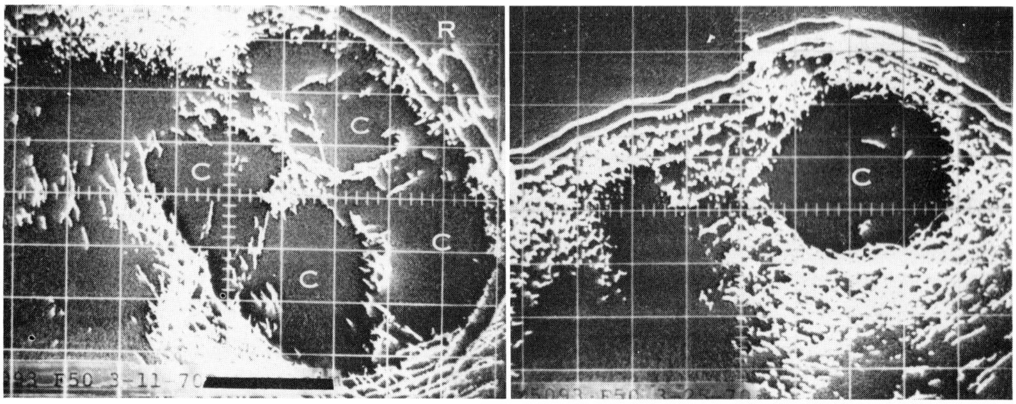

Fig. 12-3. Ultrasonic scan of right kidney area. Kidney is enlarged with diameters of 12 × 12 cm. The interlacing echo line pattern surrounding clear black areas of irregular size and shape is typical of polycystic kidney disease. The picture on the right shows a large, single cyst at the lower pole of the same kidney. *C*, Cyst.

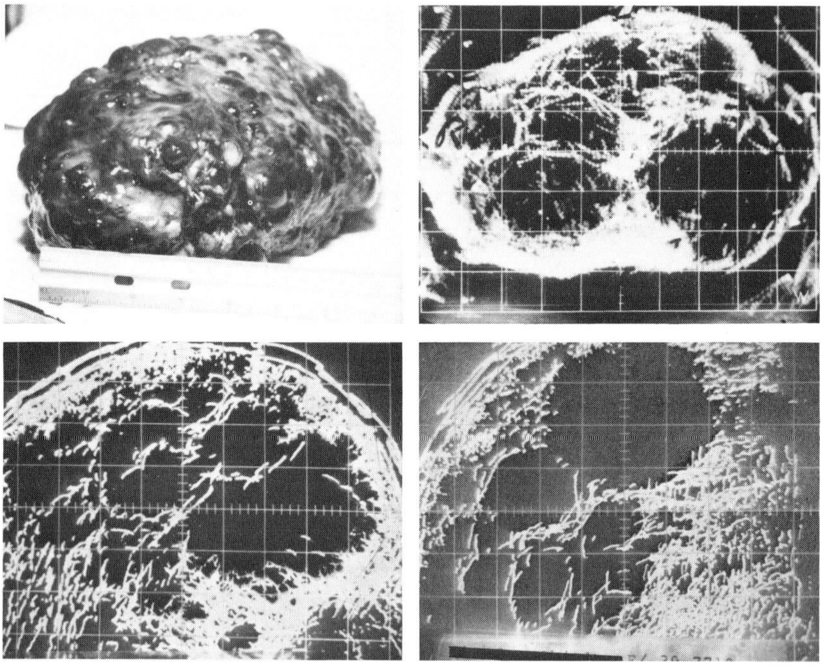

Fig. 12-4. On the upper left is a picture of a 9-pound polycystic kidney removed at surgery. The ultrasonic scan on the upper right was made on the surgical specimen. The lower left picture shows the preoperative lateral scan of the same kidney and the lower right picture is the preoperative posterior scan of the same kidney.

This polycystic pattern has been verified using our water path scanning system by examining one of these kidneys after nephrectomy. The upper left part of Fig. 12-4 shows the surgical specimen immediately after surgery. On the right is the ultrasonic scan made on this same specimen. The two lower parts show the preoperative ultrasonic scans, the one on the left being a lateral view and the one on the right a posterior scan across the right kidney area. The interlacing echo lines surrounding cysts of varying size and shape are clearly seen and are identical to the pattern obtained from the isolated kidney.

Fig. 12-5 shows a scan of the liver from a member of one of our polycystic kidney disease families. This woman has had known polycystic kidney disease since 1956 when, because of abdominal pain, exploratory surgery was done and the cysts of one kidney were punctured. Surgery and cyst puncture were done on the other kidney in 1961. In the two pictures on the left are the ultrasonic scans with an echo pattern similar to that seen for the polycystic kidneys (see Figs. 12-3 and 12-4). The upper right section shows a "gray-tone" scan that emphasizes the cystic pattern. The "gray-tone" records all echo information received at four preselected echo intensities and displays this as varying levels of "gray" on the oscilloscope screen. The right lower figure shows the isotopic scan with definite areas of decreased uptake reported as consistent with the diagnosis of polycystic liver disease.

Ultrasound may also be of value in picking up unusual complications in polycystic

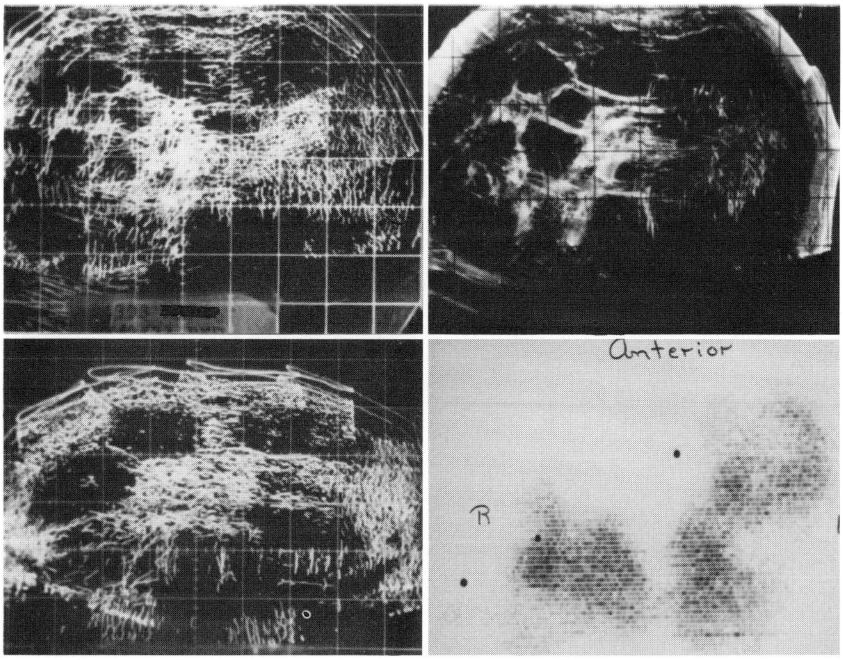

Fig. 12-5. Anterior abdominal scans of the liver area in a patient with polycystic kidney disease. The upper left picture shows an interlacing echo pattern surrounding irregular black areas, a pattern similar to that seen in a polycystic kidney. The gray tone scan on the right accentuates the display of the cyst's formation. The lower picture on the left shows the same liver at a different level. The lower right picture shows the isotopic scan.

kidney disease. We have two examples to suggest this might be feasible in some instances. The patient whose scans are shown in Fig. 12-3 developed severe hematuria. The single large cyst demonstrated in the lower portion of Fig. 12-3 showed ultrasonic evidence of increase in size. Thus if surgical intervention had been necessary, this would have been the first area to examine. Another patient developed obstruction associated with a sudden decrease in urine flow. Although this patient was on dialysis, it was possible to do an infusion intravenous pyelogram that suggested significant hydronephrosis. The ultrasound pictures (Fig. 12-6) showed an elongated, sausage-like echo pattern surrounding a sonolucent area in one part of the kidney, which was in contrast to the usual indiscriminate cystic pattern. This corresponded to the dilated calyces and pelvis seen in the surgical specimen after nephrectomy.

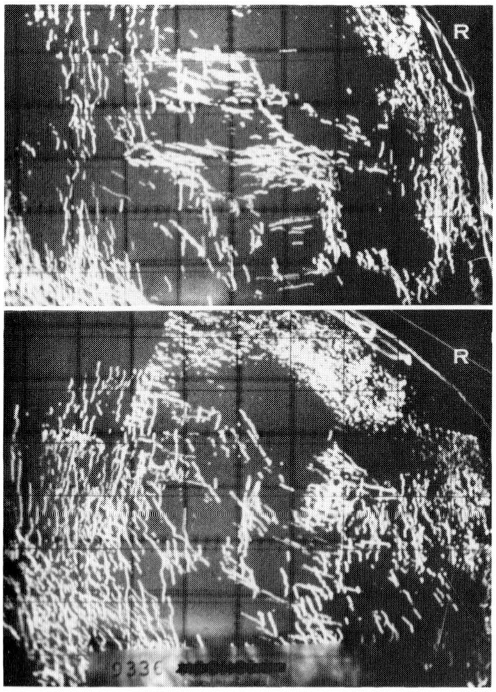

Fig. 12-6. Posterior scans of the right kidney area at two different levels in a patient with polycystic kidney disease and urinary tract obstruction. The elongated sonolucent area along the upper border corresponded to the location of dilated calyces and pelvis on the surgical specimen.

In studying polycystic kidney disease families, ultrasound appears to have several advantages. First, it is possible to pick up evidence of small cysts within the kidney before the kidney has shown any significant increase in size. Second, family members who are feeling well readily agree to having an ultrasonic examination but will refuse an intravenous pyelogram. Third, because of the ease of repeat examinations, it offers an approach to following the rate of growth of intrarenal cysts in polycystic kidney disease, which may be an important factor for managing the patient, especially in relation to prognosis. For example, some members of polycystic kidney disease families may have only several small cysts within the kidney at the age of 70 and no measurable decrease in renal function. Yet another member of the same family may have significantly enlarged kidneys and a BUN of 70 mg% at the age of 24.

Renal masses

The cross-sectional display of ultrasound has been particularly effective in providing additional information regarding the character of renal masses whose presence is suggested by intravenous pyelogram.[7] In addition to providing information about the location and contour of the renal mass, in a majority of these cases it has been possible to predict successfully whether the mass is a tumor or a cyst. The scan across the back in Fig. 12-7 illustrates the pattern of a renal cyst. The cyst is seen as a large sonolucent area (6 × 8 cm) just below the diffuse echo pattern representing back muscle. The renal cyst is usually ovoid or spherical and its echo outline is smooth and well defined. The renal echo outline is often compressed and distorted and thus not easily recognized.

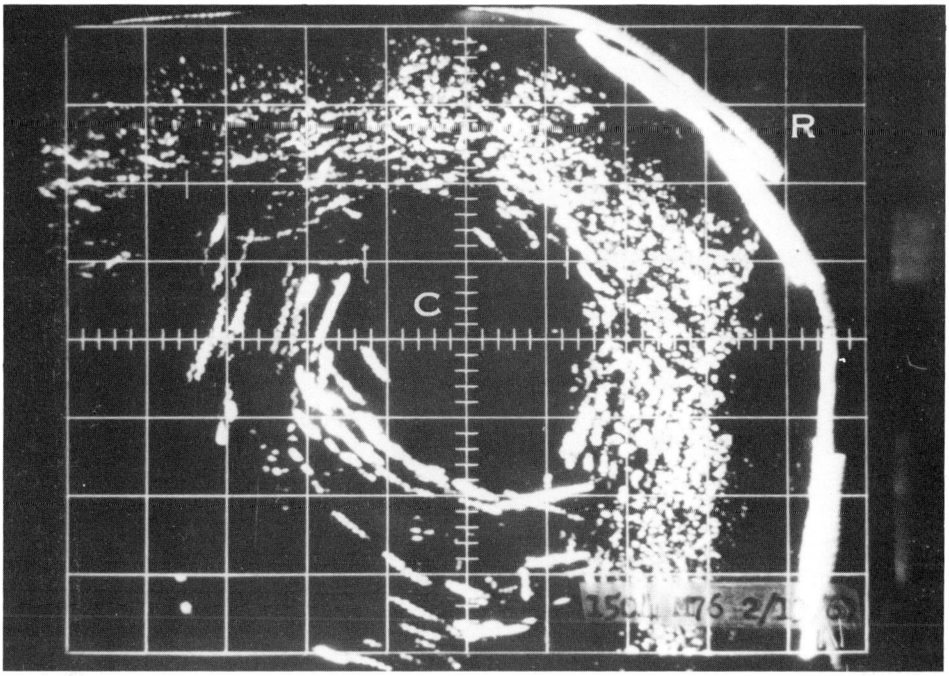

Fig. 12-7. Posterior scan of the right kidney. The kidney area is filled by a large sonolucent ovoid area surrounded by a well-defined echo pattern characteristic of renal cyst. (From Schreck, W. R., and Holmes, J. H.: J. Urol. **103:**281, 1970.)

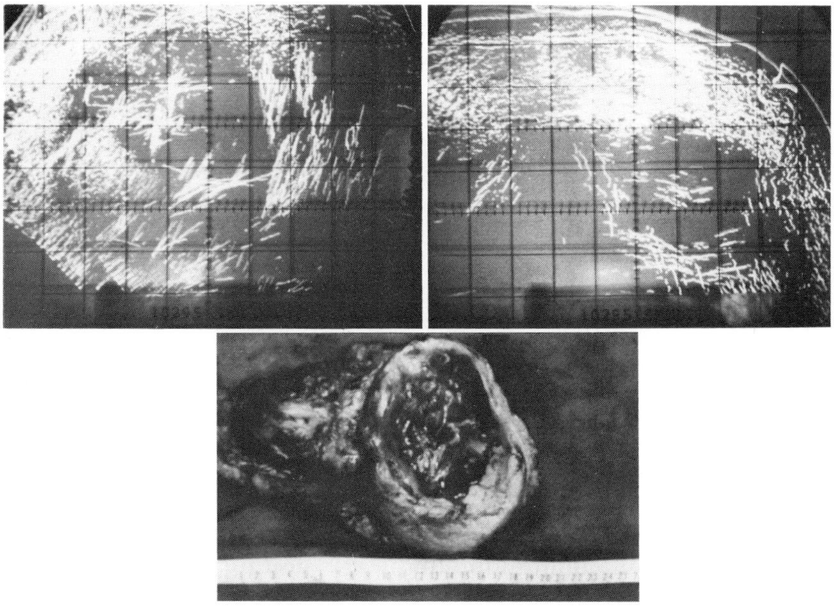

Fig. 12-8. Posterior scans of both kidneys. The picture on the upper right shows a normal configuration for the right kidney. The renal area on the upper left is filled with an enlarged 10 × 11 cm mass containing scattered echo nests between sonolucent areas. The lower picture shows the pathologic specimen of the tumor removed at surgery.

Most renal tumors at low sensitivities reflect echoes only from the surface, though occasionally a renal tumor may be visualized as a dense, solid echo mass filling the kidney area. When the tumor reflects echoes from its surface, the outline pattern will usually be irregular with frequent indentations of the echo wall, and the sonolucent area within will contain scattered echoes. This is shown in Fig. 12-8. The normal renal echo pattern is shown on the upper right for the right kidney. The left kidney area is filled by a large spherical sonolucent mass (11 × 10 cm) containing several echo nests. The surgical specimen of the tumor is seen in the lower picture. When receiver sensitivity is increased, additional echoes will appear within the previous sonolucent area, suggesting that the observed mass is a solid structure, presumably tumor. This is illustrated in Fig. 12-9. In the upper picture the left kidney area is filled by a large sonolucent mass with irregular echo borders almost triangular in shape. When receiver sensitivity is increased, the lower picture shows additional echoes within. A renal tumor was found at surgery. In contrast, if a cyst is present, the sonolucent area will not fill in with echoes when receiver sensitivity is increased.

When the physician wishes to aspirate a renal cyst, ultrasound may provide definitive information as to direction and depth for introduction of the needle. If complications should arise after aspiration, a comparison of the pictures obtained before the aspiration and those following often reveals changes in renal contour that suggest the nature of the complication.

Transplanted kidney

In the past 2 years there have been several reports describing the use of ultrasound for evaluation of complications associated with renal transplantation.[8,9] The position of the transplanted kidney makes ultrasonic scanning of this organ particularly effective. Ultrasound has been used to judge changes in size, detect obstruction, and demonstrate perirenal hemorrhages. We have found the calculation of renal volume a most useful way to assess size changes in the transplanted kidney. By relating renal size changes to changes in renal function, one can often arrive at the correct diagnosis. For example, a sudden change in size from 300 to 500 ml in renal volume over a short period certainly suggests acute rejection. We have found that measurement of size

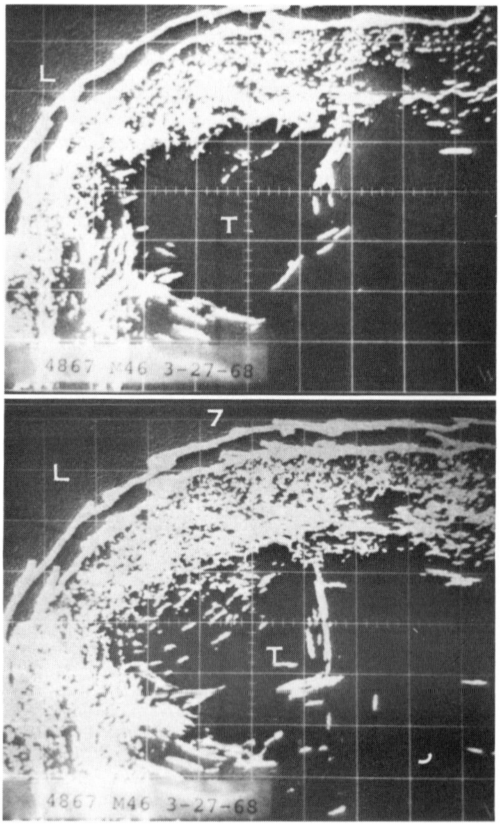

Fig. 12-9. Posterior scan of the left kidney region. In the upper picture the kidney is replaced by an irregular echo outline almost triangular in shape surrounding a sonolucent area. The lower picture shows the increase in echoes within and a weak far-wall echo when sensitivity is increased, ultrasonic criteria for tumor. *T*, Tumor. (From Schreck, W. R., and Holmes, J. H.: J. Urol. **103**:281, 1970.)

changes in the total calyceal-pelvic "echo blob" that normally occupies less than 15% of the total area of the kidney is useful in suggesting obstruction or the presence of an intrapelvic tumor, as recently observed in our series.

Fig. 12-10 shows in the upper portion a scan of the transplanted kidney made obliquely across the anterior abdomen along its longitudinal axis. The echo outline of the kidney border is clearly defined and the calyceal-pelvic "echo blob" is small and discrete. This scan was made in a 31-year-old man in 1970, shortly after his surgery. This patient had a sudden rise in serum creatinine and a decrease in creatinine clearance in March, 1973. The scan in the lower picture shows the renal size at that time to be slightly larger than the first scan. The calculated volume for the first scan was 320 ml and for the second scan 380 ml. This ruled out progressive chronic rejection resulting in a small, contracted kidney. We have not encountered in our series the complications of perirenal bleeding or abscess. These complications would be suggested by irregular sonolucent areas appearing adjacent to the renal outline.

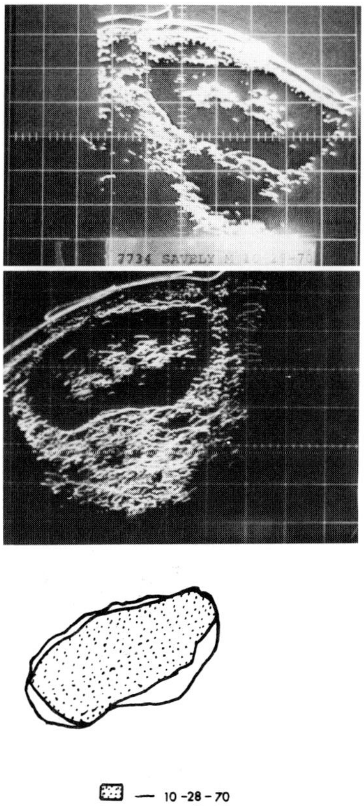

Fig. 12-10. The upper picture is an anterior abdominal scan along the longitudinal axis of the transplanted kidney made in 1970 (Picker Model 102). The middle picture shows a similar scan of the same transplanted kidney in 1973 (Unirad Sonograph II). The lower picture shows the trace outline of the two kidneys for comparison of size changes.

In our laboratory, ultrasonic examinations for changes in transplanted kidney size have been helpful in the following ways:

1. A sudden increase in size of the kidney suggests acute rejection.
2. The failure of a transplanted kidney to show the expected hypertrophy in the first 6 months has proved of value in predicting the success of a particular transplant.
3. Whenever there is a sudden increase in BUN and serum creatinine in the later posttransplant periods, the demonstration of either a large or a small kidney may be a significant aid in the differential diagnosis.
4. Changes in the area of the calyceal-pelvic "echo blob" may suggest obstruction or intrapelvic masses.

In addition, following the volume of the transplanted kidney over a period of years may contribute to the assessment of transplantation techniques, especially as new forms of treatment are developed.

Renal biopsy

Primarily because of its cross-sectional display, ultrasound has proved particularly useful in providing information to improve the performance of a renal biopsy or tapping of a renal cyst.[10] For renal biop-

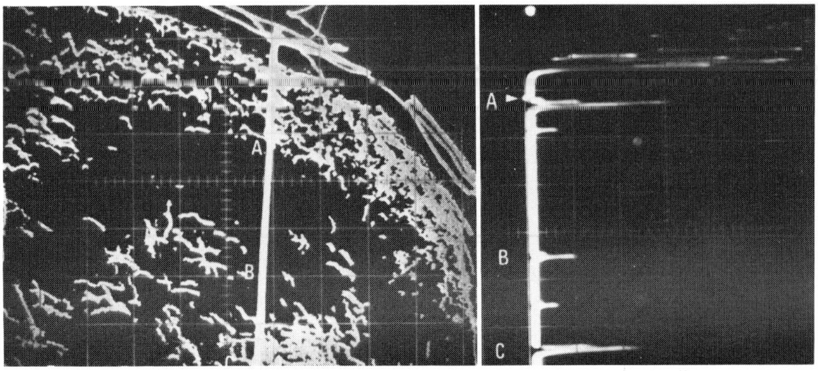

Fig. 12-11. Posterior scan of the right kidney prior to biopsy. The white line marks the point at which the A-scan display shown on the right was made. By identifying each of the A-scan points on the compound scan, precise measurements can be made for biopsy purposes.

sy, Kristensen and Holm in Copenhagen[11] and Goldberg[12] in Philadelphia have developed a transducer with a hole in the center through which the biopsy needle is inserted. After inserting the needle through the transducer, they follow the point of the needle ultrasonically. By using this technique, both groups claim a higher percentage of good specimens and fewer complications.

Our own biopsy technique includes the selection by compound scanning of the precise site for biopsy or cyst puncture, marking this on both the skin and the ultrasonic picture, and then shifting to the A-mode presentation to get a precise measurement of the depth. Fig. 12-11 illustrates our technique. The left picture shows the compound B-mode scan of the kidney with the biopsy site marked and appropriate structures identified. The A-mode presentation for more precise measurement is shown in the right. Even with a small cyst, 2 to 3 cm in diameter, this technique has been quite effective.

Hydronephrosis and renal calculi

A large hydronephrotic sac in the kidney appears ultrasonically as a large, sausage-shaped black area surrounded by a smooth echo outline. As one might suspect, the ultrasonic pattern of hydronephrosis may in some instances be difficult to distinguish from that of a renal cyst. Just like a cyst, the hydronephrotic sac remains sonolucent when receiver sensitivity is increased. Sometimes mild calyceal dilation is suggested by expansion of the total calyceal-pelvic "echo blob."

Fig. 12-12 illustrates the diagnostic value of ultrasound in hydronephrosis. This patient was referred for a suspected pancreatic cyst. The ultrasonic scan shows in its upper portion a well-defined sonolucent area on the left side that remains sonolucent when receiver sensitivity is increased. Echoes adjacent to the spine in the lower left corner suggest a compressed kidney. The barium studies shown in the lower portion of Fig. 12-12 indicate the presence of the mass. When an intravenous pyelogram was requested, the films, though inadequate, suggested that the fluid-filled mass was a hydronephrotic sac. A dye injection at surgery (shown in the lower right) demonstrated the hydronephrotic sac.

This case illustrates how ultrasound may supplement radiologic procedures in arriving at a specific diagnosis. Ultrasound demonstrated a fluid-filled mass and suggested the need for an intravenous pyelogram. However, there were no characteristics of the ultrasonic picture except

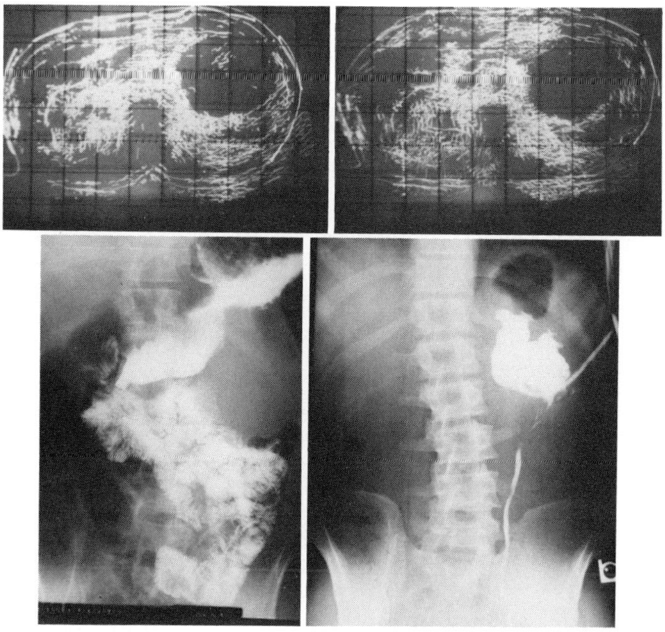

Fig. 12-12. Anterior abdominal scan with liver to the left and a dense spinal echo pattern below. Sonolucent areas representing aorta and vena cava are just above the spine. To the right in the picture is a large sonolucent area about 9 × 9 cm in size and free of echoes. The gastrointestinal series in the lower left picture suggests the presence of a large mass on the left side. The picture on the lower right shows a hydronephrotic sac injected with contrast medium at the time of surgery.

for the compressed kidney echo pattern that distinguished it from other causes of fluid-filled mass in this location.

Renal stones, whether radiopaque or nonradiopaque, will give a dense echo pattern because of reflection from the stone's surface. However, using the current equipment, this echo pattern has no specific characteristics. The stone cannot be outlined precisely because of scanning limitations, and ultrasound fails to show the posterior aspect of the stone. We have not utilized the technique described by others of placing an ultrasonic transducer directly on the external surface of the kidney at the time of surgery to help the surgeon localize stones within the kidney prior to making his initial incision. Fragmentation of renal stones by ultrasound has been described in animals, but so far the technique has not been applied routinely for humans.

Aorta

When a patient presents with acute oliguria of unknown etiology, we have found that an ultrasonic scan of the abdominal aorta is the procedure of choice to rule out aortic aneurysms or constriction of the aorta in the area of the renal arteries. Fig. 12-13 shows the echo pattern of an aortic aneurysm in the abdominal area. The longitudinal scans trace the course of the aorta and demonstrate the bulging of the aorta at the site of the aneurysm. The horizontal scan with its circular sonolucent area shows the enlarged aorta at the site of the aneurysm. A study of the aortic pulsations by T-M–mode display and the demonstration by changing receiver sensitivity of echoes along one wall suggestive of clot may help in precisely describing the aneurysm prior to surgery. Leopold has described similar studies.[13]

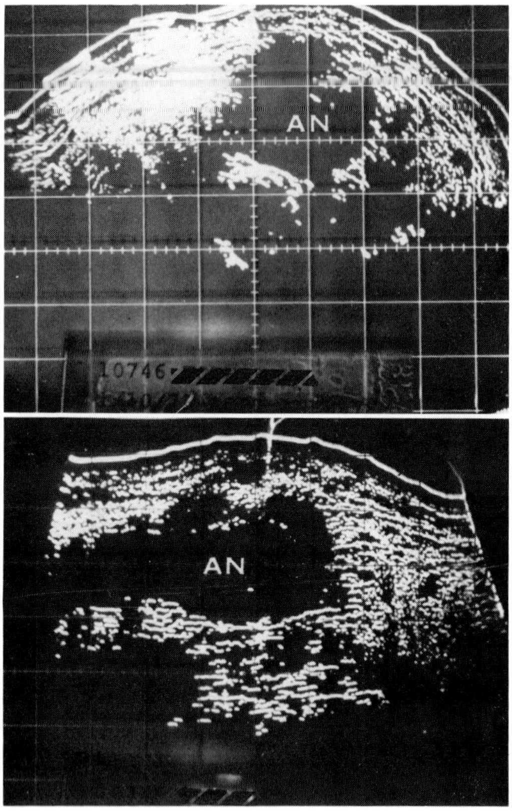

Fig. 12-13. The upper picture shows a transverse anterior abdominal scan revealing a well-defined sonolucent area that had definite pulsation. The lower picture is a longitudinal scan of the aorta showing the aneurysmal dilation. The enlarged aneurysmal area contains echoes in the upper portion. *AN*, Aneurysm.

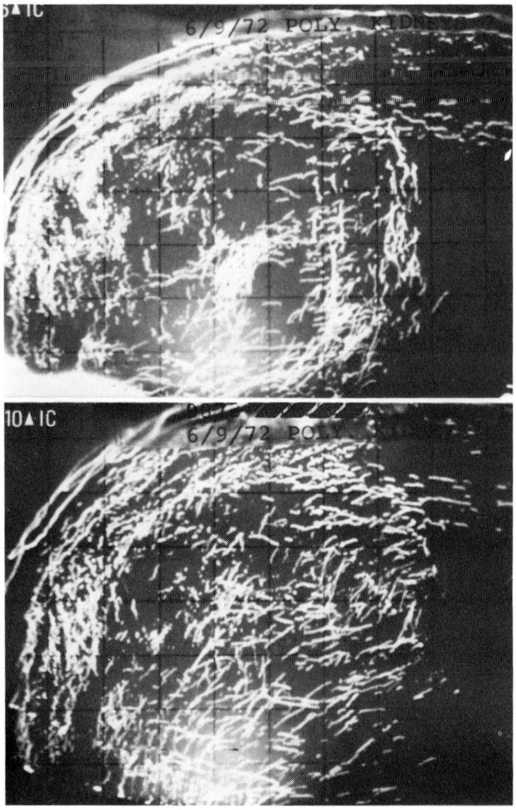

Fig. 12-14. Posterior scan of the kidney region in a 54-year-old man. The kidney is filled with a rather diffuse echo pattern, more pronounced in the lower picture, taken at a different level. There are several sonolucent areas surrounded by echo outlines of irregular size and shape, suggestive of polycystic kidney. A definite difference is noted between this pattern and those previously shown for polycystic kidney disease. The diagnosis was tuberous sclerosis.

Miscellaneous applications

Ultrasound can contribute useful information in a number of other diagnostic applications related to the kidney. In renal injury, the presence of a sonolucent area just outside the kidney outline or a sudden enlargement of the kidney at one pole indicates extrarenal or intrarenal hemorrhage, respectively. Similar patterns may be diagnostic after renal biopsy or surgery. The presence of a well-circumscribed echo area surrounding a sonolucent center adjacent to the kidney may be diagnostic of perirenal abscess. In instances of extravasation of urine or in patients with ascites, ultrasound can contribute significant diagnostic information. Lyons and associates have described its use in pediatrics.[14]

We have not yet established the significance of increased intrarenal echo patterns, nor have we developed a display to depict intrarenal echo patterns effectively. Fig. 12-14 shows an intense echo pattern within the kidney surrounding small sonolucent areas suggestive of cysts. This patient had tuberous sclerosis with multiple cyst formation as revealed by the autopsy specimen. Recently we have observed an intense echo pattern replacing the entire kidney area in a patient with multiple myeloma. Thus one could predict that as we acquire greater experience and improve our echo displays, intrarenal echo patterns will provide additional diagnostic information.

Bladder

The urine-filled bladder is readily outlined by ultrasound.[4] By using the planimeter technique previously described, one can calculate the amount of contained urine to an accuracy of ±10% when compared with catheterized volumes. In contrast to other anatomic structures, the contour of the bladder changes continually, depending on the amount of contained urine and pressure of intrapelvic structures. The upper part of Fig. 12-15 shows a horizontal scan of a bladder containing 475 ml of urine. The centrally placed sonolucent area just below the skin line and abdominal wall echoes represents the urine and the echo patterns surrounding it is the bladder wall. The two lower pictures show vertical scans of the same bladder. The middle illustration is at the midline and the lower one was made 2 cm to the right of the midline, showing the differences in contour at different positions. When the abdomen is flat over the bladder area, it is sometimes quite difficult to visualize the posterior wall.

Bladder studies have been most helpful in the following ways:

1. To determine the amount of residual urine after voiding without catheterization
2. To assess the amount of urine present in the bladder of patients with acute oliguria and, by repeat studies, to determine whether the kidney is functioning, as measured by an increase in bladder urine

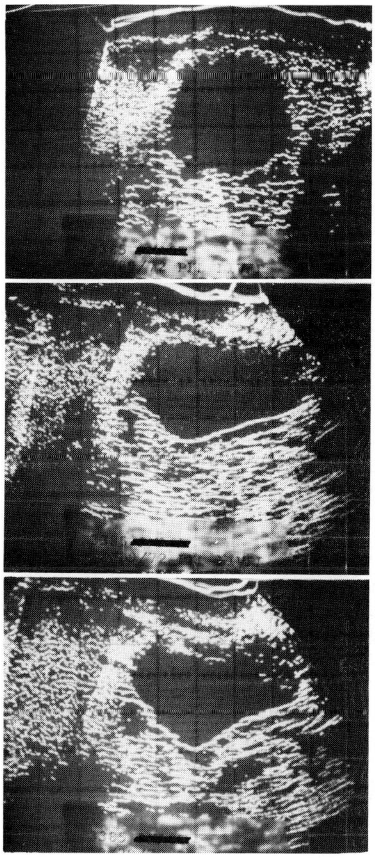

Fig. 12-15. The top picture is a horizontal scan across the abdomen 2 cm above the symphysis pubis in a healthy 24-year-old woman. The clear black area below the abdominal wall echoes represents the urine-filled bladder. The middle picture shows a vertical scan of the same bladder at the midline, and the lower picture is a vertical scan 2 cm to the right of the midline.

3. To detect and describe the invasive character of bladder tumors
4. To assess the flexibility of the bladder wall
5. To detect an intrapelvic pathologic condition when it distorts bladder contour
6. To outline the bladder prior to intravesicular taps or surgery

Residual urine

To calculate volumes, a series of scans must be taken, requiring 20 to 30 minutes.

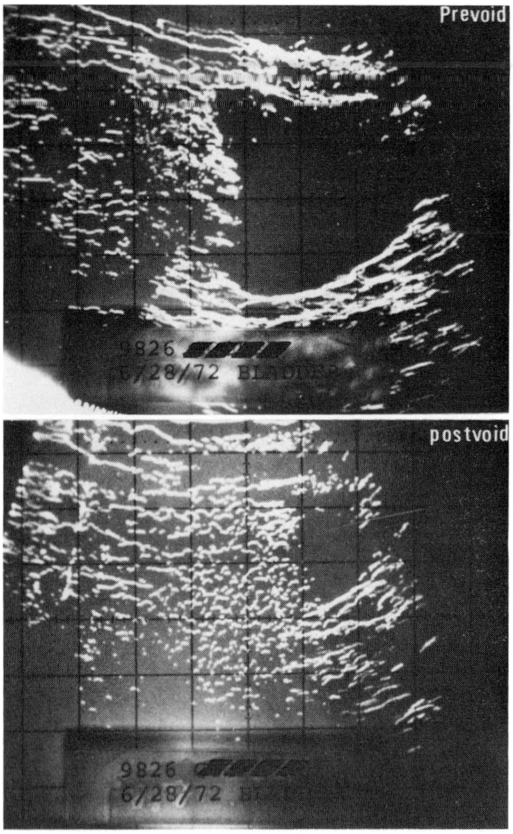

Fig. 12-16. Upper picture is a prevoiding film representing a vertical scan along the midline in the bladder area. Urine appears as a sonolucent area. The lower picture shows the postvoiding film, indicating the presence of residual urine in the bladder. (From Hinman, F. J., editor: Hydrodynamics of micturition, Springfield, Ill., 1971, Charles C Thomas, Publisher, pp. 303-319.)

An abbreviated study of two or three scans before and after voiding can be done in about 10 to 15 minutes and provides a rough estimate of the residual urine. Vertical scans are used since they more effectively depict urine under the symphysis pubis. Fig. 12-16 (upper portion) shows the outline of the urine-filled bladder prior to voiding, and the lower portion shows the presence of a significanct amount of urine after voiding. The calculated volume in the upper half was 310 ml and in the lower half 70 ml. We have used ultrasound in evaluating bladder function in all renal transplant recipients, since induced infection by catheterization is more hazardous because of the immunosuppressive therapy. In renal clearance studies, when it is not desired to catheterize, a single ultrasonic scan can be used to determine whether the patient has effectively emptied his bladder at each voiding. In patients with acute oliguria, a situation where catheterization imposes an increased risk of infection, the same information may be obtained by ultrasound. One can estimate the rate of urine flow through repeat ultrasonic studies. Tracing the outline of the bladder urine on tissue paper initially and repeating every 2 hours gives a quick visual estimate of an increase in bladder urine.

Bladder tumor

Currently, bladder tumor studies are used most often in planning therapy by assessing the extent of invasion of bladder wall and pelvic structures.[15] However, ultrasound could also have potential as a screening test, for example, on all persons over 50 or in the patient who fears catheterization or who has had previous ureteral stricture. Fig. 12-17 shows in the upper section a diffuse echo pattern involving most of the bladder cavity in a patient with confirmed extensive bladder tumor. Between the echo patches are sonolucent areas representing urine. The lower portion shows a repeat scan after partial surgical removal of the tumor. Some echoes representing tumor can still be seen; thus, ultrasound can be of value in following planned therapy without instrumentation.

Bladder contour

Assessment of bladder contour has three practical applications in our unit. The first is the detection of intrapelvic pathology by demonstration of a significant displacement of the bladder or distortion of its

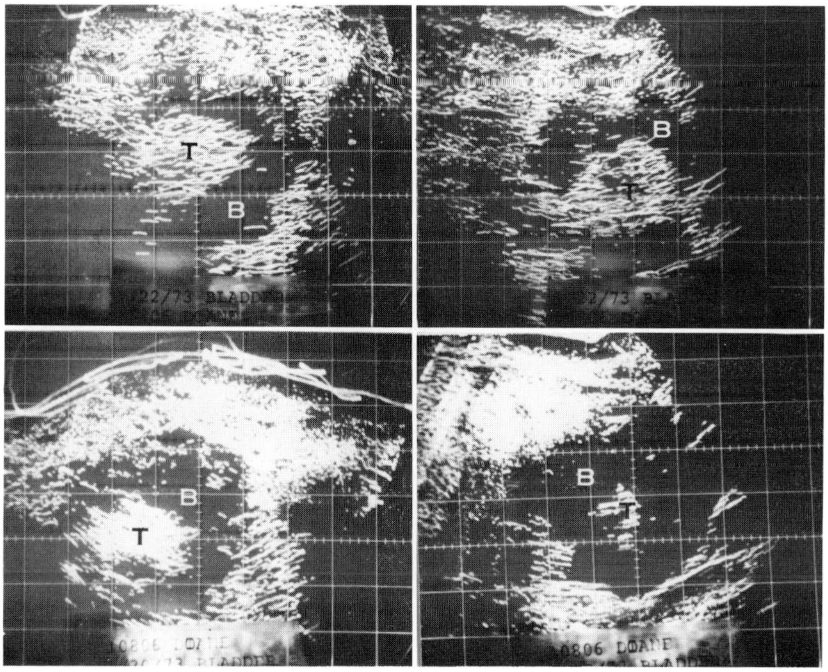

Fig. 12-17. The top pictures show on the left a horizontal scan and on the right a vertical scan of the bladder area in a man with extensive bladder tumor who had difficulty in emptying his bladder. Note the echo pattern extending into the bladder cavity and the irregular sonolucent areas representing urine surrounding the echo areas. The two lower pictures represent corresponding scans after partial resection of the tumor, showing particularly in the vertical scan that a great deal of the tumor has been removed.

contour. Demonstration of involvement of the bladder by adjacent pelvic or abdominal masses may be important in outlining more effectively that mass and, when significant bladder involvement is present, to alert the physician prior to surgical exploration or radiation therapy. The second is an assessment of bladder function in the renal transplant recipient. A well-functioning bladder that can empty completely and has normal flexibility, as demonstrated by contour changes with different urine volumes, improves the chances of a successful transplant. A third application is for assessing bladder wall involvement by infection or fibrosis.

We first described a technique of measuring the area of contained urine at each scan and then plotting the urine area versus distance from the midline.[16] This is illustrated in Fig. 12-18. Normally, the contour of these curves will vary with the contained urine volume, so they must be done at different stages of bladder filling. If there is no change in bladder contour with volume of contained urine and the bladder behaves like a rigid tube, this suggests considerable involvement of the bladder wall by previous infection or fibrosis. Furthermore, if the bladder position is significantly altered, this is also valuable information. It can localize the site of external pressure, as shown in Fig. 12-18, which also shows the best position for intravesicular tap. Ultrasound is the only method for determining the effectiveness of the triple voiding technique. After the initial voiding, if subsequent voidings demon-

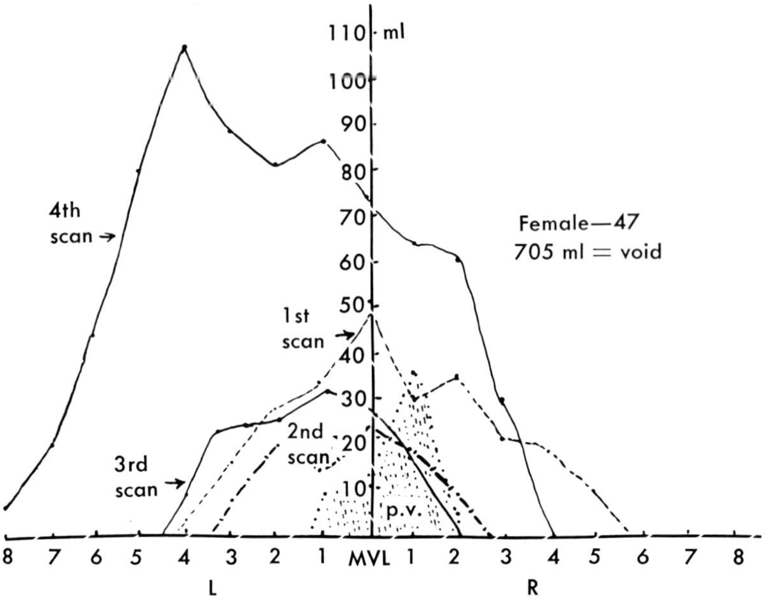

Fig. 12-18. A plot of the bladder urine versus the distance from the midline. Plots at several different urine volumes show the changes in bladder contour with filling. The shaded area represents the plot of residual urine after voiding. (From Hinman, F. J., editor: Hydrodynamics of micturition, Springfield, Ill., 1971, Charles C Thomas, Publisher, pp. 303-319.)

strate complete emptying of the bladder, the triple voiding technique is effective.

OTHER APPLICATIONS

Foreign bodies in the bladder can be detected but usually appear only as a dense echo mass and frequently cannot be completely outlined.

With genitourinary tract tumors, ultrasound can provide the radiotherapist with more effective information as to precise size and depth of the tumor, which is of inestimable value in planning radiotherapy. Even the simple expedient of providing surface contour is of help in placing the radiation source.

FUTURE APPLICATIONS

Currently the diagnostic applications of ultrasound described for the genitourinary tract and kidney provide an outline technique, which means emphasizing display of the initial echoes from organ interfaces but ignoring the smaller echoes generated from intrarenal structures of different density. For example, it should be possible to display the calyceal system in detail and to visualize the renal pyramids. In pathologic lesions, display of echoes from within a tumor may provide a characteristic pattern that can establish the type of tumor present.

One approach to this problem is the gray tone display shown in Fig. 12-5. In this technique, echoes of four preselected intensities are displayed simultaneously on the oscilloscope screen in different shades of gray. Use of a more persistent phosphor on the oscilloscope tube and photographing the afterglow is another approach to differentiating echoes of different intensities. Color coding of echoes of different intensity provides the "color mapping display" described by Baum (Chapter 15). The use of gating to focus on a specific area of the kidney offers promise, especially for studying pulsations of the renal arteries. Another approach is the study of intrarenal changes by frequency spectrum analysis.

Perhaps by learning to display echoes of different intensity more effectively one can predict ultrasonically such kidney lesions as multiple myeloma, lupus erythematosus, acute rejection of the transplanted kidney, and periarteritis nodosa. In addition, it might be possible to establish specific echo patterns that will predict the type of renal tumor present. Tissue studies on liver slices containing tumor have shown that by measuring velocity of sound transmission, attenuation, and frequency spectrum analysis, there are significant differences between tumor and normal tissue and even betweeen different tumors. Thus the diagnostic applications presented in this chapter represent only a first step in realizing the full potential of ultrasound for diagnostic study of the kidney and genitourinary tract.

REFERENCES

1. Holmes, J. H.: Diagnostic ultrasonography, Med. Coll. Virginia Quart. **3**:139, 1967.
2. Holmes, J. H.: Ultrasonic studies of the bladder and kidney. In Grossman, C. C., and others, editors: Diagnostic ultrasound, New York, 1966, Plenum Press, Inc., pp. 249-263.
3. Holmes, J. H.: The use of ultrasound for diagnosis of intra-abdominal lesions with special reference to the kidney and bladder, Proceedings of First International Congress of Ultrasonic Diagnosis in Medicine, Vienna, June, 1969, 1971, Vienna, Verlag der Wiener Medizinischen Akademie, pp. 1-22.
4. Holmes, J. H.: Ultrasonic studies of the bladder, J. Urol. **97:**654, 1967.
5. King, D. L.: Renal ultrasonography, Radiology **105:**633, 1972.
6. Igawa, K., Miyagishi, T.: The use of scintillation and ultrasonic scanning to disclose polycystic kidneys and liver, J. Urol. **108:**685, 1972.
7. Schreck, W. R., and Holmes, J. H.: Ultrasound as a diagnostic aid for renal neoplasms and cysts, J. Urol. **103:**281, 1970.
8. Winterberger, A. R., Palma, L. D., and Murphy, G. P.: Ultrasonic testing in human renal allografts, J.A.M.A. **219:**475, 1972.
9. Leopold, G. R. Renal transplant size measurement by reflected ultrasound, Radiology **95:**687, 1970.
10. Bahlmann, J., and Otto, P.: In Cameron, J. S., editor: Proceedings of the Ninth Conference of European Dialysis and Transplant Association, New York, 1972, Pitman Medical Books.
11. Kristensen, J. K., and others: Ultrasonically guided percutaneous puncture of renal masses, Scand. J. Urol. Nephrol. **6**(Suppl. 15):1972.
12. Goldberg, B. B., and Pollack, H. M.: Ultrasonic aspiration—biopsy transducer, Radiology **108:**667, 1973.
13. Leopold, G. R.: Ultrasonic abdominal aortography, Radiology **96:**9, 1970.
14. Lyons, E. A., and others: Nephrosonography in infants and children: a new technique, Br. Med. J. **2:**689, 1972.
15. Kyle, K. F., and others: Ultrasonography of the urinary tract, Br. J. Urol. **43:**709, 1971.
16. Holmes, J. H.: Ultrasonic studies of bladder filling and contour. In Hinman, F. J., editor: Hydrodynamics of micturition, Springfield, Ill., 1971, Charles C Thomas, Publisher, pp. 303-319.

13 Abdominal ultrasonography

GEORGE R. LEOPOLD, M.D.

Exploration of the upper abdominal structures by ultrasonic methods is of more recent origin than obstetric and gynecologic ultrasonography. In the pelvis the number of organs and their usual abnormalities are relatively few. In the upper abdomen the multiplicity of structures, normal variations in shape and consistency, and presence of significant sources of artifact all combine to make abdominal ultrasonography a challenging procedure to perform and interpret. Nevertheless, with perfection of scanning technique and a thorough knowledge of normal anatomy, significant information can be gained in a wide variety of clinical disorders.

The scope of such studies has been continuously expanding. Pioneer efforts included the early works of Holmes[1] and Howry,[2] primarily in the study of the kidney, and Lehman,[3] in the study of the liver. With the accumulation of experience, however, it is now commonplace to study the pancreas, gallbladder, spleen, aorta, and retroperitoneal space when the clinical situation dictates.[4,5] While conventional radiologic procedures remain the mainstay for diagnosis of intraluminal disease process in the abdomen, ultrasound studies are now readily recognized as a safe and accurate technique for evaluation of extraluminal disease processes.

TECHNIQUE

Although A-mode (amplitude modulation) studies in which the returning echoes are displayed as vertical spikes along a horizontal baseline are sometimes used in the study of abdominal disorders, they are usually more helpful when performed in conjunction with a B-scanning procedure. Their principal usefulness is in assessing the internal structure of a lesion found by palpation, x-ray, or B scan. This is done chiefly by varying the sensitivity setting of the instrument. At higher sensitivity, or "gain" settings, those masses that are solid will reveal internal echo formation because of their multiple tissue planes, while fluid-filled masses will remain echo-free (Figs. 13-1 and 13-2). Experience with this technique allows differentiation of cystic and solid masses with a 95% accuracy rate.[6]

A-mode studies are also occasionally used when increased accuracy in measuring the diameter of an object is desired. Early papers report serial A-mode measurements along the course of the abdominal aorta to determine its precise external diameter.[7] It may also be employed to detect accumulations of ascitic fluid in the flanks.[8] Changes in size of the accumulation with change in position of the patient are helpful indicators of the presence of free fluid within the abdomen.

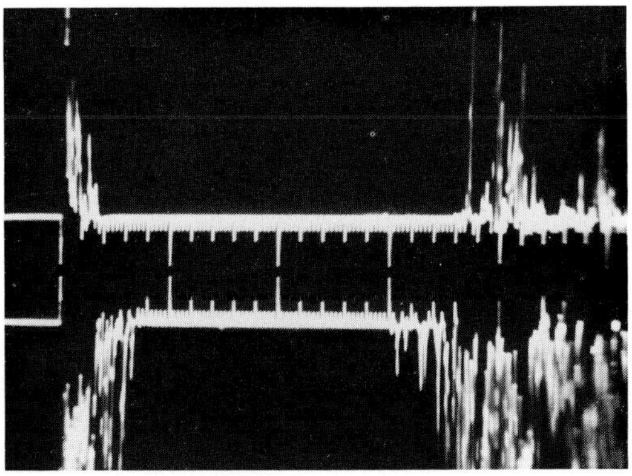

Fig. 13-1. A-mode study of typical cystic mass. The top line is the low gain setting; the higher gain study (bottom) shows no internal echoes, indicating the cystic nature of the mass.

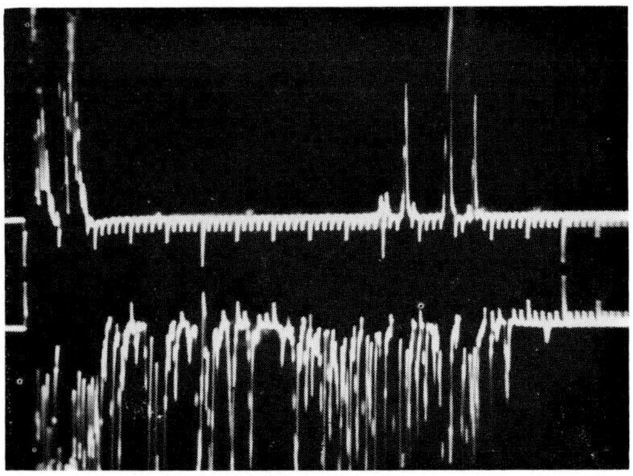

Fig. 13-2. A-mode study of solid mass. Although devoid of echoes at low gain (top), multiple internal echoes appear at high gain (bottom).

For a more complete anatomic depiction of the intraabdominal and retroperitoneal structures, the B-scanning technique is essential. Most commercially available units employ the contact method, wherein the transducer is applied directly to the patient's skin after coating it with a suitable coupling material such as mineral oil or aqueous jelly. The transducer is then manually guided with a gentle rocking motion across the plane to be examined. The purpose of the to-and-fro rocking motion during the scan is to achieve perpendicularity to a greater number of interfaces beneath the surface, since only those interfaces are recorded.

B scanning, like the M mode used in echocardiography, uses the B mode (brightness or intensity modulation) of data analysis. The returning echoes are displayed as dots of varying brightness. Through a system of potentiometers, their correct spatial orientation is recorded on the oscilloscope screen. Data accumulated may be recorded either by a storage (persistence) type of oscilloscope or by time-exposure photography of the nonstorage oscilloscope screen. Most upper abdominal studies are performed by making a series of transverse and longitudinal scans at 1- to 2-cm intervals over the area of interest. In general, the most posteriorly located structures (kidneys, retroperitoneal space) are studied in the prone position, while anterior structures, including those in the immediate prevertebral area, are best studied with the patient supine. While oblique scans are occasionally useful, the distortions of anatomy so produced often make interpretation considerably more difficult.

By far the most significant barrier to upper abdominal scanning is the presence of excessive gas within the gastrointestinal tract (Fig. 13-3).[9] Since air (and bone) are virtually complete reflectors of the ultrasonic beam, all structures located directly behind a gas collection will not be visible. Gentle pressure applied with the transducer during the course of the scan may help to displace interfering gas-filled loops. If this is unsuccessful, however, it may be necessary to postpone the study until a more favorable time.

Likewise, the presence of significant amounts of barium within the gastrointestinal tract causes serious deterioration of the image when examining in the supine position.[10] For this reason, it is always desirable to perform ultrasonic studies before conventional barium examinations.

Significant difficulty may also be caused by the rib cage in certain individuals (Fig. 13-4). Excessively knobby ribs frequently give rise to reverberation artifacts within the liver and spleen that may be confused with pathologic processes. They are usually recognizable by the predictable regularity with which they occur. Slight transducer obliquity to the scanning surface may alleviate this problem.

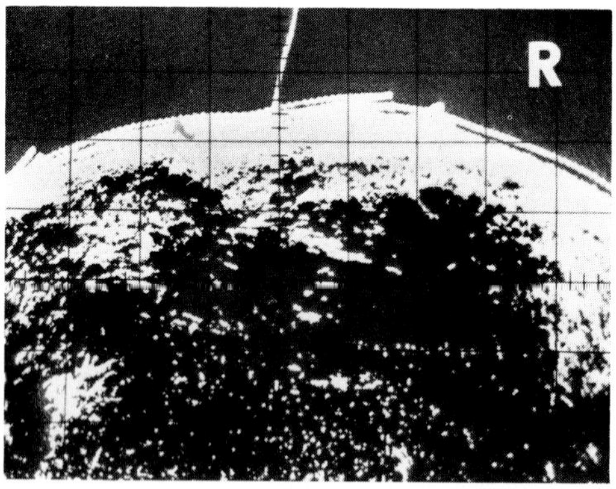

Fig. 13-3. Transverse B scans of the abdomen in the presence of large amounts of intestinal gas. Note that the spine and posteriorly located organs cannot be seen, and the scan is therefore nondiagnostic. *R*, Right side of patient in this and all subsequent transverse scans. Scale is 3 cm per square on superimposed grid.

ANATOMY

A survey study of the upper abdomen is usually initiated with transverse scans of the patient in the supine position. The umbilicus serves as a convenient starting point from which to reference all subsequent transverse scans. Some individuals prefer to use the plane of the iliac crest as a reference, since it may more easily be related to routine radiographs. These planes are usually identical, however, and correspond roughly to the level of the fourth lumbar vertebral body.

The following scans are intended to show average anatomy in the transverse plane as it is visualized ultrasonically. They were made at "normal" gain levels, usually intermediate between the "high" and "low" gain settings that have been determined useful by experience with that particular instrument.

It is helpful to have a concept of transverse anatomic relationships as gained from standard anatomic texts such as

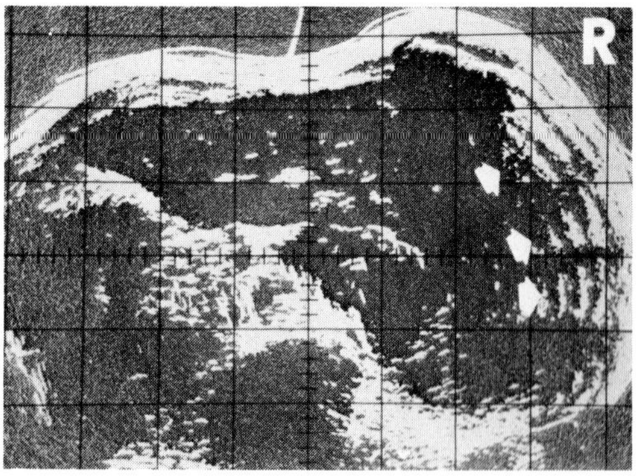

Fig. 13-4. Transverse scan of upper abdomen showing prominent rib artifacts (arrows) projected over the liver. Notice their regularity.

Eycleshymer and Schoemaker.[11] Unfortunately, detailed texts of longitudinal cross-sectional anatomy are not available. In addition, once experience is achieved with B scanning, the operator soon realizes that all such drawings are only rough guides because of the enormous variability of shape and position of the structures concerned.

Transverse scans

Umbilicus (Fig. 13-5). The most prominent structures are the spine, sonolucent psoas muscle masses, and the prevertebral vessels. The inferior vena cava is less frequently seen than the aorta because of its thinner walls and its collapse with respiration. Visualization of the spine is considered necessary before the scan can be called diagnostic, since it ensures that sound has passed through all portions of the abdomen without interference from bowel gas.

U + 5 (5 cm cephalad) (Fig. 13-6). The lower pole of the right lobe of the liver makes its appearance at this level. The fluid-filled gallbladder can frequently be seen embedded in its medial aspect. The right kidney is always well visualized because of the sonolucent liver overlying it. The calyces and other structures in the renal sinus produce central echoes and help to differentiate the kidney from the psoas muscle masses seen in the previous example.

U + 10 (Fig. 13-7). Scans made at this approximate level show a much larger portion of liver, usually including its left lobe. Central echoes are invariably present within the liver and are thought to arise from the large veins and ducts in the hilus. A

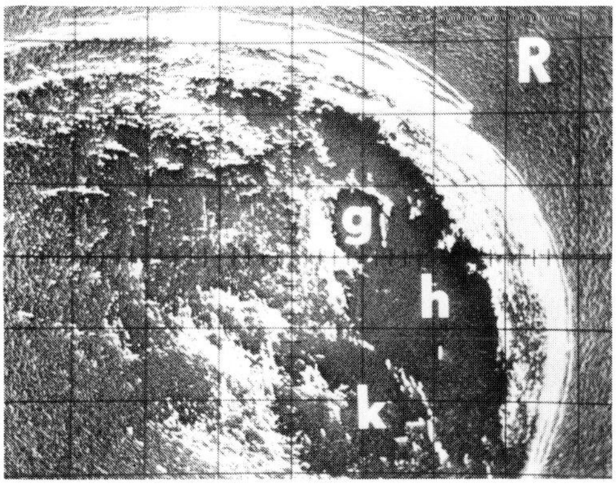

Fig. 13-6. Transverse scan 5 cm above the umbilicus in a fasting, normal patient. The relationships of the liver *(h)*, gallbladder *(g)*, and right kidney *(k)* are clearly seen.

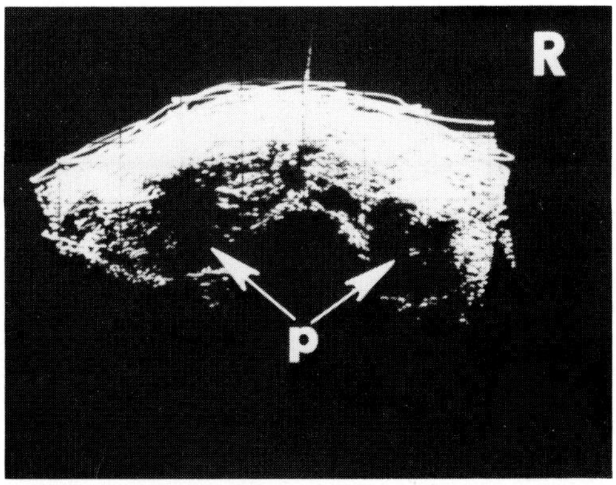

Fig. 13-5. Transverse scan at the level of the umbilicus in a normal patient. The psoas muscle bundles *(p)* are seen in paraspinous location. The circular sonolucencies just anterior to the spine are the aorta and inferior vena cava.

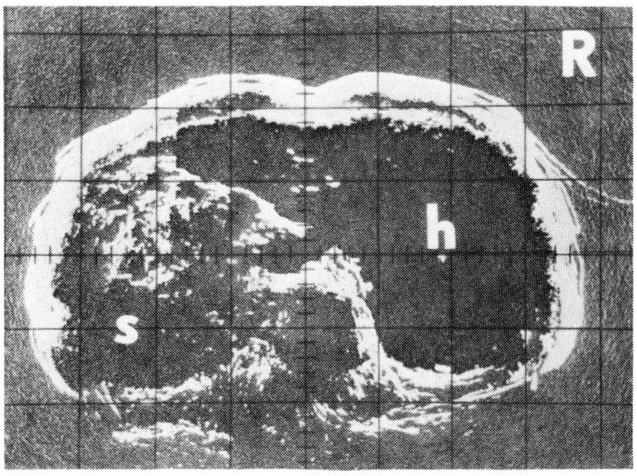

Fig. 13-7. Transverse scan 10 cm above the umbilicus. Large segments of the liver *(h)* and spleen *(s)* are now apparent. The aorta is also well seen just anterior to the spine.

collection of echoes is also frequently identifiable within the left lobe just beneath the midline. It has been speculated by some that these are artifacts caused by reverberation from the rectus sheath, but their exact origin remains obscure. A significant portion of the spleen usually appears along the left lateral flank at this level. The stomach is identified by a C-shaped echo structure placed between the liver and spleen. The contour of the stomach is incomplete posteriorly because the intraluminal gas that is normally present rises to its highest point and precludes visualization beyond.

U + 15 (Fig. 13-8). This level marks the endpoint of useful transverse scanning since the lower aspect of the lungs prevents delineation of the abdominal contents in most areas except those located very centrally (aorta, anterior margin of vertebral body).

Longitudinal scans

Midline (Fig. 13-9). The longitudinal or sagittal scan made in the midplane demonstrates well the left lobe of the liver and the abdominal aorta. The aorta will be noted to end at approximately the level of the umbilicus, since bifurcation occurs at that point, and the iliac branches lie within a different plane. A clear space will occasionally be noted between the liver and the aorta. While this may represent a diseased pancreas, a dilated, fluid-filled gastric antrum or duodenum can also present in this location. The levels of the umbilicus (L4) and the xiphoid process of the sternum (T10) are customarily marked electronically on the scan as reference points.

R − 3 (3 cm to the right of midline) (Fig. 13-10). Scans made in this longitudinal

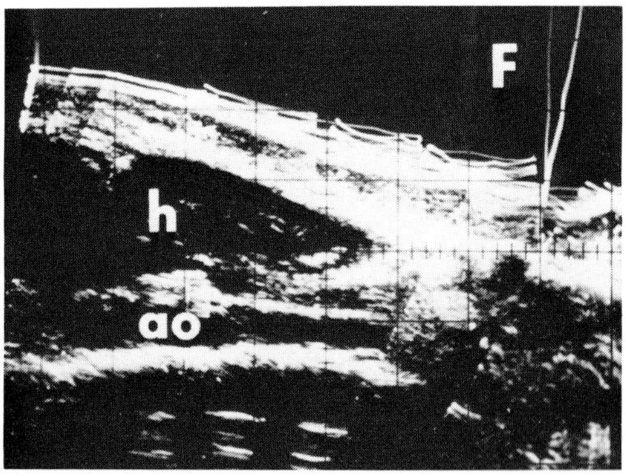

Fig. 13-9. Longitudinal (sagittal) midline scan showing normal anatomy. The liver *(h)* and aorta *(ao)* are usually the most prominent structures. *F*, Direction of patient's feet in this and all subsequent longitudinal scans.

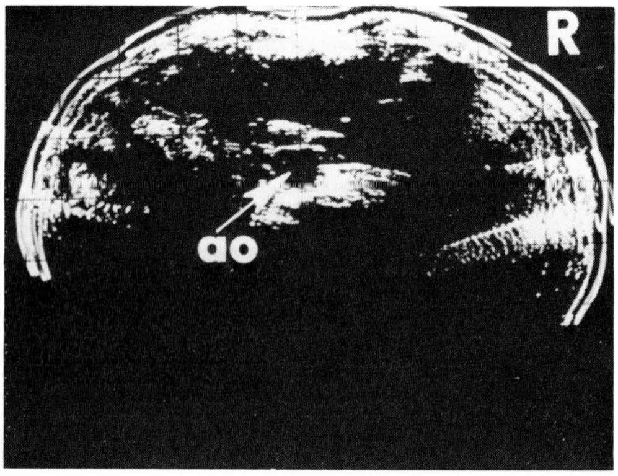

Fig. 13-8. Transverse scan 15 cm above the umbilicus. At this level, the lower aspects of the lungs preclude good visualization of the laterally placed viscera. A segment of the aorta *(ao)* may still be seen centrally.

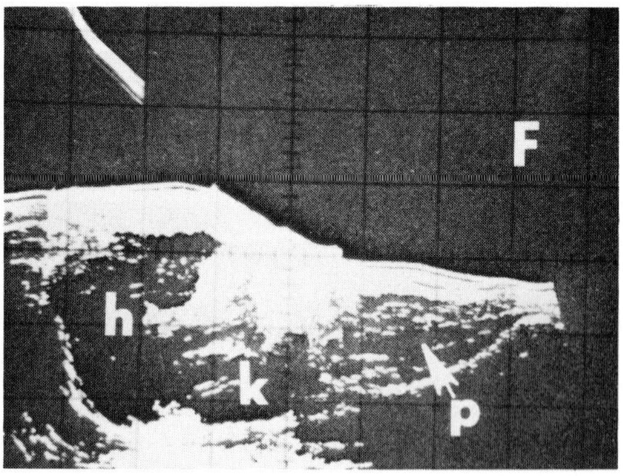

Fig. 13-10. Longitudinal scan 3 cm to the right of midline in a normal child. The liver *(h)*, right kidney *(k)*, and psoas muscle *(p)* are shown in their normal relationship.

plane demonstrate a larger segment of liver and, more posteriorly, the medial portion of the right kidney. The superior aspect of the liver and diaphragm, which are not demonstrable on transverse scans, may be seen by depressing the abdominal wall beneath the liver and angling the transducer sharply toward the patient's head.

R − 6 (Fig. 13-11). As the longitudinal scans proceed more laterally, slight tilt of the scanning head back toward the midline is often necessary to maintain contact with the skin. In this approximate area, the gallbladder is most often found lying closely adherent to the undersurface of the liver. By scanning at slightly higher than normal gain levels, the interface between the liver and the anterior wall of the gallbladder becomes much more apparent. Because of the degree of medial tilt introduced, the kidney is still visualized posterior to the liver and gallbladder. If the gallbladder is somewhat distended, long segments of the inferior vena cava will frequently be visualized immediately posterior to it.

L − 3. Longitudinal scans to the left of midline are seldom of much help in demonstrating the normal anatomy, since gastric air can obscure a significant portion of the left upper quadrant. If, however, the disease process is centered there, they are frequently helpful in determining its nature and extent.

CLINICAL APPLICATIONS

Liver

Parenchymal abnormalities of the liver may be recognized, but care must be used in selecting proper gain settings for the examination.[3] In order to recognize solid lesions within the liver, very *low* sensitivities are necessary to accentuate the acoustic impedance mismatch with normal tissue. One recognizes an abnormal focus of strong echoes in locations where ordinarily there are none. Unfortunately, the pattern produced is not specific for metastatic disease and may be simulated by scar, benign tumor, cirrhosis (Fig. 13-12), or even an infectious process that has not yet progressed to frank abscess formation. To further complicate the problem, not all metastatic disease produces enough impedance change to be detectable by this method in its current form. It is likely that a solid mass must be 3 to 4 cm in size before it can be detected with current instruments. Clinical studies suggest that by

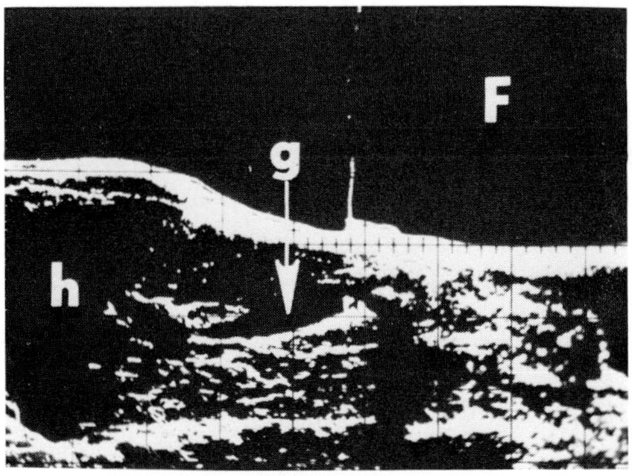

Fig. 13-11. Longitudinal scan 6 cm to the right of midline in a normal fasting patient. The liver *(h)* and gallbladder *(g)* are visible. The contour of the diaphragm is clearly outlined along the superior border of the liver.

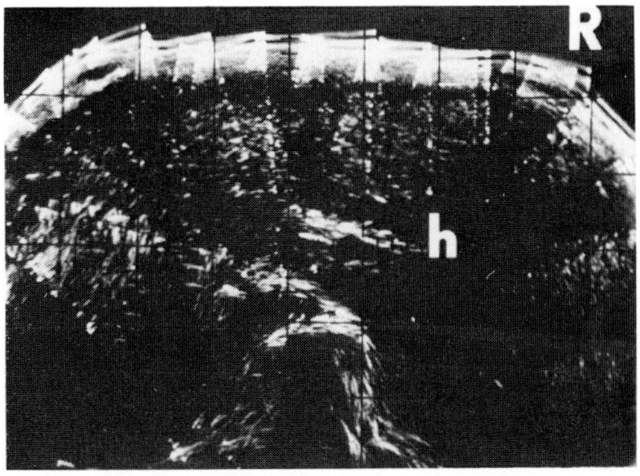

Fig. 13-12. Transverse scan of upper abdomen in patient with proved cirrhosis. The liver *(h)* is enlarged and contains many peripheral abnormal echoes, even at moderately low gain levels.

combining the conventional radioisotope scan of the liver with the ultrasonic scan, the overall accuracy in the detection of metastatic disease is increased.[12] Certainly, if percutaneous liver biopsy is contemplated, the spatial coordinates obtained from the ultrasonic scan are of considerable help in indicating the proper site, direction and depth of needle placement into a suspicious area. While advanced cirrhosis is easily recognizable by its diffuse peripheral pattern, milder degrees of this disorder may pass unnoticed.

In the detection of cystic lesions within the liver, ultrasound is a superb and unrivaled clinical tool. To detect such lesions,

A

B

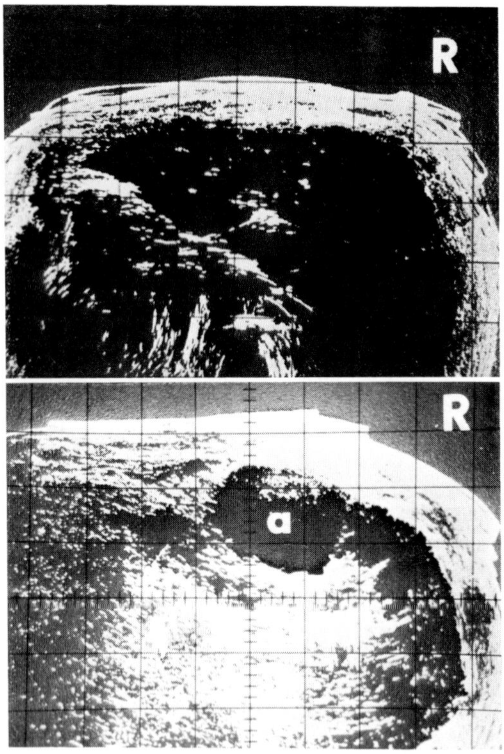

Fig. 13-13. A, Transverse scan of liver made at low or normal gain. No abnormalities are apparent. **B,** Same section as in **A,** but employing high gain. A fluid-filled cavity *(a)* (which proved to be an abscess) is seen at the junction of the right and left lobes of the liver. The echoes arising within the abscess are not unusual and probably represent debris.

high gain scanning is necessary to emphasize the fluid-filled nature of the defects (Fig. 13-13). We have seen cysts as small as 1.5 cm in the liver of a patient with polycystic disease. With an appropriate series of transverse and longitudinal scans, liver abscesses are readily detectable. Such a method is also helpful in the follow-up of these lesions during therapy. Interestingly, the abscess defect seen on ultrasonic scan shrinks much more rapidly than on the isotope scan, probably an indication of the fact that tissue around the lesion remains hypovascular for a significant period following the injury.

Fluid collections in the subhepatic space and along the lateral aspect of the liver (abscess, hematoma) are readily demonstrable on transverse scans. However, when the collection is interposed between the liver and the diaphragm, only longitudinal scans will demonstrate it. One must be careful not to misinterpret free fluid at the right lung base as subphrenic abscess. The decubitus position may aid in making this differentiation.

Gallbladder

The gallbladder is readily visible in at least 75% of patients when scans are performed in the fasting state.[3,13,13a] The gallbladder is characterized by thin walls and lack of internal echoes.

When internal echoes are noted that are repeatable from scan to scan (including one or two with suspended respiration), the chances of having cholelithiasis are quite high. Most series, however, indicate only a 50% accuracy in the ultrasonic determination of patients with radiographically evident calculi. Failure to visualize the gallbladder is not helpful, however, since many will eventually prove normal. It is apparent that good visualization without internal echoes is a very accurate indicator of the lack of disease.

In the presence of neoplastic obstruction of the common bile duct, the gallbladder may dilate to enormous proportions. Since the differentiation of intrahepatic and extrahepatic jaundice on the basis of chemical values is often difficult and routine radiographic methods do not visualize the biliary system, the ultrasonic scan assumes a very significant role in this situation. The dilated gallbladder is an easy ultrasonic target (Fig. 13-14). One must recognize, however, that the normal gallbladder is capable of attaining significant dimensions in the fasting state. It is therefore important to use secondary measures such as observing contraction after a fatty meal or detecting the obstructing mass itself before one concludes that the gallbladder is pathologically enlarged.

A

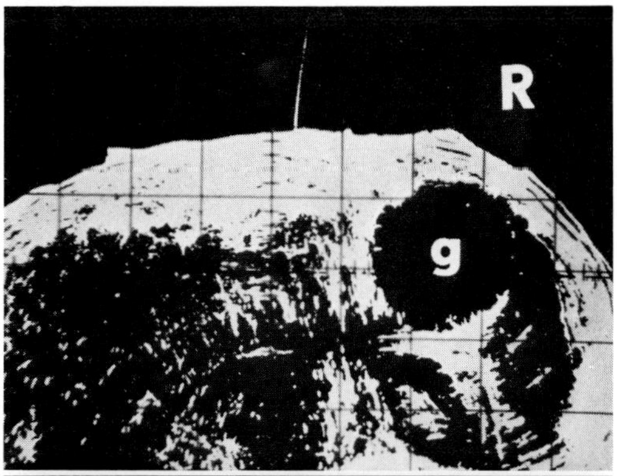

B

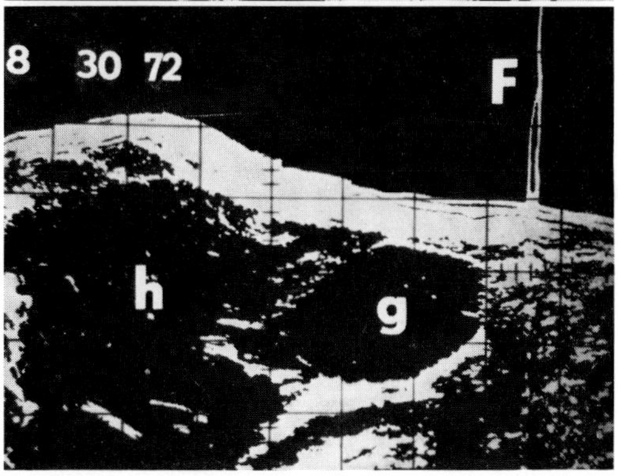

Fig. 13-14. A, Transverse, high gain scan 8 cm above the umbilicus showing a markedly dilated gallbladder *(g)* in a patient with hydrops. **B,** Longitudinal scan of same patient as **A.** The distended gallbladder *(g)* is easier to appreciate because it retains the shape of that organ.

One may frequently make a more perfect longitudinal scan of the gallbladder by noting and marking on the skin its position from a number of transverse scans. By making the final scans along these marks, the true long axis of the organ can be determined.

Pancreas

Since the pancreas lies obliquely in the upper abdomen, a single transverse scan usually does not include a long segment of the gland. It is not widely recognized how far anterior in the abdomen the pancreas lies. It is therefore necessary to carefully examine the anatomy to determine the most likely sites for the organ. Usually, the head of the pancreas lies just anterior to the right kidney and medial to the lower aspect of the right lobe of the liver and gallbladder. The body of the gland is seen several centimeters cephalad, just anterior to the aorta, and the tail is still higher and just anterior to the left kidney.

In the presence of pancreatitis, the normally invisible gland becomes edematous, enlarged, and more sonolucent, allowing its contours to be visualized (Fig. 13-15).[14] Any or all of the segments noted above may be visualized. If the enlargement

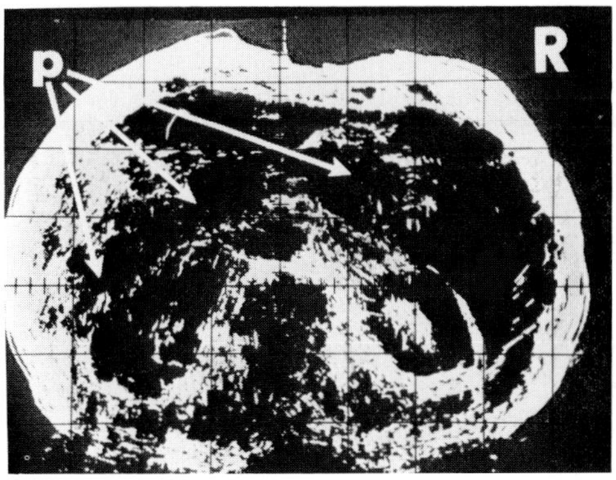

Fig. 13-15. Transverse scan 6 cm above the umbilicus in a patient with chronic pancreatitis. The entire pancreas *(p)* is edematous, thereby rendering it visible ultrasonically.

of the gland is sufficient, transverse or slightly oblique scans may succeed in demonstrating the entire gland. Frequently, the head will be disproportionately enlarged when compared to the body and tail. The enlarged head is often strikingly sonolucent and may be difficult to distinguish from pseudocyst formation. In this case, to make the distinction, one must rely on the detection of slight irregularity of the posterior margin and failure to transmit sound as well as would be expected through a totally fluid-filled mass of the same size. Patients with chronic pancreatitis tend to retain the diffuse sonolucent pattern whether they are symptomatic or not. This finding makes the technique very useful in evaluating patients with chronic upper abdominal pain of unknown etiology, even when serum and urinary enzyme levels may be normal. In patients with acute pancreatitis, the associated ileus often makes study impossible during the first few days of hospitalization. The examination should be repeated or delayed until the patient's overall condition, including his state of hydration, improves.

If pancreatitis progresses to pseudocyst formation, detection is even easier (Fig. 13-16).[15] Again, the position of the gland involved determines in a large part both the radiographic and the ultrasonic appearance. When the body of the gland is involved, care must be taken to rule out a dilated, fluid-filled stomach as a possible source of the echo abnormality. Aspiration of gastric contents and rescanning then become essential. Serial examinations in patients with pseudocyst may show either increase or decrease in size. Pseudocyst collections may be multiple, and they are frequently somewhat irregular in contour, since they have no true capsule and readily adapt to conform with the surrounding viscera.

Carcinoma of the pancreas may be identified if a solid mass is recognized in one of the expected locations of the pancreas (Fig. 13-17). Lesions of the head of the gland are more easily detected since they may be sharply contrasted with the liver and right kidney. In addition, the abnormal gallbladder dilation that is frequently present provides a useful secondary sign. Tumors of the body and tail are more difficult to diagnose because of the gas-filled

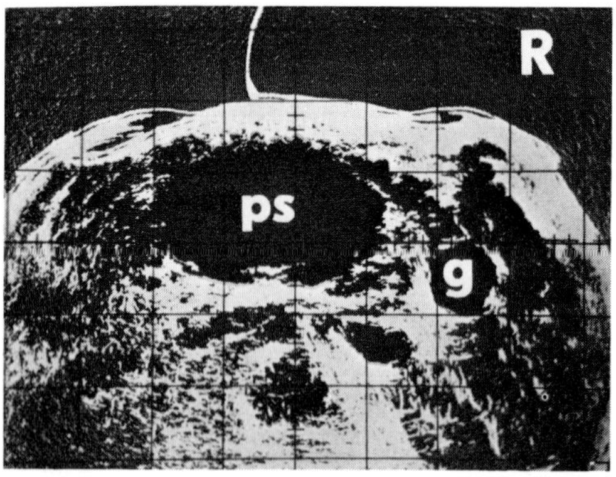

Fig. 13-16. High gain transverse scan of patient with proved pseudocyst of the head of the pancreas. Note the anterior location of the pseudocyst *(ps)* and the prominent gallbladder echoes *(g)*. In this case, the apparent dilation of the gallbladder was simply the result of prolonged fasting.

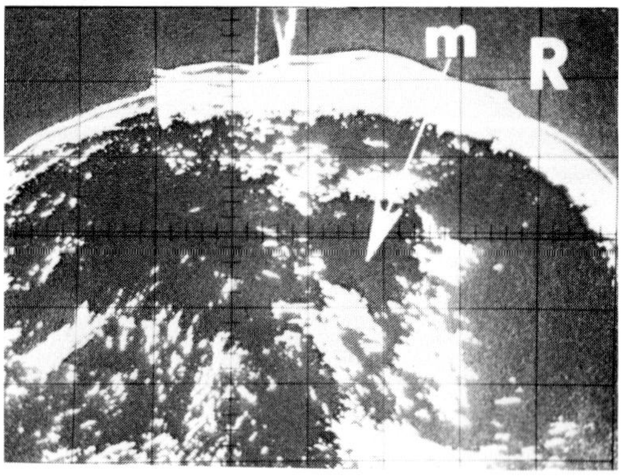

Fig. 13-17. Transverse scan of upper abdomen showing an irregularly contoured mass *(m)* interposed between the right kidney, liver, and spine. This is the expected location of the head of pancreas, and at surgery, a tumor of these dimensions was found arising in that site.

stomach and small bowel. Prone scans are occasionally useful in these situations, particularly with tumors of the pancreatic tail. When a solid mass is present in the region of the head of the pancreas, the possibility of enlarged lymph nodes should still be included in the differential diagnosis, since the porta hepatis contains a rich lymphatic bed that is frequently involved by lymphoma or metastatic spread from other primary organs. Differentiation of an enlarged, inflamed head of pancreas from tumor may be difficult or impossible, and frequently one must rely heavily on the clinical history to separate the two entities.

Despite the obvious limitations of ultrasonic scanning in carcinoma of the pancreas, it is frequently helpful enough to recommend its routine use in evaluating such cases. We have now seen several cases where the ultrasound study was the only positive preoperative test in this disorder.

Spleen

Although the spleen is usually well visualized in the supine position (Fig. 13-18), a more complete evaluation is possible when the patient is scanned prone. While variations in contour from patient to patient may be considerable, enlargement is usually obvious. It will be noted that considerably higher gain settings are necessary to produce echoes within the parenchyma of the spleen than in the liver. The spleen is the most "cystic" appearing of all the abdominal organs, since its composition is nearly 60% to 70% blood at all times.

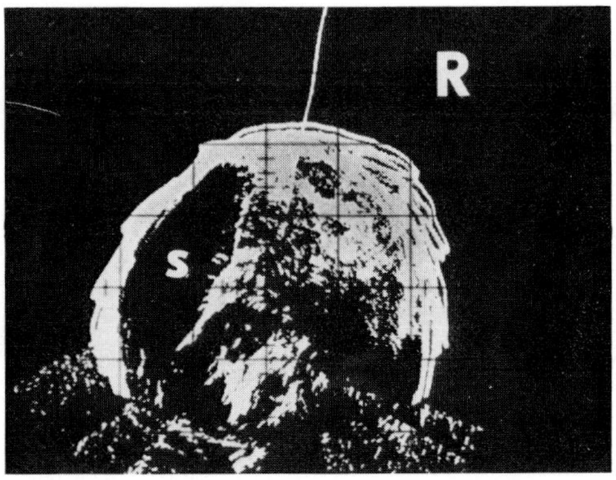

Fig. 13-18. Transverse scan of 4-month-old child with biliary cirrhosis. Marked splenomegaly *(s)* secondary to portal hypertension is present. The liver is not shown in this scan.

Ultrasonically, size variations and trauma have been the major areas of interest to date. In addition to detection of splenomegaly, the response of the spleen to chemotherapy or radiation can accurately be assessed noninvasively in hematologic disorders being so treated. Schemes for calculation of an actual splenic volume have already been proposed. When blunt trauma to the left flank occurs, the method is often capable of revealing loss of integrity of the spleen. If splenic subcapsular hematoma is present, a "double contour" of the organ may frequently be observed. While other entities such as infarction, congenital cysts, and primary and secondary tumors should theoretically be recognizable, their occurrence is sufficiently rare, and there is therefore little accumulated experience in the literature with them.

Aorta

Because of its highly elastic walls, the aorta is the easiest intra-abdominal organ to demonstrate. In most circumstances, the abdominal aorta can be traced from the level of the tenth dorsal vertebra to the bifurcation in a single longitudinal scan. Ordinarily, gain settings somewhat lower than normal are employed to produce very sharp outlines of this strong echo-producing structure. Most individuals beginning ultrasonic scanning are surprised to note the relatively anterior location of the aorta near the umbilicus. If the aorta is unduly tortuous, its size and position must be plotted from a series of transverse scans performed in the usual manner. Numerous studies in the literature indicate the accuracy of this method in the detection of abdominal aortic aneurysm.[17-19] Although some have used A mode studies alone, most have located the widest external diameter by B scanning and then measured with A mode. In this respect, it should be noted that in some aneurysms, the transverse diameter exceeds the anteroposterior diameter and therefore transverse scans as well as longitudinal scans should accompany each study. The superiority of this method, which shows the true outer contour of the aneurysm, in comparison with the conventional aortogram showing only the lumen, seems clearly established. Although the major emphasis has been in the detection of aneurysms (Fig. 13-19), it has become apparent that serial studies are capable of providing much information in those patients who are not considered operative candidates.

Periaortic lymphadenopathy may simulate aortic aneurysm if careful scanning in both longitudinal and transverse directions is not performed (Fig. 13-20).[20] This phenomenon has been called the "echo silhouette" sign, and it is believed to be caused by similarity in density between nodal tissue and the elastic wall of the aorta. On transverse scan, periaortic nodes frequently exhibit a transonic mantle in the prevertebral area. Nodes from metastatic carcinoma, on the other hand, tend to preserve the borders between the two structures.

A

B

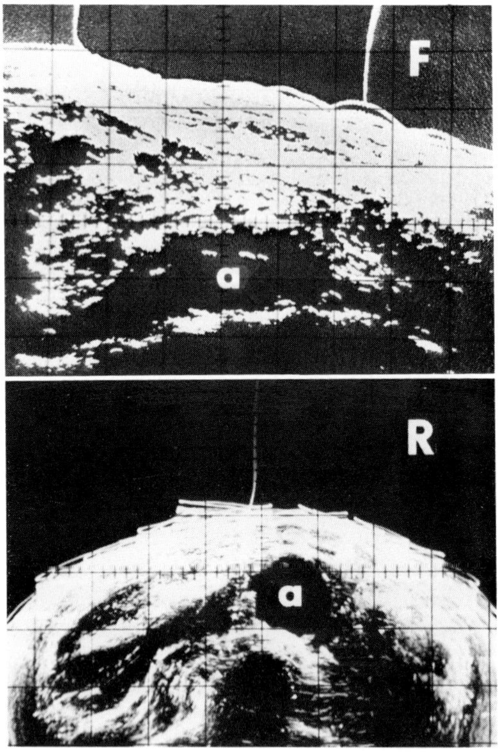

Fig. 13-19. A, Midline longitudinal scan of a patient with an abdominal aortic aneurysm *(a)*. A thin line of thrombus echoes can be identified anteriorly within the aneurysm. **B,** Transverse scan of another patient with an abdominal aortic aneurysm. Note that the aneurysm presents on the right side of the abdomen.

Extraorgan, intra-abdominal lesions

Ultrasound is particularly well suited for the study of extraluminal masses within the abdomen. Primary tumors and lymph node metastases within the leaves of the mesentery are usually easy to demonstrate and prove a valuable adjunct to conventional radiographic studies.

Ascites may be recognized by either A-mode or B-scan techniques. In general,

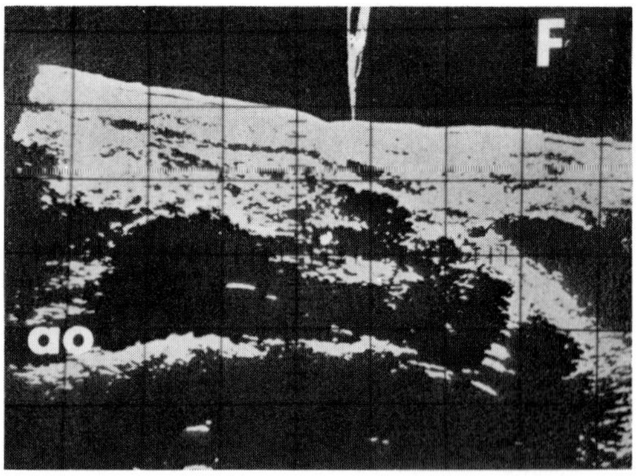

Fig. 13-20. Midline longitudinal scan of a patient with preaortic lymphadenopathy that obliterates the anterior aortic wall. Note the resemblance to the patient shown in Fig. 13-19, *A*.

there are two recognizable patterns of ascitic fluid on B scan. The usual serous ascites tends to collect symmetrically in the posterior aspect of both flanks (Fig. 13-21). In the upper abdomen the liver and spleen may be separated from the abdominal wall. Longitudinal scanning reveals large fluid-filled areas in the pelvis that tend to have sharp, angular borders rather than the rounded contours usually associated with pelvic masses. There is also an ascitic pattern that shows irregular loculations of fluid and clumping of the normal bowel echoes. The appearance, unlike that of serous effusions, is relatively unchanged with alteration of the patient's position. While some authors believe that this appearance is virtually diagnostic of malignant ascites, it can also be seen in adhesive peritoneal inflammatory disease such as tuberculosis.

The recognition of intra-abdominal abscesses by this technique is also an extremely valuable application, since standard diagnostic methods have so little to offer in this regard. Varying amounts of ileus may make the study difficult, but persistence with scans in multiple planes and position is frequently rewarding. In the postoperative period, the study is often complicated by drains, retention sutures, and bandages, and each study must be appropriately tailored to obtain the maximum amount of information possible.

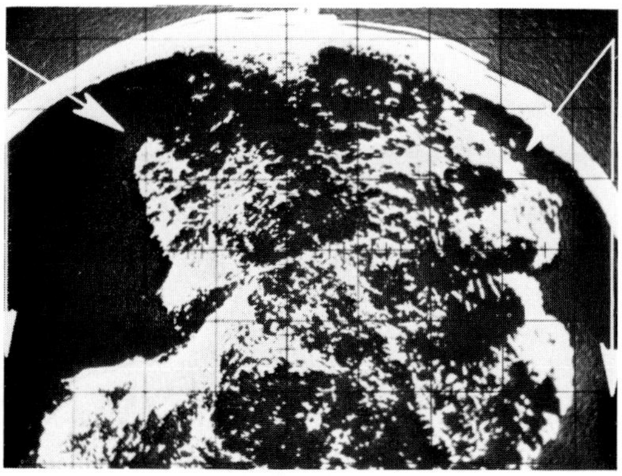

Fig. 13-21. Transverse scan at the level of the umbilicus in a patient with ascites (arrows). Fluid accumulates in the lateral and posterior aspects of both flanks, while the bowel loops are displaced toward the center of the abdomen.

SUMMARY

Abdominal ultrasonography has become a valuable technique for visualization of intra-abdominal organs and disease processes. Larger space-occupying masses of the liver may be seen, as well as the normal and dilated gallbladder. Pancreatic tumor, pseudocyst, and pancreatitis may often be diagnosed by ultrasonography. In addition, aortic aneurysms, periaortic lymphadenopathy, and extraorgan tumors and abscesses may be visualized. As a noninvasive and apparently harmless imaging procedure, ultrasonography should be utilized early in the evaluation of patients suspected of having these conditions.

REFERENCES

1. Holmes, J.: Ultrasonic studies of the bladder and kidney. In Grossman, C., and others, editors: Diagnostic ultrasound, New York, 1966, Plenum Press, p. 465.
2. Howry, D., and Bliss, W.: Ultrasonic visualization of soft tissue structures of the body, J. Lab. Clin. Med. **40:**579, 1952.
3. Lehman, J.: Ultrasound in the diagnosis of hepatobiliary disease, Radiol. Clin. North Am. **4:**605, 1966.
4. Freimanis, A.: Echographic exploration of abdominal structures, Crit. Rev. Radiol. Sci. **1:**207, 1970.
5. Holm, H.: Ultrasonic scanning in the diagnosis of space occupying lesions of the upper abdomen, Br. J. Radiol. **44:**24, 1971.
6. Ostrum, B., Goldberg, B., and Isard, H.: A-mode ultrasound differentiation of soft tissue masses, Radiology **88:**745, 1967.
7. Goldberg, B., Ostrum, B., and Isard, H.: Ultrasonic aortography, J.A.M.A. **198:**353, 1966.
8. Goldberg, B., Goodman, G., and Clearfield, H.: Evaluation of ascites by ultrasound, Radiology **96:**15, 1970.
9. Freimanis, A., and Asher, W.: Development of diagnostic criteria in echographic study of abdominal lesions, Am. J. Roentgenol. **108:**747, 1970.
10. Leopold, G., and Asher, W.: Deleterious effects

of gastrointestinal contrast material on abdominal echography, Radiology **98:**637, 1971.

11. Eycleshymer, A., and Schoemaker, D.: A cross section anatomy, ed. 2, New York, 1970, Appleton-Century-Crofts.
12. Leyton, B., Halpern, S., and Leopold, G.: Correlation of ultrasound and colloid scintiscan studies of the normal and diseased liver, J. Nucl. Med. **14:**27, 1973.
13. Hublitz, U., Kahn, P., and Sell, L.: Cholecystosonography: an approach to the nonvisualized gallbladder, Radiology **103:**645, 1972.

13a. Leopold, G., and Sokoloff, J.: Ultrasonic scanning in the diagnosis of biliary disease, Surg. Clin. North Am. **53:**1043, 1973.

14. Filly, R., and Freimanis, A.: Echographic diagnosis of pancreatic lesions, Radiology **96:**575, 1970.
15. Leopold, G.: Pancreatic echography: a new dimension in the diagnosis of pseudocyst, Radiology **104:**365, 1972.
16. Engelhart, G., and Blauenstein, U.: Ultrasound in the diagnosis of malignant pancreatic tumors, Gut **11:**443, 1970.
17. Leopold, G.: Ultrasonic abdominal aortography, Radiology **96:**9, 1970.
18. Leopold, G., Goldberger, L., and Bernstein, E.: Ultrasonic detection and evaluation of abdominal aortic aneurysms, Surgery **72:**939, 1972.
19. Nusbaum, J., Freimanis, A., and Thomford, N.: Echography in the diagnosis of abdominal aortic aneurysms, Arch. Surg. **102:**385, 1971.
20. Asher, W., and Freimanis, A.: Echographic diagnosis of retroperitoneal lymph node enlargement, Am. J. Roentgenol. **105:**438, 1969.

14 Ophthalmic ultrasonography

D. JACKSON COLEMAN, M.D.

Ultrasonic techniques provide the sole means of identifying intraocular pathology in the presence of opaque media. In addition, orbital changes involving soft tissue can be identified with this method, and it may be the only means of preoperatively identifying, localizing, and evaluating orbital neoplasms.

Diagnostic application of ultrasound in ophthalmology was first reported by Mundt and Hughes in 1956.[1] Early techniques involved the use of A-scan, or one-dimensional time-amplitude ultrasound, and were pioneered by Oksala[2] of Finland, Jannson[3] of Sweden, Ossoinig[4] of Austria, Gernet[5] of Germany, and Bronson[6] of the United States. B-scan, or two-dimensional ultrasonic imaging, of the eye and orbit was described by Baum in 1958.[7] Clinical B-scan diagnostic changes were first documented by Purnell[8] and Coleman.[9] M-scan, or time-motion, techniques for use in opthalmology were first described by Coleman and Weininger in 1967.[10] All three methods have found specific application in ophthalmology for delineation of ocular and orbital abnormalities.

Various techniques for use of the A-scan, B-scan, and M-scan alone or in combination have evolved. Most notably, Ossoinig[11] has described specific techniques using A-scan alone, some of which demonstrate the location as well as internal movement of lesions. He has also utilized compression of the lesion and A-scan observation of the resultant acoustic change. Others, including Baum,[12] Purnell,[13] and Coleman,[14,15] have depended more on the use of the B scan to provide a topographic display of anatomy that aids diagnosis so uniquely.

This research was supported by National Institutes of Health Grant EY-00275-08.

The preferred technique involves the use of B scan *combined* with simultaneous A-scan and M scan monitoring. In this system, a water bath is mandatory in order to provide maximum resolution of anterior ocular structures and to allow serial scanning in a systematized manner similar to that used in tomographic radiography. Routinely, the globe and orbit are scanned at 2-mm intervals in the horizontal plane. Horizontal sections rather than vertical are used because the bony rim of the orbit does not invade the scan path as much in the horizontal meridian as it does in the vertical. Vertical sections may be required in certain instances and can easily be obtained by rotating the scanning carriage through 90 degrees.

OCULAR DIAGNOSIS

A normal globe is shown in Fig. 14-1. The ultrasonographic tomogram of the globe clearly differentiates tissue separated by more than 0.2 mm when frequencies of 15 and 20 MHz are used. The section shown is through the lens and clearly outlines all the major structures and compartments of the globe.

The prime use of ultrasound in the evaluation of the globe involves four main areas of diagnosis: retinal detachment, vitreous hemorrhage, ocular tumor, and foreign bodies. Other applications, such as the determination of choroidal detachment, dislocated lens, and traumatic change, are also important.

Retinal detachment. Retinal detachments are easily seen on the B scan as a membrane displaced anteriorly from the posterior globe wall. The constant anatomic attachment of the retina at the ora serrata and the optic nerve, even when the retina is detached elsewhere, helps to delineate this disorder from an inflammatory membrane, which may resemble detached retina. It is important to remember that the subretinal space cannot be seen visually in the presence of retinal detachment. With ultrasound this area can be methodically and carefully searched for the presence of ocular tumors or other abnormality. A tumor underlying a retinal detachment is shown in Fig. 14-2.

Vitreous hemorrhage. Ultrasonography can clearly demonstrate the extent and density of vitreous hemorrhages (Fig. 14-3). In these situations, where light visualization is impossible, not only the type of hemorrhage, with its indication of prognosis for the globe, but also secondary structural changes such as retinal detachment or dislocated lens can be seen acoustically. Even more important, ocular tumors can usually be differentiated from vitreous hemorrhage. Recent studies of the prognostic ability of ultrasonography to relate the density and extent of hemorrhage to visual outcome have resulted in indispensable guidelines for evaluating these patients for possible surgery.[16]

Ocular tumors. Ocular tumors such as malignant melanoma, metastatic carcinoma, and hemangioma require not only

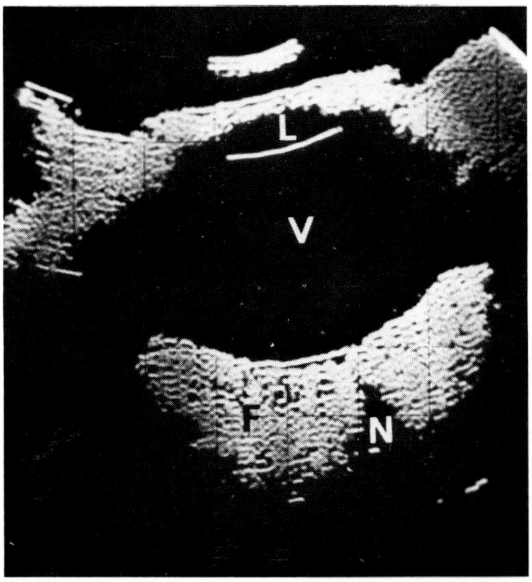

Fig. 14-1. B-scan ultrasonogram of a globe and orbit with normal lens *(L)*, vitreous *(V)*, optic nerve *(N)*, and orbital fat *(F)*.

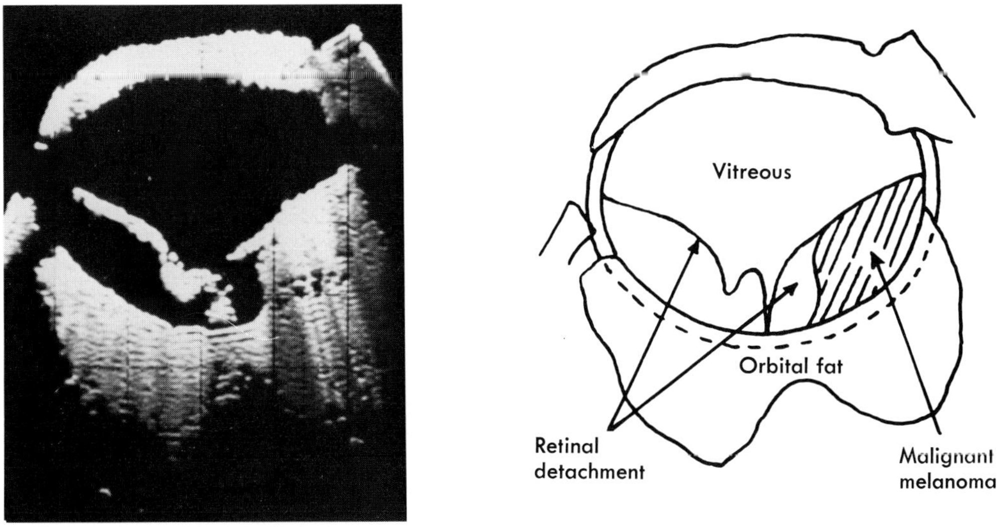

Fig. 14-2. Total retinal detachment secondary to a malignant melanoma of the choroid. (From Coleman, D. J.: Am. J. Ophthalmol. **74**[6]:1057-1065, 1972.)

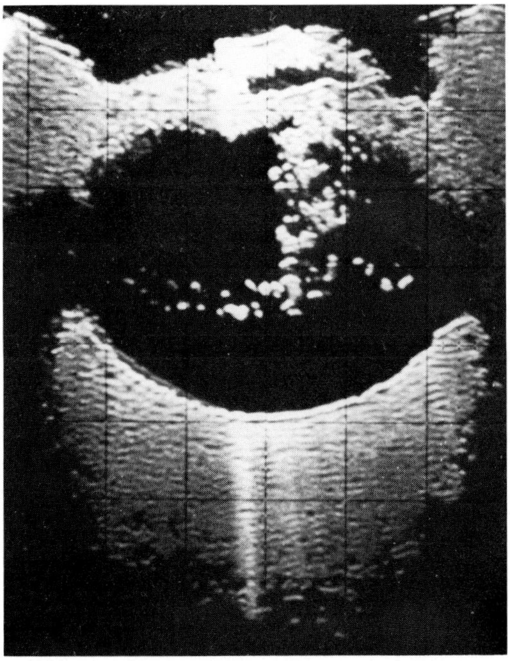

Fig. 14-3. Hemorrhage into the anterior solid vitreous appears ultrasonically as white flecks in the normally black anechoic area of the vitreous.

detection but also differentiation, since their treatment varies. Many studies by Ossoinig,[11] Purnell,[8] and Coleman,[17] among others, have shown the advantages of ultrasound in ocular tumor diagnosis and demonstrated the reliability of such diagnosis to be greater than 96%. Specific characteristics used to differentiate these tumors acoustically include the quantitative attenuation of sound through the solid lesion seen within the eye, choroidal excavation (or replacement of the choroid by tumor), the presence of an acoustically quiet zone at different frequencies, the position, morphology, and kinetic changes of echoes, and the size of the tumor. These last measurements can be of immense value in determining growth or regression of the tumor and can aid in determining the size of cobalt plaque to be applied when the tumor is amenable to such therapy.

Foreign body. Foreign body localization is relatively easily performed by ultrasonography, but in the case of metallic foreign bodies, it is less reliable for initial detection than radiographic techniques.

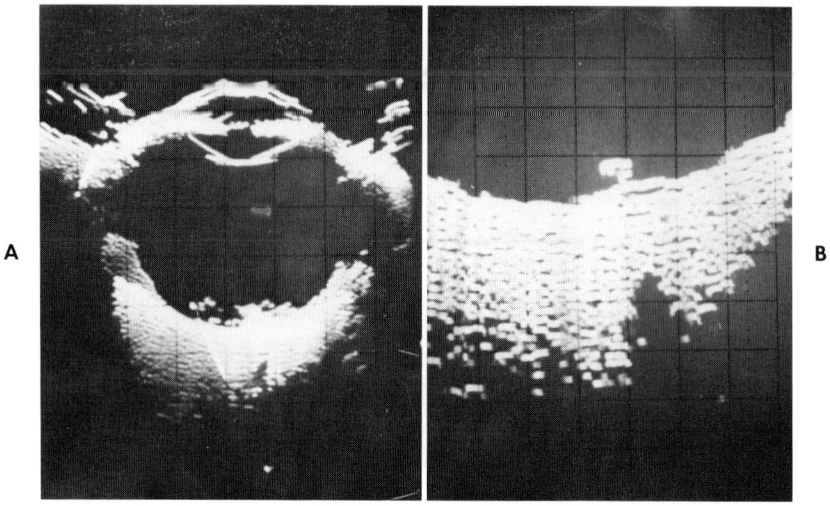

Fig. 14-4. A, A metallic foreign body at the posterior pole, partially surrounded by fibrin. B, An electronically enlarged view of the foreign body that shows shadowing in the retrobulbar echo pattern because of acoustic absorption by the foreign body. (From Coleman, D. J.: Am. J. Ophthalmol. 73[4]:501-506, 1972.)

For this reason, we prefer to first identify the foreign material by radiographic techniques and then to utilize ultrasound for precise localization in reference to other ocular structures.[18] An intraocular foreign body is shown in Fig. 14-4.

The degree of foreign body response to a magnetic field, as well as the strength with which it is embedded in the eye, can be graphically portrayed by A or M scan.[19] At the time of surgical removal of the foreign body, ultrasound can be of major importance in precise localization and extraction.[6]

Trauma. In numerous posttraumatic situations, intraocular contents are obscured by hemorrhagic changes or opacities of the cornea or lens. Ultrasound is uniquely able to delineate choroidal detachment, dislocation of the lens (Fig. 14-5), vitreal changes, and retinal aberrations.[20] The technique is thus an indispensable tool in evaluating all ophthalmic trauma.

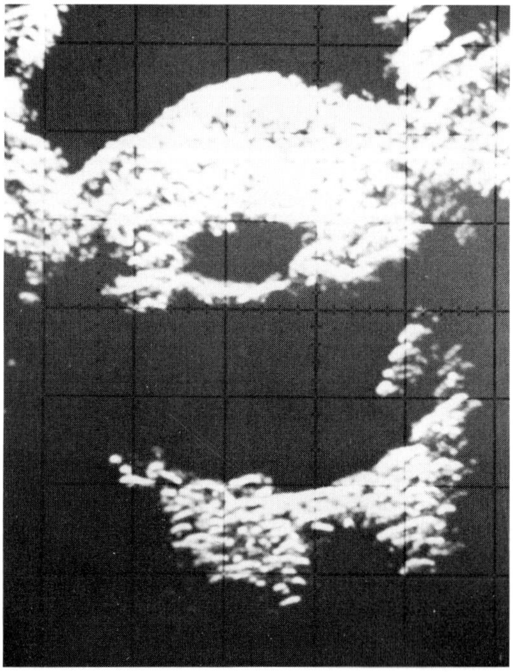

Fig. 14-5. A traumatic anterior chamber hemorrhage appears acoustically as dense white echoes obscuring visualization of the lens that is dislocated posteriorly into the acoustically clear vitreous.

ORBITAL DIAGNOSIS

Orbital evaluation with ultrasound is a proved, reliable, and often unique detector of orbital abnormality.[15] Because of the lack of morbidity, ultrasonography is usually the first procedure indicated when orbital pathology is suspected. Not only can it direct further studies, but it can properly direct the choice and route of surgery if this is indicated. Serial ultrasonic sectioning of the normal retrobulbar structures identifies the optic nerve, the orbital walls, and extraocular muscles as anatomic landmarks. The retrobulbar fat, as Purnell[13] pointed out, produces the major portion of the orbital echoes. Abnormalities of these echoes can easily be seen on the B scan picture. Accentuation of the orbital wall, with thickening of the muscle, is a highly reliable and useful indication of Graves' disease.[21]

Tumors, either neoplastic or benign, have been classified in terms of outline and ability to transmit ultrasonic waves. A flow chart used for identifying orbital lesions is shown in Fig. 14-6.[9] Mass lesions of the orbit are described as encapsulated (rounded) or irregular, and each of these categories is further subdivided into acoustically solid or cystic textures.

Solid lesions. Solid lesions of the orbit with encapsulation are most typically the neurogenic tumors.[22] These tumors show a rounded outline adjacent to or surrounding the nerve. Kinetic scans demonstrate whether or not a mass moves with the nerve or whether it remains fixed and immobile. They are performed by asking the patient to rotate the globe in different directions while movement of the optic nerve is monitored acoustically. In general, the solid lesion will have a textured quality and show relatively poor transmission (Fig. 14-7).

Cystic lesions. Cystic lesions of the orbit[23] show (1) rounded contours typical of encapsulation, (2) few internal echoes, indicative of high fluid content, and (3) marked accentuation of the postcystic or-

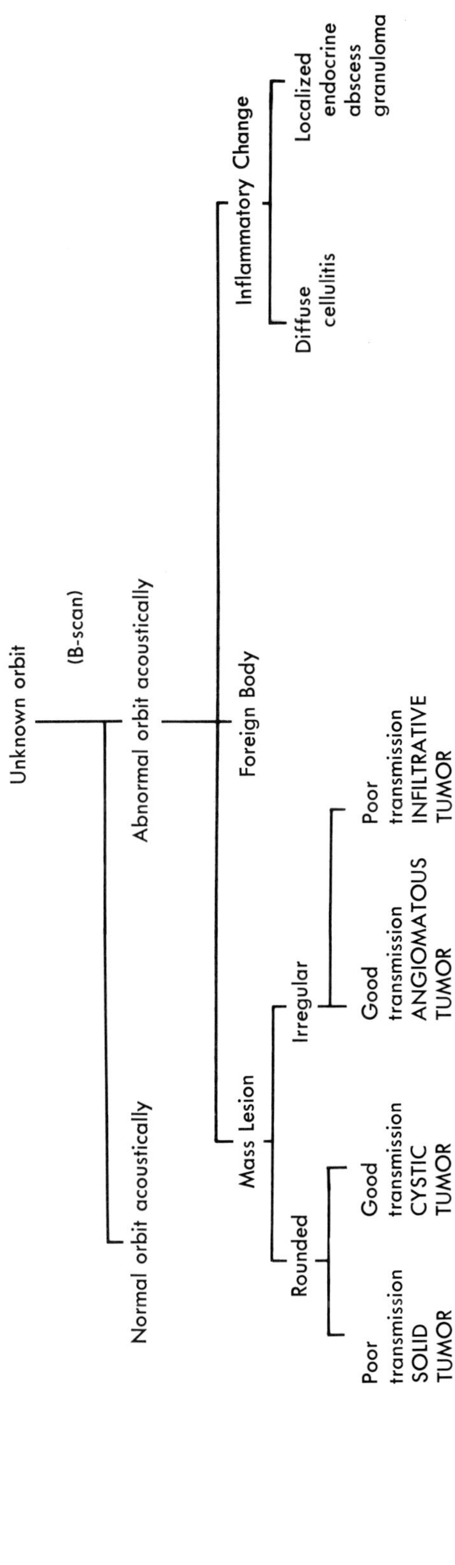

Fig. 14-6. Ultrasonic characterization of patients referred for orbital evaluation.

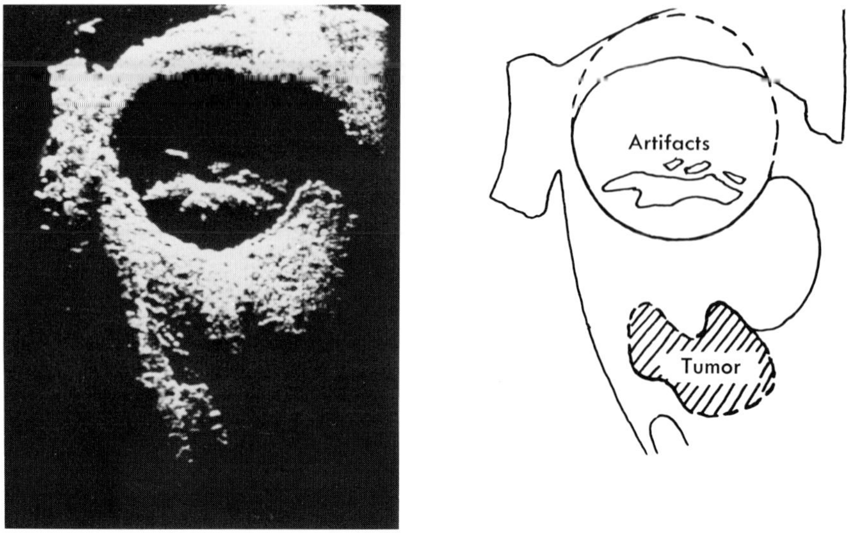

Fig. 14-7. B-scan ultrasonogram of a lymphoma of the orbit, an acoustically solid tumor with an irregular outline which transmits sound poorly. (From Coleman, D. J.: Am. J. Ophthalmol. **74**[4]:704-718, 1972.)

bital wall areas. This tumor pattern is seen most typically in the presence of mucocele, dermoid cyst, and cavernous hemangioma. The exact B-scan localization of the lesion within the orbit, when correlated with radiographic findings, is most helpful in selecting the surgical approach.

Vascular tumors. An irregularly outlined lesion with the good transmission indicative of fluid contents signals the presence of lymphangioma[24] or nonencapsulated hemangioma. The finger-like projections of these tumors may be transected, giving the appearance of multiple cystic structures in the retrobulbar fat (Fig. 14-8).

Infiltrative lesions. Irregularly outlined mass lesions with poor acoustic transmission and internal acoustic echoes are solid lesions such as lymphoma,[25] metastatic carcinoma, and pseudotumors[26] or granulomas. The presence of myositis or inflammatory edema surrounding the nerve or in Tenon's space usually differentiates pseudotumor from the neoplastic tumor categories. An example of an inflammatory tumor is seen in Fig. 14-9.

Orbital foreign bodies. Orbital foreign bodies are often difficult to localize acoustically unless previous radiographic location has been obtained. The inability to differentiate the echo amplitude of a foreign material from the surrounding orbital fat is responsible for this difficulty. Lowering the gain often will help identify the foreign body echo as one of greater amplitude than fat. Wood or other vegetable material is often identified by the presence of a clear outline of the wood produced by surrounding purulence or edema. An example of wood foreign material in the orbit is shown in Fig. 14-10.

Inflammatory disease. Distinguishing neoplasms from orbital inflammatory lesions such as pseudotumor and Graves' disease constitutes the major difficulty in orbital diagnosis. However, the eye changes of Graves' disease are characterized by thickening of the muscle and marked accentuation of the muscle-orbital wall boundary. It is suspected that mucopolysaccharide infiltration causes a change in the acoustic properties of the muscle,

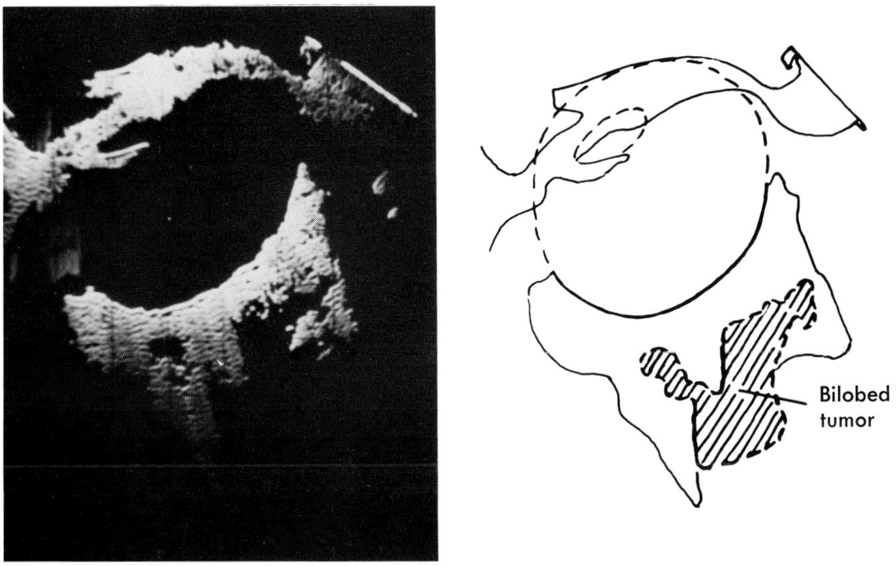

Fig. 14-8. Lymphangioma of the orbit demonstrating irregular outline with good sound transmission. (From Coleman, D. J.: Am. J. Ophthalmol. **74**[4]:704-718, 1972.)

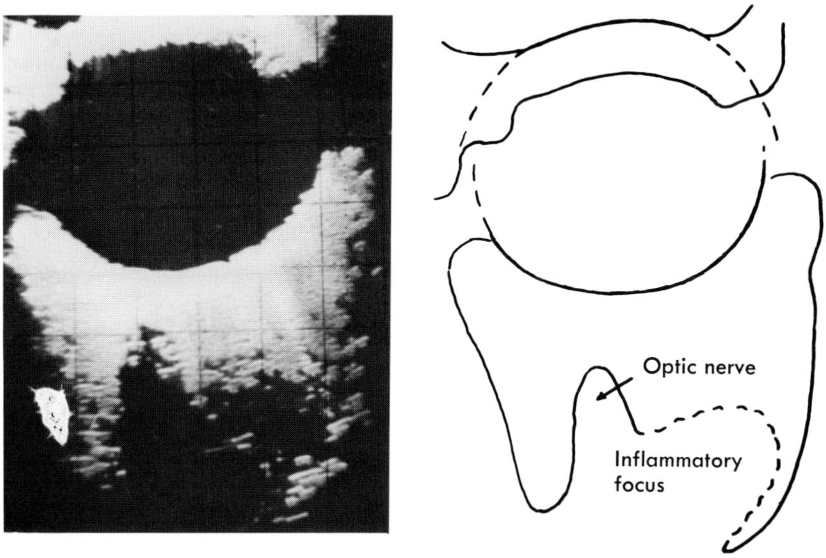

Fig. 14-9. This granuloma at the orbital apex demonstrates moderate acoustic transmission with some internal echoes indicating solidity and a rounded outline. This type of inflammatory lesion is often indistinguishable acoustically from neoplasms. (From Coleman, D. J.: Am. J. Ophthalmol. **74**[4]:704-718, 1972.)

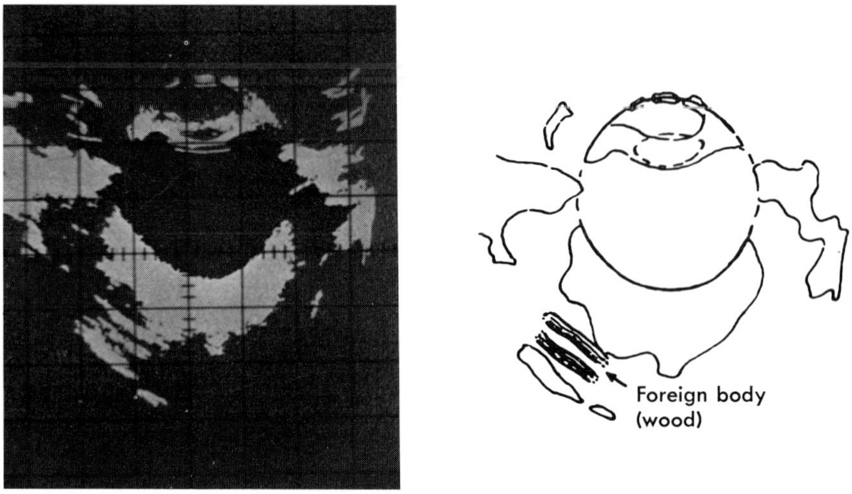

Fig. 14-10. A nonradiopaque orbital foreign body located anterior to the orbit wall. This wood splinter is shown here on a storage type of oscilloscope display. (From Coleman, D. J.: Am. J. Ophthalmol. **74**[4]:704-718, 1972.)

enhancing the muscle-orbit boundary. The thickness of the muscle can usually be accurately delineated with both A and B scan.

SUMMARY

Ultrasonography of the eye and orbit, using one- and two-dimensional imaging and kinetic techniques, is indispensable for adequate evaluation of eyes with opaque media. It permits evaluation of retinal detachment, vitreous hemorrhage, ocular tumors, and foreign bodies and may also be of use with choroidal detachment, dislocated lens, and traumatic injuries. Ultrasonography is also uniquely valuable in evaluation of abnormalities of the orbit and may direct further studies as well as the choice and route of surgical intervention. It aids localization of foreign bodies, may differentiate tumor types, and helps distinguish inflammatory conditions from neoplasm. Being without morbidity, ophthalmic ultrasonography is an essential new diagnostic technique for examination of the eye and orbit.

Acknowledgments

I thank Emil Bethke for the illustrations, Margaret Cubberly for the photography, and Heinz Rosskothen for machine work on the scanner.

REFERENCES

1. Mundt, G. H., and Hughes, W. F.: Ultrasonics in ocular diagnosis, Am. J. Ophthal. **41:**488-498, 1956.
2. Oksala, A., and Lehtinen, A.: Diagnostics of detachment of the retina by means of ultrasound, Acta Ophthal. **35:**461-467, 1957.
3. Jannson, F.: Measurements of intraocular distance by ultrasound, Acta Ophthal. **74**(Suppl.):1-51, 1963.
4. Ossoinig, K.: Ultrasonic diagnosis of the eye: an aid for the clinic. In Oksala, A., and Gernet, H., editors: Ultrasonics in ophthalmology, Basel, 1967, S. Karger, pp. 116-133.
5. Gernet, H., and Franceschetti, A.: Ultrasound biometry of the eye. In Oksala, A., and Gernet, H., editors: Ultrasonics in ophthalmology, Basel, 1967, S. Karger, pp. 175-206.
6. Bronson, N. R.: Techniques of ultrasonic localization and extraction of intraocular and extraocular foreign bodies, Am. J. Ophthal. **60**(4):596-603, 1965.
7. Baum, G., and Greenwood, I.: The application of ultrasonic locating techniques to ophthalmology. II. Ultrasonic slit lamp in the ultrasonic visualization of soft tissues, Arch. Ophthal. **60:**263-279, 1958.
8. Purnell, E. W.: Ultrasound in ophthalmological diagnosis. In Grossman, C., and others, editors: Diagnostic ultrasound, New York, 1966, Plenum Press, pp. 95-110.

9. Coleman, D. J., Konig, W. W., and Katz, L.: A hand-operated ultrasound scan system for ophthalmic evaluation, Am. J. Ophthal. **68**(2):256-263, 1969.
10. Coleman, D. J., and Weininger, R.: Ultrasonic M-mode technique in ophthalmology, Arch. Ophthal. **82:**475-479, 1969.
11. Ossoinig, K.: Clinical echo-ophthalmolography. In Blodi, F. C.: Current concepts in ophthalmology, St. Louis, 1972, The C. V. Mosby Co., pp. 110-130.
12. Baum, G.: A reappraisal of orbital ultrasonography, series II, Trans. Am. Acad. Ophthal. Otolaryngol., Sept.-Oct., 1965, pp. 943-958.
13. Purnell, E. W.: Ultrasonic interpretation of orbital disease. In Gitter, K. A., and others, editors: Ophthalmic ultrasound, St. Louis, 1969, The C. V. Mosby Co., pp. 249-259.
14. Coleman, D. J.: Reliability of ocular and orbital diagnosis with B scan ultrasound. Part I: Ocular diagnosis, Am. J. Ophthal. **73**(4):501-516, 1972.
15. Coleman, D. J.: Reliability of ocular and orbital diagnosis with B scan ultrasound. Part II: Orbital diagnosis, Am. J. Ophthal. **74**(4):704-718, 1972.
16. Coleman, D. J.: Vitreous surgery—ultrasonic evaluation and procedure, presented at the American Medical Association's 122nd Annual Convention, New York, 1973.
17. Coleman, D. J.: Reliability of ocular tumor diagnosis with ultrasound, Trans. Am. Acad. Ophthal. Otolaryngol., Sept.-Oct., 1973.
18. Coleman, D. J., and Trokel, S. L.: A protocol for B scan and radiographic foreign body localization, Am. J. Ophthal. **71:**84-89, 1971.
19. Coleman, D. J., and Franzen, L. A.: Demonstration of magnetic properties of foreign bodies with M scan ultrasound, presented at the American Institute of Ultrasound in Medicine, Philadelphia, 1972.
20. Coleman, D. J., Jack, R. L., and Franzen, L. A.: Ultrasonography in ocular trauma, Am. J. Ophthal. **79**(2):279-288, 1973.
21. Coleman, D. J., and others: High resolution B-scan ultrasonography of the orbit. Part V: Eye changes of Graves' disease, Arch. Ophthal. **88:**465-471, 1972.
22. Coleman, D. J., Jack, R. L., and Franzen, L. A.: High resolution B-scan ultrasonography of the orbit. Part IV: Neurogenic tumors of the orbit, Arch. Ophthal. **88:**380-384, 1972.
23. Coleman, D. J., Jack, R. L., and Franzen, L. A.: B-scan ultrasonography of orbital mucocoeles, Eye Ear Nose Throat Mon. **51:**25-30, 1972.
24. Coleman, D. J., Jack, R. L., and Franzen, L. A.: B-scan ultrasonography of orbital lymphangiomas, Br. J. Ophthal. **57**(3):193-198, 1973.
25. Coleman, D. J., Jack, R. L., and Franzen, L. A.: High resolution B-scan ultrasonography of the orbit. Part III: Lymphomas of the orbit, Arch. Ophthal. **88:**375-379, 1972.
26. Coleman, D. J., and others: High resolution B-scan ultrasonography of the orbit. Part VI: Pseudotumors of the orbit, Arch. Ophthal. **88:**472-480, 1972.

15 Color ultrasonography for tissue differential diagnosis

GILBERT BAUM, M.D.

One of the most recent advances in ultrasonographic differential diagnosis is the use of color, the acoustic analogue of histologic staining. The instrumentation characteristics, the methods used to standardize the staining technique, and the data processing that such staining makes possible are described. Clinical application of the technique to images of the eye, orbit, and breast is demonstrated.

Staining is just as essential to ultrasonographic differential diagnosis as it is to histopathologic diagnosis. Staining is of value in histopathology because the staining pattern is reproducible from tissue to tissue and from slide to slide. In the absence of such reproducibility, the mere conversion to color is of no value and may actually prove to be more confusing than a black and white ultrasonogram. Reproducible staining makes it possible for the eye to recognize and identify patterns that would escape detection when viewed on the black and white ultrasonograms, for reasons that will be explained subsequently.

Ultrasonographic staining is essential for the tissues of the orbit, the breast, and potentially the parenchyma of the liver, kidney, spleen, and ovary. The orbit and breast lack a definitive anatomy, so mere distortions in anatomic outline may prove to be inconclusive.

Supported by grant GM 12460-03, American Cancer Society Grant CI #27, and National Breast Cancer Task Force–National Cancer Institute contract N01-CB-23872.

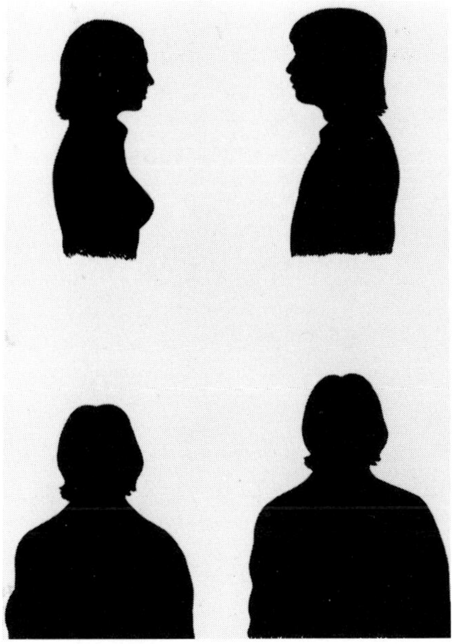

Fig. 15-1. A silhouette of a boy and girl with long hair. Only in the lateral position is it possible to distinguish male from female on this silhouette figure.

Most commercial ultrasonographic systems display only a silhouette of the observed tissue, so gross anatomic distortions must be present for the disease processes to be visualized. Prior to the onset of anatomic distortion—that is, when the lesion is small—only echo amplitude changes may be present. A silhouette would fail to show these amplitude changes. An analysis of a very simple silhouette will clarify this point (Fig. 15-1).

Boys and girls wear their hair approximately the same length today so that in an anteroposterior silhouette view it may be extremely difficult to distinguish male from female. However, if we view these same two people in a lateral view, the male is very readily distinguished from the female. Distinguishing male from female is very simple in an anterior view snapshot even if the image is defocused (Fig. 15-2).

Similarly, in an organ such as the eye, which possesses precisely defined anatomic "landmarks," valuable diagnostic information may be obtained when a dis-

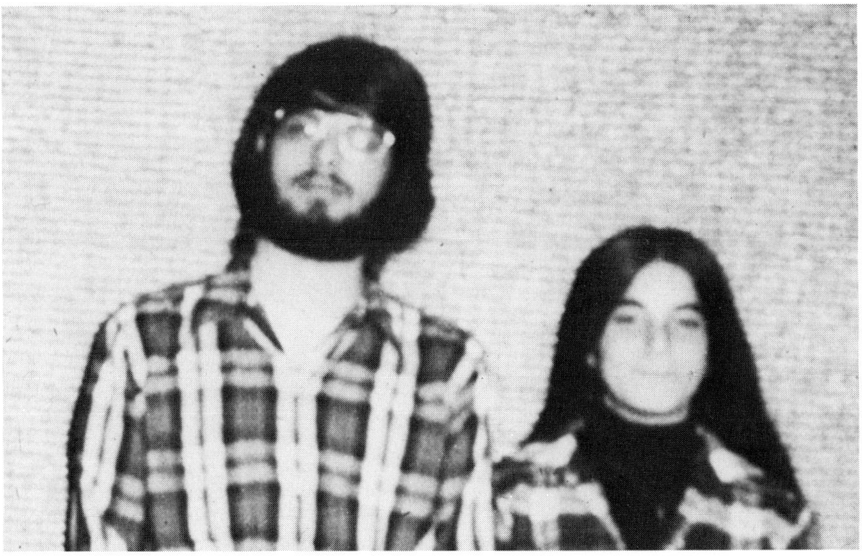

Fig. 15-2. A gray scale photograph of a boy and girl with long hair. It is now possible to distinguish male from female by a second set of characteristics despite the orientation of the male and female figures.

ease uniformly produces a classic distortion of its anatomy.

Fig. 15-3 is a compound scan of a silhouette ultrasonogram of a normal eye. This silhouette very precisely follows the anatomic cross-section through the eye.

Fig. 15-4 is an eye containing a total retinal detachment. The distortion produced in the silhouette by the retinal detachment is so classic that this is all the information that is needed to arrive at a diagnosis.

In organs lacking such a well-defined anatomy, such as the breast or orbit, or in instances where the disease process has not disrupted the usual anatomy, a snapshot or gray scale capability is essential

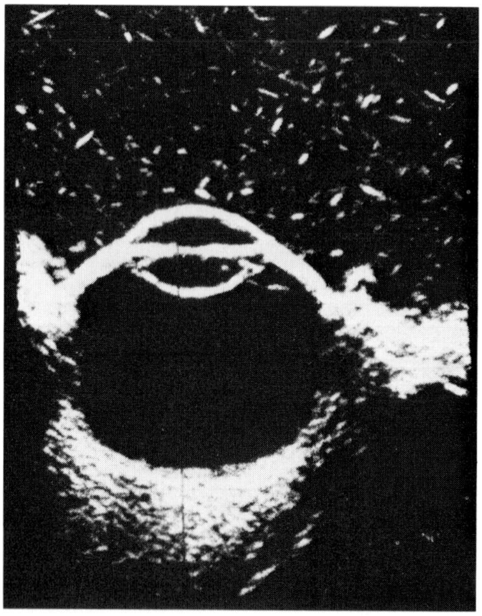

Fig. 15-3. A compound scan of the human eye.

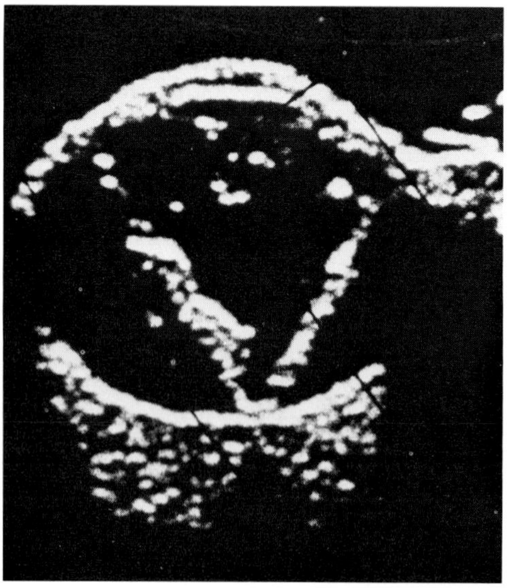

Fig. 15-4. A silhouette ultrasonogram of an eye containing a total retinal detachment.

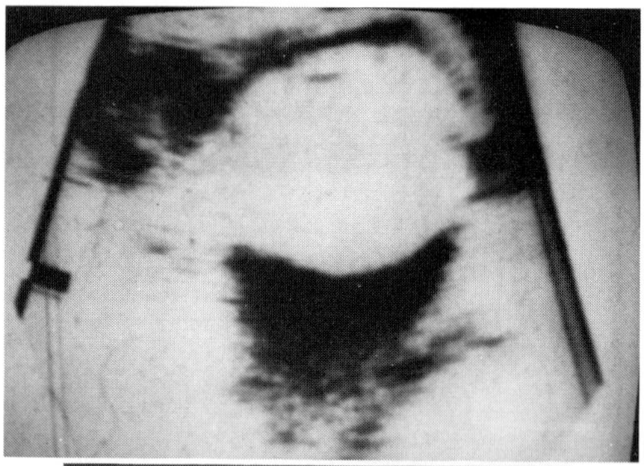

A

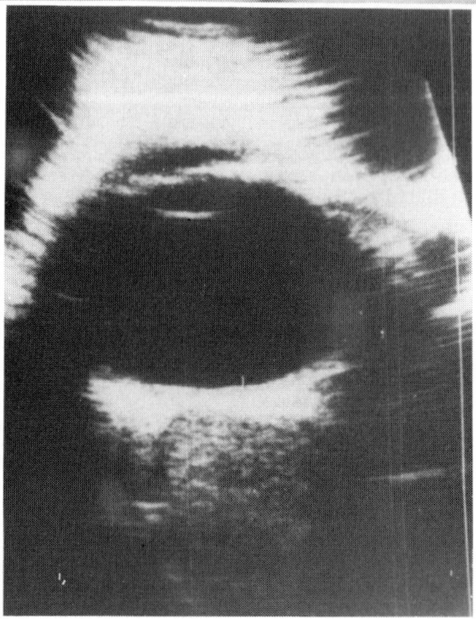

B

Fig. 15-5. A, An ultrasonogram of an eye containing an orbital tumor. **A,** It is impossible to detect the textural changes produced by the tumor unless gray scale and the correct contrast gradient are present in the ultrasonogram. **B,** An ultrasonogram similar to **A,** wherein a change in contrast gradient makes it possible to visualize the orbital tumor.

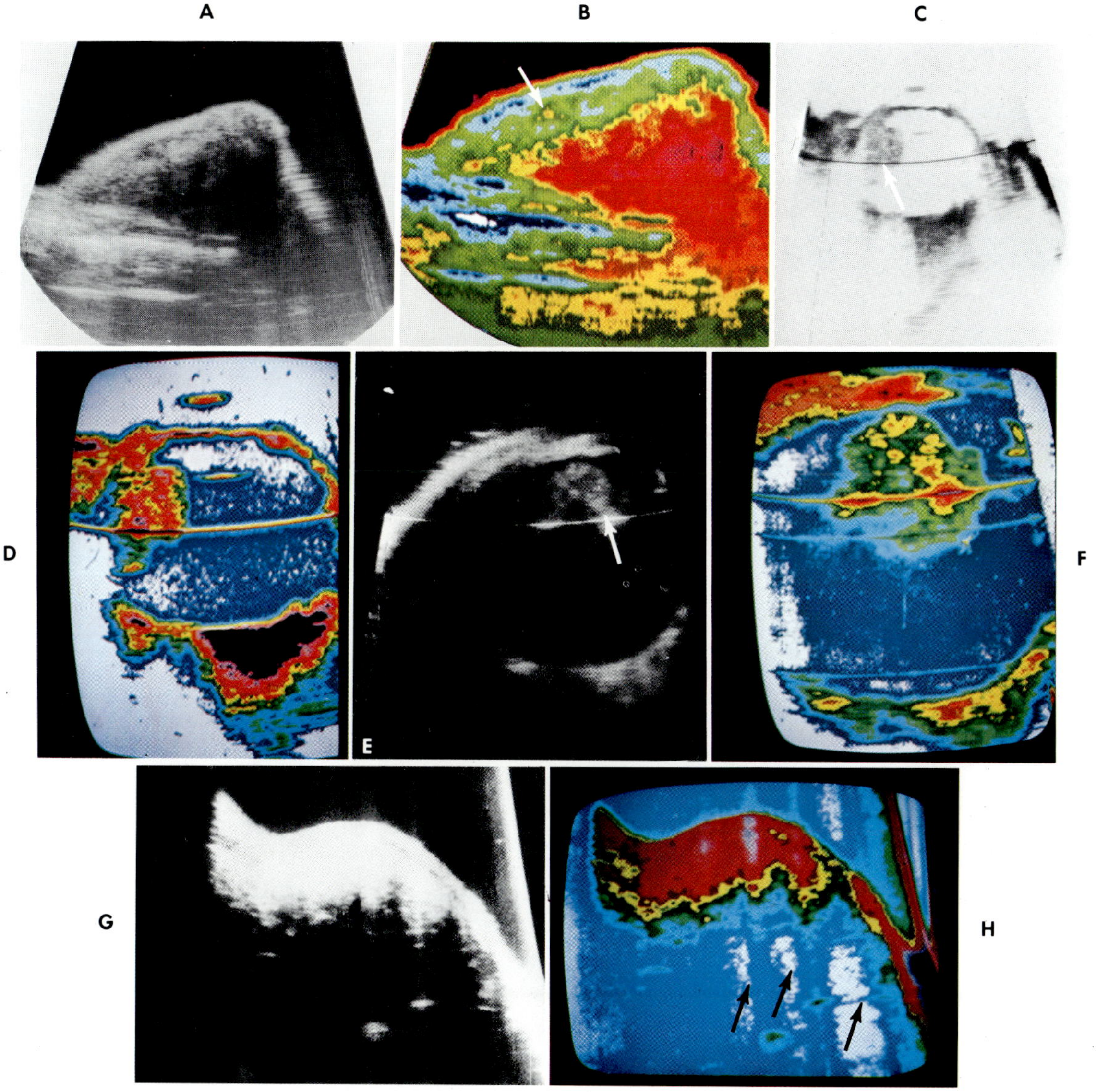

Plate 2. A, An ultrasound mammogram of a breast containing metastatic carcinoma. **B,** A color-coded isodensitometric print-out of **A.** Note that the addition of color makes it possible to distinguish an area of acoustic discontinuity (arrow) that initially escapes detection in **A. C,** A high-resolution gray scale ultrasonogram of a malignant melanoma of the eye (arrow). **D,** A color-coded isodensitometric print-out of **C** (see text). **E,** A high-resolution gray scale ultrasonogram of an eye containing a retinoblastoma (arrow) in essentially the same position. **F,** A color-coded isodensitometric print-out of **E** (see text). **G,** The distortion produced by vibration of the transducer is shown. **H,** A color-coded isodensitometric print-out of **G.** The amplitude distortion produced by mechanical vibration is more pronounced on the color-coded isodensitometric print-out (arrow).

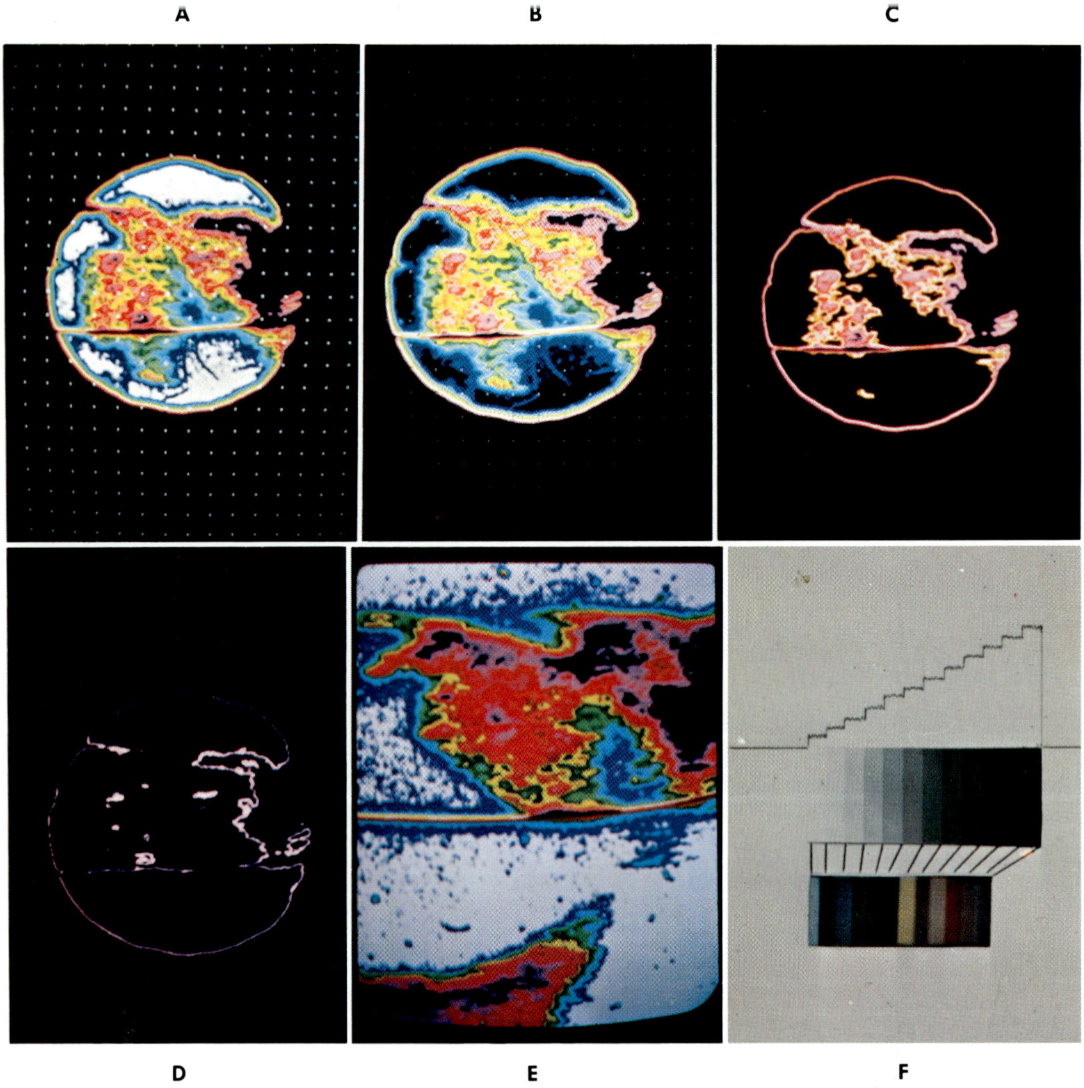

Plate 3. A, A color-coded isodensitometric print-out of Plate 2, *C* and *D*. A mask surrounds the portion of the eye containing the malignant melanoma in Plate 2, *C* and *D*. An electronically inserted grid is superimposed over the image of the tumor so that the acoustic characteristics of equal volumes of tissues may be compared. **B,** The distribution of a single level of amplitude within the malignant melanoma, namely, all the white areas have been replaced by black. **C,** The distribution of several different amplitude levels within the tumor (white, blues, and greens). **D,** The distribution of a single level of amplitude within the tumor. **E,** Optic magnification of a portion of the ultrasonogram containing the tumor makes it possible to study the amplitude pattern of the tumor in greater detail. **F,** The interrelationships between A mode, B mode, and isophotodensitometry. Each film density represents an amplitude of known value. A specific color is then assigned to each density value.

for diagnosis. Fig. 15-5, *A*, versus Fig. 15-5, *B*, illustrates how critical gray scale and correct contrast are for the visualization of an orbital tumor.

Although the addition of gray scale increases the informational content of the ultrasonogram by 50%, it also introduces the problems of gray scale compression and the inability of the eye to handle excessive gray scale, especially when the gray scale is randomly scattered or distributed.

It is fairly simple for the eye to distinguish density steps on an optical density wedge where the steps of gray are adjacent to each other with a sharp dividing line between each step. At the extreme dark and light ends of the scale, the eye may encounter some difficulty in distinguishing between steps (Fig. 15-6). When many shades of gray are randomly distributed (Plate 2, *A*), judging steps of gray becomes extremely difficult. It is a simple matter for the eye to distinguish different levels of randomly distributed densities when a color code is substituted for the various shades of gray (Plate 2, *B*).

Fig. 15-6. An optical density wedge covering three density units. The figure demonstrates the limited range of gray scale which the eye is capable of distinguishing under one set of viewing conditions. This range is reduced when the changes in gray scale among adjacent spots are minimal and the changes are randomly distributed.

One of the factors contributing to the difficulty in distinguishing these shades of gray is the compression required to display the 80-dB dynamic range of the acoustic echoes inherent in the tissue on the 30-dB gray scale available on the face of the cathode ray tube.

The term "dynamic range" refers to the range of echo amplitudes from the front surface of the skin and depths of tissues. These generally cover an amplitude range of approximately −20 to −85 dB. Ultrasonographic staining facilitates differential diagnosis and data processing as well as the localization faculty just demonstrated.

Plate 2, *C*, is a high-resolution gray scale ultrasonogram of a malignant melanoma of the eye. Plate 2, *E*, is a similar ultrasonogram of an eye with a retinoblastoma in essentially the same location. Because of the anterior location of these tumors, absorption plays a minimal role.

Plate 2, *D*, is a color-coded isodensitometric print-out of Plate 2, *C*, namely, the malignant melanoma, Plate 2, *F*, is a similarly processed print-out of the retinoblastoma shown in Plate 2, *E*. The difference between these tumors is minimal on the black and white ultrasonogram but pronounced on the stained ultrasonogram. It is the difference on the stained or color-coded ultrasonogram that makes improved ultrasonographic differential diagnosis possible. However, this end result can only be achieved if the staining process is reproducible and the required information is recorded on the black and white ultrasonogram.

Thus far, it has been shown why staining is essential and some of its advantages have been demonstrated. The remaining portions of this paper describe the data processing that may be carried out when stained or color-coded ultrasonograms are used. Also, the properties that the ultrasonograms must contain for successful staining and data processing, the equipment required to produce this type of ultrasonogram, the instrumentation used to stain the ultrasonograms, and the way in which reproducibility is achieved will be discussed.

Ultrasonographic staining simulates histologic staining because the position of the cell is represented by anatomic distortion of echoes. Changes in the amplitude of the tissue echoes correspond to the staining characteristics of the tissue. Hence, the method used to produce ultrasonographic staining makes it possible to carry out five types of data processing of these ultrasonograms:

1. Comparison of the difference in color pattern of the total or selected portions of the ultrasonogram
2. Histogram analysis of a diseased area, for example, the tumor area
3. Subtraction of a signal at a single or at multiple levels of amplitude
4. Display of the amplitude distribution of a signal at a single or at different intensity levels
5. Sequential or stepwise analysis and comparison of tumor structure

Thus Plate 2, *C* to *F*, gives comparisons of the total eye that contained a malignant melanoma and a retinoblastoma, respectively.

In Plate 3, *A*, a mask has been placed around the malignant melanoma shown in Plate 2, *C* and *D*. Superimposed over this masked area is an electronically inserted grid that makes it possible to measure the size and extent of the tumor. The use of a mask ensures the measurement and comparison of equal tissue volumes. Since the diameter of the acoustic beam is constant, histograms of the amplitude characteristics of equivalent volumes of different types of tissues may be carried out as shown in Fig. 15-7. This histogram of the amplitude characteristics of the malignant melanoma versus the retinoblastoma shows that the former possesses more strong echoes and fewer weaker echoes than a corresponding volume of retinoblastoma. These histograms are more significant than a single, isolated A scan through the tissue because the effect of the angle of incidence or viewing angle is averaged out.

Plate 3, *B*, shows the distribution of a single level of amplitude within the total pattern; white is removed. Plate 3, *C*, shows the distribution of several levels of amplitude and Plate 3, *D*, that of a single level. The foregoing shows that it is possible to sequentially remove in a stepwise fashion each color or amplitude. This enables one to compare the distribution of the various echo levels within different tumors and to determine the amplitude construction of the tumor.

It is also possible to magnify a portion of the ultrasonogram prior to isophotodensitometric study so that the amplitude structure of a tumor may be studied in minute detail of 0.3 to 1 mm (Plate 3, *E*).

The stained ultrasonogram or the color-coded isodensitometric print-out may be viewed as a colored relief map of the observed tissues. The data processing that I have just described enables us to determine the characteristics of this relief map.

The preparation of such a map requires ultrasonograms on which the precise position and amplitude of the reflecting tissue components are recorded. Unless these data are recorded on the film, data processing cannot recover it. The preparation of ultrasonograms that possess the necessary resolution, tonal scale, and contrast requires special equipment.

Such an ultrasonographic system makes it possible to observe, ultrasonographically, features in tissue that were heretofore invisible. When viewed with this system, the

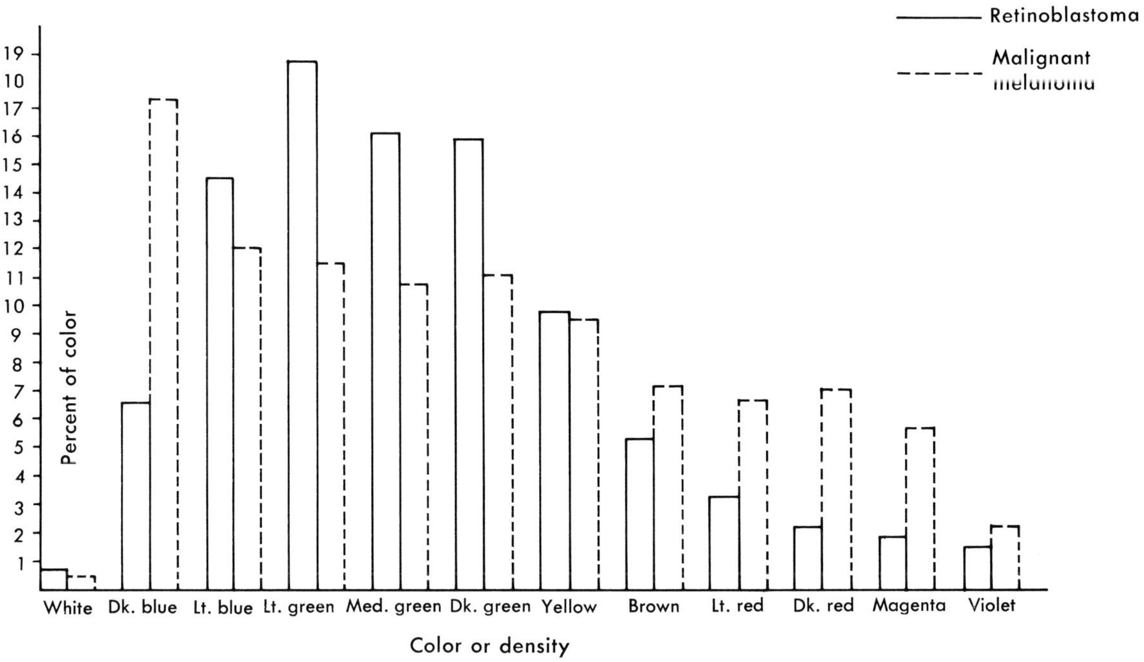

Fig. 15-7. A histogram of the amplitude characteristics of malignant melanoma versus a retinoblastoma.

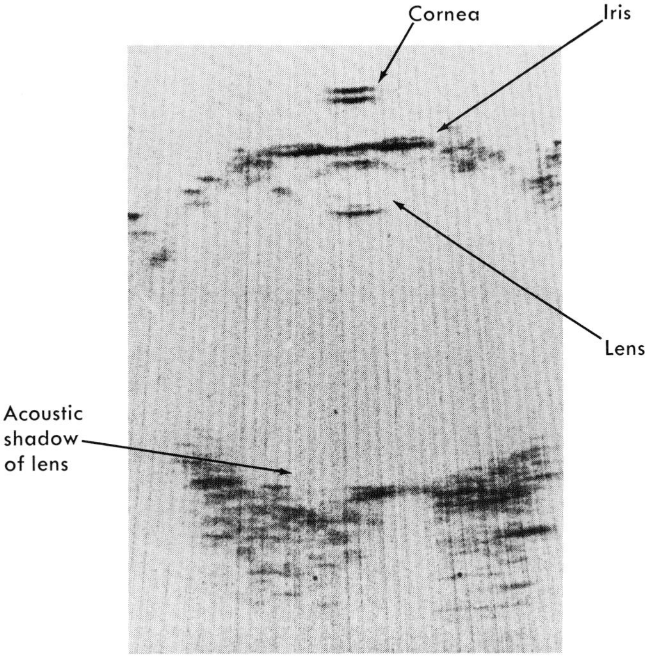

Fig. 15-8. A high-resolution gray scale ultrasonogram of a human eye.

eye shows the anterior and posterior layers of the cornea and iris as well as the clear intervening stroma. The optically transparent lens, the clear vitreous body, and the acoustic shadow of the lens are also shown (Fig. 15-8). The entrance of the blood vessels into the eye is now routinely observed (Fig. 15-9).

For the first time, we have also been able to observe fluid in Tenon's space, which is normally collapsed behind the eye, and fluid surrounding one of the muscles attached to the eye (Fig. 15-10). This patient has a pseudotumor of the orbit.

Similar improvements in the ultrasonographic visualization of other tissues viewed by this system can be demonstrated.

The equipment characteristics necessary to produce these ultrasonograms include the following:

1. The ultrasonographic system must have an amplitude stability of 1% and a dynamic range in excess of two density units. Then there is enough gray scale available so that a specific shade of gray can be assigned to each significant step in intensity, for example, 3 dB per shade of gray.
2. A constant velocity electromechanical scanner must be used so that each point on the surface of the tissue receives an equivalent amount of ultrasonographic radiation (Plate 2, *G*). Failure to observe this constraint produces the distortion shown in Plate 2, *H*.

Ultrasonographic staining is accomplished by converting the black and white high-resolution, gray scale–containing ultrasonograms into colored isodensitometric print-outs by the use of a closed-circuit color television isophotodensitometer. A standard color code is achieved by representing a given film density by a specific color of the isophotodensitometer (Plate 3, *F*). The film densities are standardized by producing an optical density step wedge on the film that is used to examine the patient. The optic density step is produced

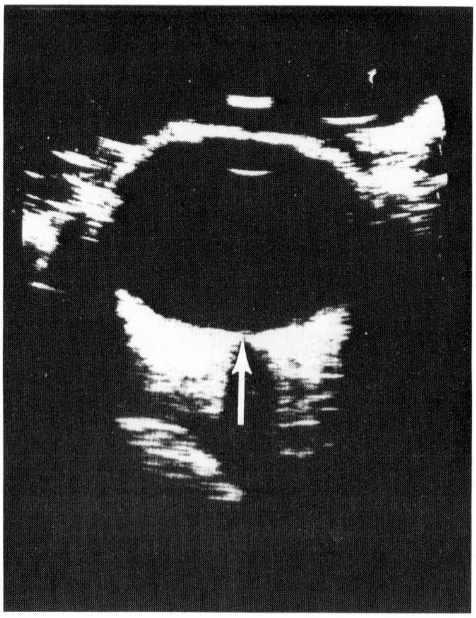

Fig. 15-9. The entrance of a central retinal vessel into the eye is shown at the arrow.

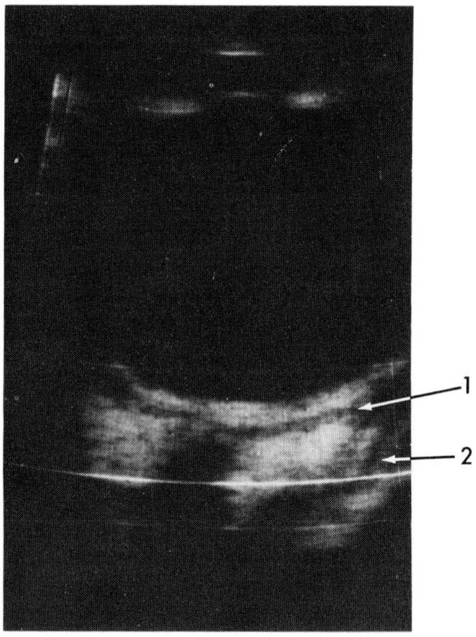

Fig. 15-10. A high-resolution ultrasonogram showing fluid in Tenon's capsule (arrow 1) and around the lateral rectus muscle (arrow 2) in a patient with pseudotumor of the orbit.

in the following fashion. The geometry between a glass test block and the transducer is first optimized to produce the maximal obtainable signal. Then sequential scans of the glass test block are taken as 3-dB steps of attenuation are introduced between each scan. This results in a sequential series of film densities; each density on the film corresponds to an echo of known amplitude from a glass test block. These densities are then used to calibrate the color code of a closed-circuit television isophotodensitometer so that each color corresponds to an echo of known amplitude. This procedure results in a color-coding system that is as reproducible and faithful as staining used in histopathology. Compensation for absorption and viewing angle results in color coding that is reproducible from patient to patient. It is this careful control of the color-coding process that makes this procedure valuable. Without the use of these constraints the mere conversion to color would be of dubious value.

In summary, this chapter has shown why staining is desirable for ultrasonographic differential diagnosis and the advantages it offers. Ultrasonographic staining facilitates data processing and makes it possible to study the amplitude and anatomic characteristics of the tissue simultaneously. The need for ultrasonograms possessing good resolution, tonal scale, and contrast has been shown. The methods used to achieve ultrasonographic staining have been described. Most important of all, the need for the methods of achieving reproducible staining have been stressed.

The tools and techniques for achieving the acoustic analogue of histopathologic staining developed at our laboratory open new vistas in ultrasonographic differential diagnosis. But to be of value, very rigid quantitative control of this process must be maintained so that consistent reproducible staining is achieved.

REFERENCES

1. Baum, G.: Instrumentation problems in ophthalmic ultrasonography, Ultrasonics **1:**43-47, 1968.
2. Baum, G.: Aids in ultrasonographic diagnosis. In Bock, J., and Ossoinig, K., editors: Ultrasonographica medica, Proceedings of the First World Congress in Ultrasonic Diagnostics in Medicine and SIDUO III, Vienna Academy of Medicine, pp. 203-208, 1971.
3. Baum, G.: Standardization in B-mode ultrasound equipment. In Bock, J., and Ossoinig, K., editors: Ultrasonographica medica, Proceedings of the First World Congress in Ultrasonic Diagnostics in Medicine and SIDUO III, Vienna Academy of Medicine, pp. 61-70, 1971.
4. Baum, G.: Problems in ultrasonographic diagnosis of retinal disease, Am. J. Ophthal. **71:**723-739, 1971.
5. Baum, G.: Quantized ultrasonography, Ultrasonics **10:**1, 1972.
6. Baum, G.: Ultrasonics and ophthalmology, Eye Ear Nose Throat Mon. **51:**43, 1972.
7. Baum, G.: Fundamentals of medical ultrasonography, New York, 1974, G. P. Putnam's Sons.

16

Biologic effects of diagnostic ultrasound

DONALD L. KING, M.D.
PADMAKAR P. LELE, M.D., D.Phil. (Oxon.)

Over the past 20 years the possibility of injury by ultrasonic energy has been a primary concern of physicians, scientists, and engineers developing and applying diagnostic ultrasound. The tragic sequelae to the early unguarded use of x-irradiation were foremost in the minds of these investigators. Consequently, in the development of diagnostic ultrasound there was a conscious, deliberate effort to utilize a minimum of ultrasonic energy, to observe for clinical evidence of side effects, and to experimentally determine the parameters of safe exposure. Today our knowledge of these parameters and of the biologic effects of ultrasound is inevitably incomplete. Nevertheless, up to the present time it has been impossible to substantiate any evidence of harmful effects of diagnostic ultrasound. Accumulated clinical and experimental evidence suggests that there is a large safety margin for current diagnostic ultrasound techniques.

A wide range of energy levels is utilized in the many medical and nonmedical applications of ultrasound. Those used in diagnostic ultrasound are at the low end of this energy spectrum. Ultrasound at somewhat higher average intensity levels has been used for over 30 years in physiotherapy to produce localized deep heating of tissue.[1] Aside from the local effects of heat, no short- or long-term effects from this practice have been demonstrated.[2] Higher energy levels are utilized for ablation of nerve endings in the treatment of

Meniere's disease.[3] In experimental neurosurgery high-intensity focused ultrasound has been used to produce trackless intracerebral tissue destruction.[4] High levels of ultrasonic energy are widely used in cleaning devices and for industrial drilling and polishing of metals. Clearly, the possibility of hazard from exposure to ultrasound depends upon the physical characteristics of the energy being utilized. To reasonably evaluate the probability of harmful effects, one must understand as fully as possible the biologic effects at different physical parameters and dosage regimens of ultrasonic irradiation.

ULTRASONIC ENERGY

Ultrasonic energy is mechanical energy, not electromagnetic radiation. It consists of vibratory motion of particles of a transmitting medium. The oscillations of these particles in simple harmonic motion produce regions of alternating compression and rarefaction transmitting the energy through the medium in the form of a wave. When the direction of wave propagation is the same as the direction of particle motion, these waves are called longitudinal waves. The particles transmitting the energy are periodically displaced from their mean positions, reaching maxima of velocity and displacement and undergoing forces of acceleration and deceleration many thousands of times the force of gravity.[5,6] The motion of the particles is resisted by elastic forces of the medium. There is no net movement of the medium. Measurement of the energy flux in an ultrasonic beam, the radiation force, is accomplished by means of a radiation balance. This device, similar to a chemical microbalance, measures the rate of momentum transfer from the beam to the surface of the balance.[7,8] The product of the measured force and the sound wave velocity yields the power intercepted in watts. The intensity of the beam is the power per unit cross-sectional area, or watts per square centimeter. As an alternative to direct measurement, the power or intensity of an ultrasound beam has often been calculated from the electric input to the generating transducer. Such a calculated intensity is probably an unreliable indicator of effective energy flux within the sound beam, since the efficiency of transducers may vary in time. The sound beam intensity undergoes complex variations because of differences in pulse shape and spatial distribution of energy within the beam.

ULTRASONIC FIELD

The typical unfocused diagnostic ultrasound beam is in the shape of a narrow cylinder. The diameter of the cylinder is approximately the diameter of the generating transducer crystal, 1 to 2 cm, and its length is 15 to 20 cm. Because of the physical characteristics of the transducer and the nature of sound waves, there is a nonhomogeneous distribution of energy within the sound beam. This heterogeneity is an important factor when considering the possibility of harmful effects of diagnostic ultrasound. The variations in spatial distribution of energy within the beam occur longitudinally along the axis of the beam as well as transversely across the beam diameter. The cylinder of a continuous-wave (as opposed to pulses used in pulse-echo diagnostic equipment) ultrasound beam can be divided into two distinct regions, the Fresnel zone, or the near field, and the Fraunhofer zone, or the far field. The length of the near zone varies directly with frequency of the beam and with the square of the transducer radius. For diagnostic ultrasound beams, the transition from the near to far fields occurs at a distance of 5 to 20 cm from the transducer, depending upon the frequency and transducer diameter. In the near zone the axial intensity distribution goes through several maxima and minima with increasing distance from the transducer. Transversely across the beam there also are a series of intensity maxima and minima producing a varying beam pattern.[9] In the far field the beam begins to diverge and the intensity gradually decreases with increasing distance from the transducer and from the central axis of the beam. With the diagnostic systems currently in use, the tissues generally lie within the near field.

Since the spatial intensity distribution in the near field of an ultrasound beam is nonuniform, measurement of total intensity alone does not yield a most significant physical parameter, the peak intensity. The spatial distribution of beam energy, the beam profile, may be evaluated or observed by the schlieren (shadow) method[10] (Fig. 16-1), by plotting direct intensity measurements using a miniaturized omnidirectional piezoelectric probe,[7] or by plotting isoecho amplitude curves. The schlieren technique, in which the sound beam is visualized by the change it produces in the refractive index of the transmitting water medium, is not suitable for quantitative analysis. In general, however, the brightness of the schlieren image is proportional to the intensity of the sound beam. The piezoelectric probe is probably the most useful technique currently available. Examples of isoecho beam profiles obtained by Gordon[11] and Wells[12] are shown in Fig. 16-2. The peak intensity in the sound beam appears to occur over relatively small areas along the central axis. Further discussion of the various techniques for measurement of intensity is to be found in Reid and Sikov.[13]

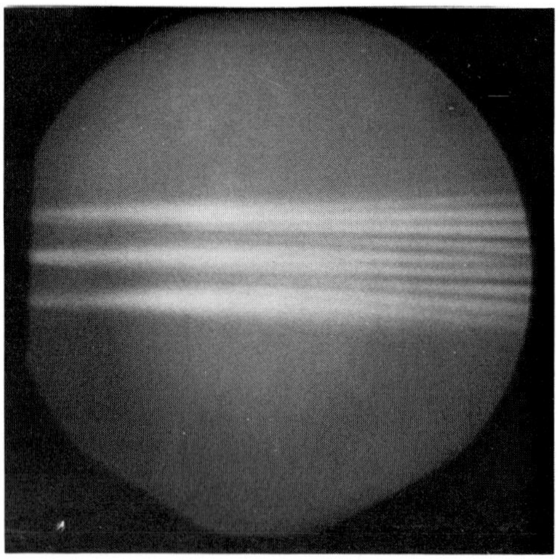

Fig. 16-1. Schlieren (shadow) photograph of the beam pattern produced by three 1-mm transducers spaced 3 mm apart. This illustrates in exaggerated form the heterogeneity of ultrasound beams. The white areas of the beam indicate areas of higher ultrasound intensity arising from the additive effects of phase interference.

ULTRASONIC DOSIMETRY

The essential variables in irradiation regimes with ultrasound of any given frequency are the intensity of the beam (energy incident upon a target tissue per unit area per unit time), the instantaneous peak intensity at any point in the beam, and the effective exposure time (total time a target tissue is exposed to a specified ultrasonic energy). The average intensity of a beam of ultrasound is determined by a number of factors, including the total energy input to the transducer, the energy conversion efficiency of the transducer, and the coupling efficiency of the trans-

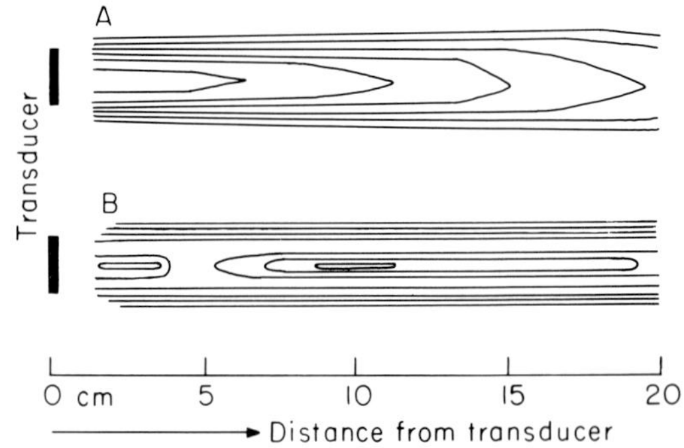

Fig. 16-2. Isoecho beam profiles obtained by two different investigators.[11,12] The contours indicate the areas within the sound beam over which echoes will be recorded from a standard spherical target at increasing levels of amplification. The nominal beam width is increased by increasing system amplification.

ducer when applied to the body. In addition to the near-field intensity variations discussed above, further local variations may occur within the tissues from absorption, reflection, and the formation of standing waves and interference patterns. The interference phenomena may produce localized instantaneous peak intensities well in excess of the spatial average intensity as determined by the radiation microbalance. Peak intensities have been stated to exceed spatial average intensities by as much as two and a half to three times.[14,15] Peak intensity is probably a more significant parameter for evaluating possible clinical hazard than spatial average intensity. The intensity of a beam may also be markedly increased by the use of acoustic lenses to produce focusing of the sound waves. Hill[16] has stated that the effect of focusing on peak intensity is a function of pulse shape and transducer dimensions and has suggested that the intensity in tissues from diagnostic instruments may thus be increased by a factor of 10. Peak intensity is also dependent on the lens characteristics.[17] While focusing transducers have not generally been used in diagnostic ultrasound, efforts to increase lateral resolution and instrument sensitivity may lead to their wider use in the future.

The interaction of the sound beam with transmitting tissues also affects its intensity. Adventitious focusing of the beam may occur as the waves pass through various tissue interfaces. In general, however, as the beam traverses the tissues it undergoes attenuation, or decrease in intensity, by several different mechanisms.[18] Divergence of the waves from a parallel beam beyond the near zone gradually reduces the energy of the beam per unit cross-sectional area. Attenuation of intensity also occurs by scattering and reflection or refraction at discontinuities within the medium so that energy no longer moves in the original direction of propagation. Lastly, the beam intensity is diminished by true absorption, the conversion of energy from its vibrational form to other forms such as heat. Absorption in soft tissues is determined by a number of variables including tissue viscosity, temperature, and sound wave frequency. Absorption increases with increasing frequency of the sound waves.

Time factors play an important role when considering ultrasound beam intensity and its possible biologic effects. Aside from Doppler fetal heart motion detectors and some imaging system, which are continuous-wave instruments, diagnostic ultrasound instruments utilize intermittent short pulses of sound waves. The pulse repetition rate used is often 1,000 pulses per second, although there is considerable variation among commercially available instruments. The pulse duration is also probably equally varied but is assumed, for purposes of discussion, to be 1 μsec in length. The duty factor, the proportion of time the instrument is actually producing sound waves, is therefore 1 μsec/msec, or 0.1% of the time. Thus the time-averaged intensity of a pulsed ultrasound beam is of the order of one one-thousandth of the same beam in continuous operation. The effective exposure time is the sum of the pulse durations, or one one-thousandth of the exposure period. Thus the average intensity and the integral energy dose are markedly reduced by the short duty cycle of pulsed instruments, while the instantaneous peak intensities remain unaffected. Another time factor related to the pulse repetition frequency is the pulse separation interval. The ratio of the pulse duration to separation may also significantly influence the production of biologic effects of ultrasound.

Currently used commercial pulsed diagnostic instruments produce time-averaged intensity levels of 5 to 20 mw/cm^2.[19,20] The instantaneous peak intensities of these instruments are 5 to 10 w/cm^2,[16,21] though peak intensities as high as 100 w/cm^2 have been reported from commercial pulse-echo diagnostic instruments.[22] The continuous wave Doppler fetal heart detection instruments produce a beam with an intensity of 10 to 30 mw/cm^2.[16,23,24] The continuous wave treatment ultrasound beams used in physiotherapy operate at intensities of 3 to 5 w/cm^2.[21,25]

In practical application the effective exposure time or integral energy dose to any given target tissue is further decreased by another time factor, the scanning motion of the ultrasound beam during the examination. In 800 pregnant patients examined ultrasonically, Hall[26] found that the transducer was in contact with the skin for approximately 5 minutes in pulse-echo examinations and for 2 minutes in examinations with the Doppler fetal heart detector. In any examination a particular volume of tissue will be exposed for only a small portion of this total irradiation time.

Let us consider the examination of an 8 to 10-week intrauterine gestation to exclude the diagnosis of ectopic pregnancy. A series of twenty cross-sections might typically be made longitudinally and transversely over the uterus. Each cross-section takes approximately 2 seconds of scanning time to complete. The fetus, about 3 to 4 cm in length, would be exposed, let us assume, in ten of those cross-sections for half of the time required for each, or a total of 10 seconds. Considering a duty factor of 0.1%, the effective exposure time of the fetus would have been 0.01 second. Assuming the examination had been very inefficiently performed and 200 cross-sections through the fetus were made, the effective exposure time of the fetus would still have been only 0.1 second, and that would have been spread over a 10- to 20-minute examination period. By comparison, exposure to similar intensities in physiotherapy may last 10 minutes or more.

MECHANISMS OF BIOLOGIC ACTION

Little is known of the mechanisms of action of diagnostic ultrasound.[27] An experimental system sensitive enough to repeatedly demonstrate any harmful effect of diagnostic ultrasound has not yet been specified. At significantly higher intensity levels the mechanisms of action of ultrasound may be classified as thermal effects, cavitational effects, and "other" effects.[28] Thermal or heating effects of ultrasound on a macroscopic scale are related to the average ultrasonic intensity.[27] In living organisms the heat capacity and thermal conductivity of the blood most probably obviate whatever minimal heating might occur from the low intensity levels of diagnostic instruments.

Cavitation refers to the formation of microbubbles in the tissues from dissolved gases during the negative pressure phase of the sound wave. At appropriate intensity levels cavitation can be a very violent and destructive process and is utilized in a number of applications of ultrasonic energy. In the 1- to 4-MHz frequency range cavitation may occur in the liquid state above the threshold intensities of 0.2 to 5.0 w/cm^2.[27] Stable (resonant) cavitation appears to occur with continuous ultrasound exposure and is probably inhibited by pulsing with short durations and duty factors as in current pulse-echo instruments. Collapse, or unstable cavitation, in which the bubbles collapse completely during the compression phase of the wave, occurs at significantly higher intensity thresholds in liquids, 300 w/cm^2 at 1 MHz.[28] The threshold for cavitation in soft tissues is generally presumed to be higher than in liquids, but recent work suggests that this may not necessarily be true.[29] Nonetheless, no cavitation, stable or unstable, was found to occur in the brain of the cat (in vivo) or in blood plasma at intensities below 250 w/cm^2, even with pulse durations of 0.1 second or longer.[29]

Other effects of ultrasound may occur, although their nature is not well understood and their existence in organized mammalian tissues in vivo has not been demonstrated even at intensity levels much higher than those used diagnostically.[31] Direct mechanical effects on the particles of the medium may take place. Under certain circumstances microstreaming, tissue movement not subject to reversal every half wave, and circulation of particles in the transmitting medium have been described.[32,33] Such a direct effect can produce disruption of macromolecules and may, under appropriate circumstances, produce disruption of chromosomes. Chemical changes may be induced in tissues by ultrasound, possibly as a secondary effect of other mechanisms. Chemical reactions may be accelerated, as may enzymatic action. Free radicals may form by the collapse of cavitation bubbles and initiate other chemical reactions.[34] Other phenomena, such as shearing,[35] particle agglomeration,[36] and changes in the surface charge and the electrophoretic mobility of cells[37] have also been described, but the magnitude of these effects in vivo are yet unknown.

Most probably the mechanisms of action of ultrasound vary with the experimental conditions, the target tissue, and the irradiation parameters and variables. Extreme caution is necessary in interpretation of experimental results and their extrapolation to clinical conditions.

BIOLOGIC EFFECTS OF DIAGNOSTIC ULTRASOUND

Damaging biologic effects of high-energy level ultrasound have been amply documented in the literature.[9,32,34] Unfortunately, much of the early work lacked adequate measurement and documentation of ultrasonic parameters and dosimetric variables. Its usefulness is therefore limited. Recently, improved calibration techniques have provided better definition of beam parameters in vitro. Techniques for measuring ultrasonic dosage in vivo, however, remain to be developed and applied. In spite of these difficulties, both epidemiologic and experimental studies have been undertaken to determine the biologic effects of diagnostic ultrasound.

An extensive retrospective clinical study of obstetric patients by Hellman, Duffus, Donald, and Sunden[38] has revealed no evidence of fetal or maternal injury. Their review of 1,114 normal obstetric patients undergoing ultrasound examination revealed no evidence of increased fetal abnormality or abortion in comparison to the general population. Bernstine,[23] reviewing a series of 720 patients who had undergone 5- to 15-minute ultrasound examination at 10 weeks' gestation or greater, found no evidence of hazard from ultrasound. At present many thousands of patients have undergone a variety of ultrasound examinations, including the brain, eye, thyroid, heart, abdominal viscera, and pregnant uterus, and so far as is known there has been no reported case of deleterious effect attributable to the use of diagnostic ultrasound.

In a similar vein, animal experiments with diagnostic ultrasound have failed to demonstrate any harmful effect. Smyth,[19] exposing mice and rats to diagnostic ultrasound, found no evidence of effect on behavior, growth, food consumption, blood chemistries, or organ histology. No evidence of congenital anomaly was found among first- and second-generation offspring. Woodward, Pond, and Warwick,[39] using peak intensities extending upward from the diagnostic range, exposed the abdomen of pregnant mice to ultrasound at various stages of gestation. At term the number of fetuses, resorption sites, and fetal abnormalities were tabulated. No significant increase in the incidence of abnormalities was found. Shimizu and Shoji,[40] on the other hand, have reported increased frequency of fetal malformation and intrauterine death in pregnant mice irradiated for 5 hours with continuous-wave ultrasound (2.25 MHz) on the ninth day of pregnancy. The work of Lele and Sofia[41] suggests that these effects may have been caused by prolonged, sustained fetal hyperthermia resulting from ultrasonic irradiation at a critical phase of organogenesis. Taylor and Pond,[25] using intensity levels and exposure durations significantly greater than those used in diagnostic ultrasound, were able to produce paresis and hemorrhage in adult rat spinal cords. They found that damaging ability decreased with increasing frequency and increased with hypoxia. At a given frequency and threshold intensity, damage occurred whenever an integrated effective dose was delivered independent of time-averaged intensity and duty factor. Extrapolating from their data, they suggest that a diagnostic examination exposure might have to exceed 3 to 6 hours before summation of dosage would produce observable damage. Ogden[42] subjected fetal and newborn rats to diagnostic ultrasound and subsequently found no alteration in brain weights or chemical analyses.

In 1970 Macintosh and Davey[43] reported an increased number of chromosomal aberrations after exposure of human leukocyte cultures to diagnostic levels of ultrasound. In a subsequent study[44] they confirmed their earlier work and reported that under their experimental conditions chromosomal aberrations did not occur below a threshold intensity of 8.2 mw/cm². Several other groups of workers have attempted to duplicate or verify their findings without success. Boyd,[24] attempting to repeat and extend the experiment, could not produce any increase in chromosomal aberrations over controls. Buckton,[14] Watts,[21] and Bobrow,[45] using ultrasound in the diagnostic levels and above, each failed to demonstrate any damaging effect on leukocyte chromosomes. Abdulla[46] insonated fetuses for 10 hours with diagnostic ultrasound prior to hysterotomy and found no increase in chromosomal aberrations of either the mother or the fetus compared to controls. Coakley and associates[47] also attempted to reproduce the work of Macintosh and Davey and extend the exposure parameters to much higher levels and longer intervals. They also used focused ultrasound waves at an intensity of 100 w/cm² for 30 minutes, as well as pulsed ultrasound waves at peak intensities up to 350 w/cm² for 5 minutes. In every instance they were unable to produce an increase in chromosomal aberrations over control levels. In related experiments on hamster cells, Hill[16] and Bleaney[48] were unable to show any deleterious effects with the parameters used. Of note is the fact that Hill utilitzed focused ultrasound intensities of 150 to 200 w/cm², a pulse duration of 50 μsec, and a pulse repetition frequency of 1,000 for exposures of 1 or 2 hours.

Coakley and Slade[49] have suggested that the results of Macintosh and Davey may be caused by the release of toxic products from the polyethylene used to contain the cell cultures. In addition, their slides were not scored blind, and Buckton and Baker[14] have suggested that their positive findings based primarily on chromatid aberrations should be interpreted with caution, since the number of chromatid aberrations seen in blood cultures is extremely variable and mostly the result of technical artifact.

CONCLUSION

Ultrasound at diagnostic levels of intensity and exposure delivers energy to the tissues and must have some biologic action. The nature and clinical significance of this action remain to be discovered. The available evidence indicates that there is most probably no significant somatic effect of diagnostic ultrasound. The more critical question of possible genetic effect, immediate or delayed, remains unanswered. The accumulating evidence suggests that damaging effects of diagnostic ultrasound on genetic tissue, in contrast to x-irradiation, if present at all, are going to be extremely difficult to document.

In spite of the apparent safety of diagnostic ultrasound, continuing efforts must be made to minimize the energy levels used consistent with diagnostic accuracy. Average and peak intensities of the sound beam must be kept as low as possible. The pulse duration and pulse repetition frequency should be maintained at minimum practical levels. The integral effective dose to genetic tissue and the developing fetus should be kept as low as possible. Clinical application must continue to be guided by judgements based upon an awareness of the uncertainties involved.

REFERENCES

1. Lehmann, J. F., and Guy, A. W.: Ultrasound therapy. In Reid, J. M., and Sikov, M. R., editors: Interaction of ultrasound and biological tissues: workshop proceedings, U. S. Department of Health, Education, and Welfare Publication FDA 73-8008, BRH/DBE 73-1, Washington D. C., 1973, U. S. Government Printing Office, pp. 121-128.
2. Patrick, M. K.: Ultrasound in physiotherapy, Ultrasonics **4:**10-14, 1966.
3. Pennington, C. L., Stevens, E. L., and Griffin, W. L.: The use of ultrasound in the treatment of Meniere's disease, Laryngoscope **80:**578, 1970.
4. Lele, P. P.: Ultrasound in biology and medicine. In Stanley, H. E., editor: Biomedical physics and biomaterial science, Cambridge, Mass., 1972, M. I. T. Press, pp. 257-299.
5. Connolly, C., and Pond, J.: The possibility of harmful effects in using ultrasound for medical diagnosis, Biomed. Eng. **2:**112-115, 1967.
6. O'Brien, W. D., and others: On the assessment of risk to ultrasound, 1972, Ultrasonics Symposium Proceedings, IEEE-72 CHO-708-850, 1972.
7. Hill, C. R.: Calibration of ultrasonic beams for bio-medical applications, Phys. Med. Biol. **15:**241-248, 1970.
8. Rooney, J. A.: Determination of acoustic power outputs in the microwattmilliwatt range, Ultrasound Med. Biol. **1:**13-16, 1973.
9. Wells, P. N. T.: Physical principles of ultrasonic diagnosis, London, 1969, Academic Press, Inc., pp. 53-72.
10. Hunter, H. H., and others: Stroboscopic schlieren system for the visual observation of pulsed ultrasonic waves, Proc. IEEE **52:**744-745, 1964.
11. Gordon, D.: Comparison of ultrasonic pulse echo apparatus used in medicine, Ultrasonics **2:**199-202, 1964.
12. Wells, P. N. T.: Some physical limitations in ultrasonic diagnosis, Biomed. Eng. **1:**390-394, 1966.
13. Reid, J. M., and Sikov, M. R., editors: Interaction of ultrasound and biological tissues: workshop proceedings, U. S. Department of Health, Education, and Welfare Publication FDA 73-8008, BRH/DBE 73-1, Washington, D. C., 1973, U. S. Government Printing Office, pp. 153-214.
14. Buckton, K. E., and Baker, N. V.: An investigation into possible chromosome damaging effects of ultrasound on human blood cells, Br. J. Radiol. **45:**340-342, 1972.
15. Hill, C. R., and others: Biophysical effects of cavitation in a 1 MHz ultrasonic beam, Ultrasonics for Industry Conference Papers, 26-30. Quoted in Macintosh, I. J. C., and Davey, D. A.: Relationship between intensity of ultrasound and induction of chromosome aberration, Br. J. Radiol. **45:**320-327, 1972.
16. Hill, C. R., Joshi, G. P., and Revell, S. H.: A search for chromosome damage following exposure of Chinese hamster cells to high intensity, pulsed ultrasound, Br. J. Radiol. **45:**333-334, 1972.
17. Robinson, T. C., and Lele, P. P.: An analysis of lesion development in the brain and in plastics by high-intensity focused ultrasound at low-megathertz frequencies, J. Acoust. Soc. Am. **51:**1333-1351, 1972.
18. Wells, P. N. T.: Physical principles of ultrasonic diagnosis, London, 1969, Academic Press, Inc., pp. 19-25.
19. Smyth, M. G.: Animal toxicity studies with ultrasound at diagnostic power levels. In Grossman, C. C., and others, editors: Diagnostic ultrasound, New York, 1966, Plenum Press, pp. 296-299.
20. Dewhurst, C. J.: The safety of ultrasound, Proc. R. Soc. Med. **64:**996-997, 1971.
21. Watts, P. L., Hall, A. J., and Fleming, J. E. E.: Ultrasound and chromosome damage, Br. J. Radiol. **45:**335-339, 1972.
22. Dunn, F., and Fry, F. J.: Ultrasonic threshold dosages for the mammalian central nervous system, IEEE Trans. Bio-med. Eng. **BME-18:**253-256, 1971.
23. Bernstine, R. L.: Safety studies with ultrasonic Doppler technic: a clinical follow-up of patients and tissue culture study, Obstet. Gynecol. **34:**707, 1969.
24. Boyd, E., and others: Chromosome breakage and ultrasound, Br. Med. J. **2:**501-502, 1971.

25. Taylor, K. J. W., and Pond, J. B.: A study of the production of haemorrhagic injury and paraplegia in rat spinal cord by pulsed ultrasound of low megaHertz frequencies in the context of the safety for clinical usage, Br. J. Radiol. **45**:343-353, 1972.
26. Hall, A. J.: Ultrasonic dosimetry in obstetrics. In de Vlieger, M., White, D. N., and McCready, V. R., editors: Proceedings of the II World Congress on Ultrasonics in Medicine, International Congress Series, No. 277, Rotterdam, 1973, Excerpta Medica, Inc.
27. Hill, C. R.: Biophysical basis for possible ultrasonic hazards, Br. J. Radiol. **44**:563, 1971.
28. Wells, P. N. T.: Physical principles of ultrasonic diagnosis, London, 1969, Academic Press, Inc., pp. 222-226.
29. Lele, P. P., Senapati, N., and Hsu, W. L.: Mechanisms of tissue-ultrasound interaction. In de Vlieger, M., White, D. N., and McCready, V. R., editors: Proceedings of the II World Congress on Ultrasonics in Medicine, International Congress Series, No. 277, Rotterdam, 1973, Excerpta Medica, Inc., pp. 345-352.
30. Garrett, W. J., and Robinson, D. E.: Ultrasound in clinical obstetrics, Springfield, Ill., 1970, Charles C Thomas, Publisher, pp. 23-26.
31. Lele, P. P., and Pierce, A. D.: The thermal hypothesis of the mechanism of ultrasonic focal destruction in organized tissues. In Reid, J. M., and Sikov, M. R., editors: Interaction of ultrasound and biological tissues: workshop proceedings, U. S. Department of Health, Education, and Welfare Publication FDA 73-8008, BRH/DBE 73-1, Washington, D. C., 1973, U. S. Government Printing Office, pp. 121-128.
32. Hill, C. R.: The possibility of hazard in medical and industrial applications of ultrasound, Br. J. Radiol. **41**:561-569, 1968.
33. Gershoy, A. and Nyborg, W. L.: Perturbation of plant-cell contents by ultrasonic micro-irradiation, J. Acoust. Soc. Am. **54**:1356-1367, 1973.
34. Freimanis, A. K.: The biological effects of medically applied ultrasound and their causes, CRC Crit. Rev. Radiol. Sci. **1**:639-652, 1970.
35. Rooney, J. A.: Shear as a mechanism for sonically induced biological effects, J. Acoust. Soc. Am. **52**:1718-1724, 1972.
36. Nyborg, W. L., and Gershoy, A.: Microsonation of cells under nearthreshold conditions. In de Vlieger, M., White, D. N., and McCready, V. R., editors: Proceedings of the II World Congress on Ultrasonics in Medicine, International Congress Series, No. 277, Rotterdam, 1973, Excerpta Medica, Inc.
37. Joshi, G. P., Hill, C. R., and Forrester, J. A.: Mode of action of ultrasound on the surface charge of mammalian cells *in vitro*, Ultrasound Med. Biol. **1**:45-48, 1973.
38. Hellman, L. M., and others: Safety of diagnostic ultrasound in obstetrics, Lancet **1**:1133-1134, 1970.
39. Woodward, B., Pond, J. B., and Warwick, R.: How safe is diagnostic sonar? Br. J. Radiol. **43**:719-725, 1970.
40. Shimizu, T., and Shoji, R.: An experimental safety study of mice exposed to low intensity ultrasound. In de Vlieger, M., White, D. N., and McCready, V. R., editors: Proceedings of the II World Congress on Ultrasonics in Medicine, International Congress Series, No. 277, Rotterdam, 1973, Excerpta Medica, Inc.
41. Lele, P. P., and Sofia, J. W.: Ultrasonic teratology in mouse and man. In press.
42. Ogden, J. R.: Investigation of the effect of diagnostic ultrasound on brain growth and neurone proliferation of foetal and immature rats, a preliminary report, Br. J. Radiol. **44**:563, 1971.
43. Macintosh, I. J. C., and Davey, D. A.: Chromosome aberrations induced by an ultrasonic fetal pulse detector, Br. Med. J. **4**:92-93, 1970.
44. Macintosh, I. J. C., and Davey, D. A.: Relationship between intensity of ultrasound and induction of chromosome aberrations, Br. J. Radiol. **45**:320-327, 1972.
45. Bobrow, M., Blackwell, N., and Unrau, A. E.: Absence of any observed effect of ultrasonic irradiation on human chromosomes, J. Obstet. Gynaecol. Br. Commonw. **780**:730-736, 1971.
46. Abdulla, U., and others: Effect of diagnostic ultrasound on maternal and fetal chromosomes, Lancet **2**:829-831, 1971.
47. Coakley, W. T., and others: Examination of lymphocytes for chromosome aberrations after ultrasonic irradiation, Br. J. Radiol. **45**:328-332, 1972.
48. Bleaney, B. I., Blackbourn, P., and Kirkley, J.: Resistance of CHLF hamster cells to ultrasonic radiation of 1.5 MHz frequency, Br. J. Radiol. **45**:354-357, 1972.
49. Coakley, W. T., and Slade, J. S.: Examination of sonicated human lymphocytes for chromosome damage, Br. J. Radiol. **44**:563, 1971.

Appendix

Biparietal diameter determination of gestational age*

BIPARIETAL DIAMETER (CM)	GESTATIONAL AGE (WEEKS)	BIPARIETAL DIAMETER (CM)	GESTATIONAL AGE (WEEKS)
2.0	12.0	6.0	25.5
2.1	12.5	6.1	26.0
2.2	13.0	6.2	26.0
2.3	13.0	6.3	26.5
2.4	13.5	6.4	27.0
2.5	14.0	6.5	27.0
2.6	14.0	6.6	27.5
2.7	14.5	6.7	28.0
2.8	15.0	6.8	28.0
2.9	15.0	6.9	28.5
3.0	15.5	7.0	29.0
3.1	16.0	7.1	29.0
3.2	16.0	7.2	29.5
3.3	16.5	7.3	30.0
3.4	17.0	7.4	30.0
3.5	17.0	7.5	30.0

*This table was derived from data collected from a heterogeneous population at the Downstate Medical Center, New York City. The gestational age is given in weeks from the onset of the last menstrual period. The table has shown good clinical reliability. Users are cautioned that the table serves only as a guideline to estimation of gestational age and fetal maturity. For any biparietal measurement, the standard deviation for the corresponding gestational age is ± 1 to 2 weeks. From Hellman, L. M., and others: Sources of error in sonographic fetal mensuration and estimation of growth, Am. J. Obstet. Gynecol. **99:**662-670, 1967; and Hellman, L. M., and others: Growth and development of the human fetus prior to the twentieth week of gestation, Am. J. Obstet. Gynecol. **103:**789-798, 1969.

Biparietal diameter determination of gestational age—cont'd

BIPARIETAL DIAMETER (CM)	GESTATIONAL AGE (WEEKS)	BIPARIETAL DIAMETER (CM)	GESTATIONAL AGE (WEEKS)
3.6	17.5	7.6	30.8
3.7	18.0	7.7	31.0
3.8	18.0	7.8	31.7
3.9	18.5	7.9	32.0
4.0	19.0	8.0	32.7
4.1	19.0	8.1	33.0
4.2	19.5	8.2	33.6
4.3	20.0	8.3	34.0
4.4	20.0	8.4	34.6
4.5	20.5	8.5	35.0
4.6	21.0	8.6	35.5
4.7	21.0	8.7	36.0
4.8	21.5	8.8	36.5
4.9	22.0	8.9	37.0
5.0	22.0	9.0	37.4
5.1	22.5	9.1	38.0
5.2	23.0	9.2	38.4
5.3	23.0	9.3	39.0
5.4	23.5	9.4	39.0
5.5	24.0	9.5	39.8
5.6	24.0	9.6	40.0
5.7	24.5	9.7	40.8
5.8	25.0	9.8	41.0
5.9	25.0	9.9	41.7

Index

A

D

E

I

K

O

P

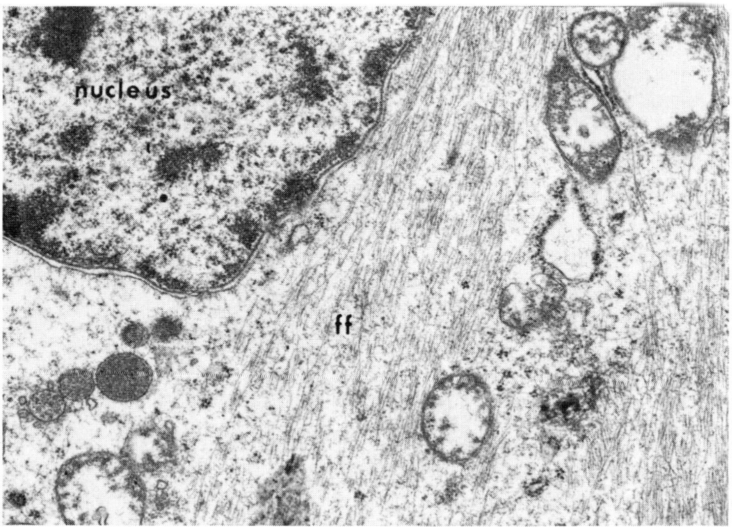

Fig. 3-3. Portion of a fibrous astrocyte in the orbital portion of human optic nerve. Many tonofilaments *(ff)* course near the nucleus. (×33,000; from Anderson, D. R., Hoyt, W. F., and Hogan, M. J. Trans. Am. Ophthalmol. Soc. **65**:275, 1967.)

plasm contains filaments, or fibrils, in addition to the other usual organelles (Fig. 3-3). These filaments are found in both the fibrous and the protoplasmic astrocyte; the distinction between the two types of astrocytes is based entirely on their three-dimensional architecture and not upon whether or not they contain these filaments.

Microtubules* are sometimes observed in astroglial cytoplasm, particularly in association with the centrioles, but this organelle is not a prominent feature of normal adult astrocytes. They have been described, however, in astrocytes of embryonic optic nerve, and are also found in tumor astrocytes of optic nerve gliomas.

Also worthy of note is that astrocytes contain glycogen. However, if there is a period of tissue anoxia before the fixative has time to act, the glycogen may be metabolized anaerobically and be absent from the section.

*Microtubules are organelles found in the cytoplasm of many cells throughout the body. They are approximately 150 nm in diameter and have a tubular appearance. They appear circular in cross section, and when cut longitudinally there are two parellel dark lines representing the opposite walls of the tube. The function of microtubules is not known, but they are found most often in cells that have some longitudinal orientation, such as the lens fibers, and it is often assumed that they play a role either in the formation of elongated cells or in the maintenance of an elongated shape. Microtubules are seen only in electron micrographs of tissue that was fixed primarily with an aldehyde fixative such as formaldehyde or glutaraldehyde, and if only osmium has been used as a fixative, filaments are seen in the places where microtubules were present.

people would not consider the most anterior extent of glia to be part of the lamina cribrosa, even though in fact the glial framework is continuous out to the margins of the optic papilla.

It was hinted above that posteriorly in the optic nerve head capillaries are within the collagenous trabeculae of the lamina cribrosa and that more anteriorly the capillaries, which here might be called disc capillaries, accompanied by a very thin sleeve of connective tissue, are within the glial columns.

The following discussion examines in some detail various anatomic units of the neuroectodermal compartment and their physiologic functions.

Astrocytes

The macroglia of the central nervous system are divided into two categories, astrocytes and oligodendrocytes. Astrocytes are classically identified on the basis of their three-dimensional architecture by light microscopy in silver-stained preparations. Astrocytes have many long branching processes, in contrast to the oligondendrocytes, which have only a few short processes. Two varieties of astrocytes are often described, the fibrous astrocyte, which has thin, long processes, and the protoplasmic astrocyte, which has shorter, broad-based processes.

By electron microscopy, both types of astrocytes are similar. The astrocyte has a larger, paler nucleus and a more abundant, paler cytoplasm than the oligodendrocyte (Fig. 3-2). Of particular note is that the astrocyte cyto-

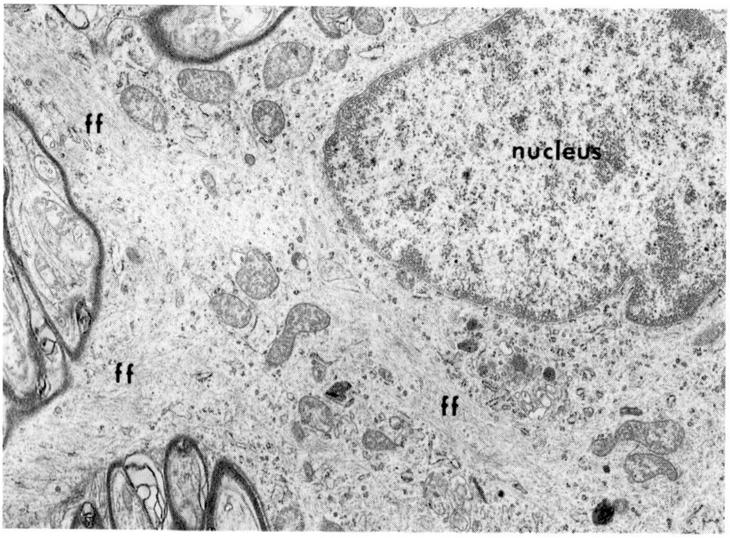

Fig. 3-2. Cynomolgous monkey optic nerve astrocyte. Tonofilaments *(ff)* fill much of the cytoplasm and extend into the processes. (×15,000; from Anderson, D. R., and Hoyt, W. F.: Arch. Ophthalmol. **82:**506, 1969.)

and presumably this is the main exit. The capillary network may also find venous exit by means of tributaries that enter the choroid and join the choroidal draniage into the vortex veins.

Electron microscopy shows the blood vessels of the optic nerve and optic nerve head to be the type seen throughout the central nervous system and retina. The endothelial cells are nonfenestrated. Adjacent endothelial cells are united by prominent, tight junctions. This is true even for the capillaries of the optic nerve head that are part of the posterior ciliary circulation. The capillaries of the choroid, although derived from the same arteries, are quite different.

NEUROECTODERMAL COMPARTMENT

In the *intraorbital portion of the optic nerve,* the neuroectodermal compartment consists of bundles of myelinated nerve fibers (axons) and glial cells (astrocytes and oligodendrocytes). Except for the presence of the connective tissue pial septa, the intraorbital portion of the optic nerve is exactly like other white matter tracts of the central nervous system. There are no ganglion cells or synapses.

Myelin ends in the region of the lamina cribrosa. Thus in the optic nerve head, the neuroectodermal compartment consists of unmyelinated axons and astrocytes. There are only these two components; there are no oligodendrocytes, ganglion cells, synapses, or other neural components.

The arrangement of the nerve fibers and the astrocytes in the optic nerve head and their relationship to the collagen sheets of the lamina cribrosa are illustrated in Plates 1 and 2. The nonmyelinated nerve fibers are grouped together in bundles and apparently remain separated as individual bundles as they pass through this region. The collagenous sheets are prominent, while astrocytes fill the space between successive sheets and surround the perforation (Plate 2). Moving anteriorly, the connective tissue becomes less prominent. Parelleling the reduction in collagenous tissue, the glial component of the lamina cribrosa becomes more prominent so that anteriorly the lamina cribrosa consists entirely of the glial tissue within which are embedded the disc capillaries.

This leads us to a semantic point. In everyday conversation we often use the term *lamina cribrosa* to refer to the perforated collagenous sheets that bridge the scleral canal. In contrast, anatomic description usually refers to two parts of the lamina cribrosa: the posterior, or scleral, part, which consists of connective tissue sheets, and the anterior, or choroidal or glial, part, which is primarily glial and begins at the level of the choroid, where the connective tissue sheets disappear. Plates 1 and 2 show how there is a gradual transiton between the two parts of the lamina cribrosa and how the glial structure then extends forward to fill the entire optic disc. The anterior boundary of the glial portion of the lamina cribrosa is indefinite, and most if it exists have been the subject of some debate. Apparently, at least in some individuals, there is a central artery of the optic nerve that runs axially through the center of the optic nerve along its entire intraorbital course in addition to the central retinal artery, which courses through the center of the nerve only in the part near the globe. Other individuals may lack such an axial blood supply or may receive, in the anterior portion of the nerve, a few branches from the central *retinal* artery.

Venous drainage from the intraorbital portion of the optic nerve is accomplished mainly if not entirely through tributaries that join the central retinal vein.

Intraocular portion of the optic nerve. The circulation at the optic nerve head (intraocular portion of the optic nerve) is considerably more complex. In this region three arterial systems and two venous systems meet. The circulatory dynamics are affected not only by the multiple supply and drainage routes but also by the difference between the tissue pressure in the orbit, in the orbital portion of the optic nerve (the cerebrospinal fluid pressure), and in the optic nerve head (intraocular pressure).

The primary blood supply to the optic nerve head is from the short posterior ciliary arteries. These arteries enter the sclera adjacent to the optic nerve and are concerned principally with the blood supply of the choroid. Branches from these arteries extend into the optic nerve head from the outer choroid and sclera at the level of the lamina cribrosa. Adjacent arterial branches often anastomose to form an arterial ring in the sclera adjacent to the optic nerve. This ring is the circle of Zinn-Haller. The circle of Zinn-Haller is sometimes incomplete or even absent in humans and it has not been observed at all in monkeys.

In direct continuity with the optic nerve head are tissues with other arterial supplies: the retina, supplied by the central retinal artery, and the orbital portion of the optic nerve, supplied by the pial arterial network and possibly also by the central artery of the optic nerve. The capillary network seems to be continuous, providing capillary anastomose between these three arterial systems in the optic nerve head.

As might be expected, there is individual variation in the territories principally supplied by these three arterial systems. This variation is illustrated particularly by the well-known occurrence of cilioretinal arteries, which are derived from the short posterior ciliary arteries, either directly or via the circle of Zinn-Haller, but supply a portion of the retina. In a similar way the central retinal artery may send retrograde branches from the retina or disc surface to supply the disc and possibly even the optic nerve behind the eye. Retrograde branches of the ciliary arteries may contribute to the pial network. Pial vessels may extend forward to supply parts of the optic nerve head.

Capillaries of the optic nerve head drain into the central retinal vein,

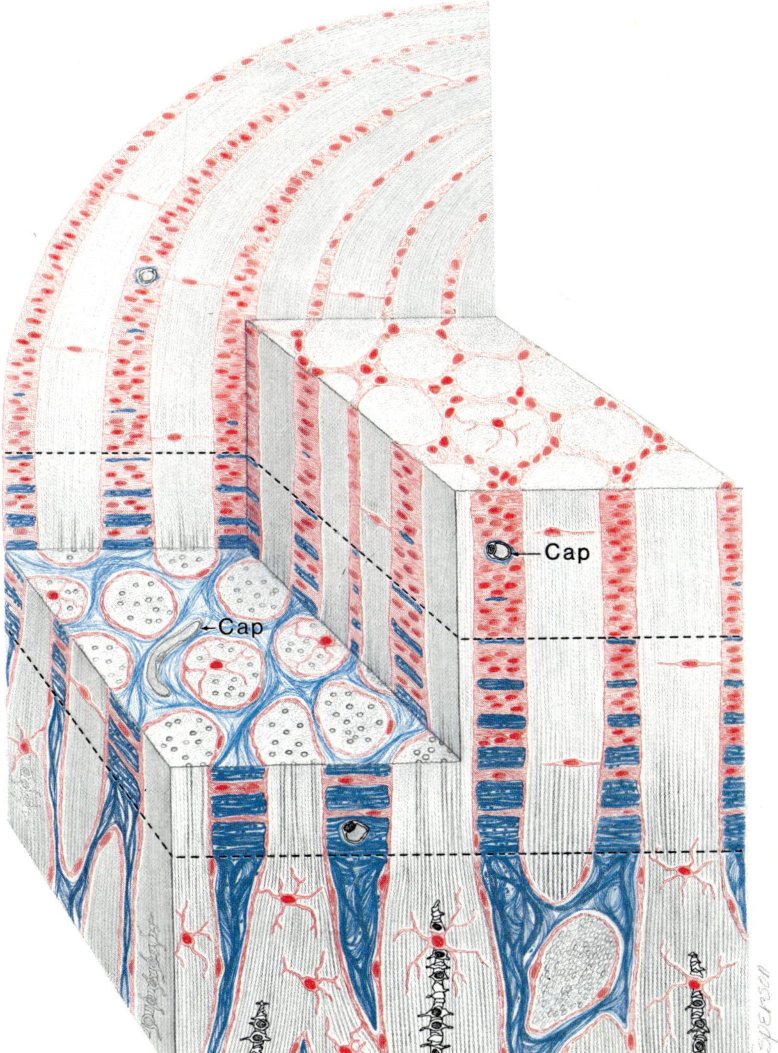

Plate 2. Schematic drawing of relationships of connective tissue (blue) and glia (red) in posterior and anterior portions of lamina cribrosa. Note the location of capillaries *(Cap)*. (From Anderson, D.R.: Arch. Ophthalmol. **82:**800, 1969.)

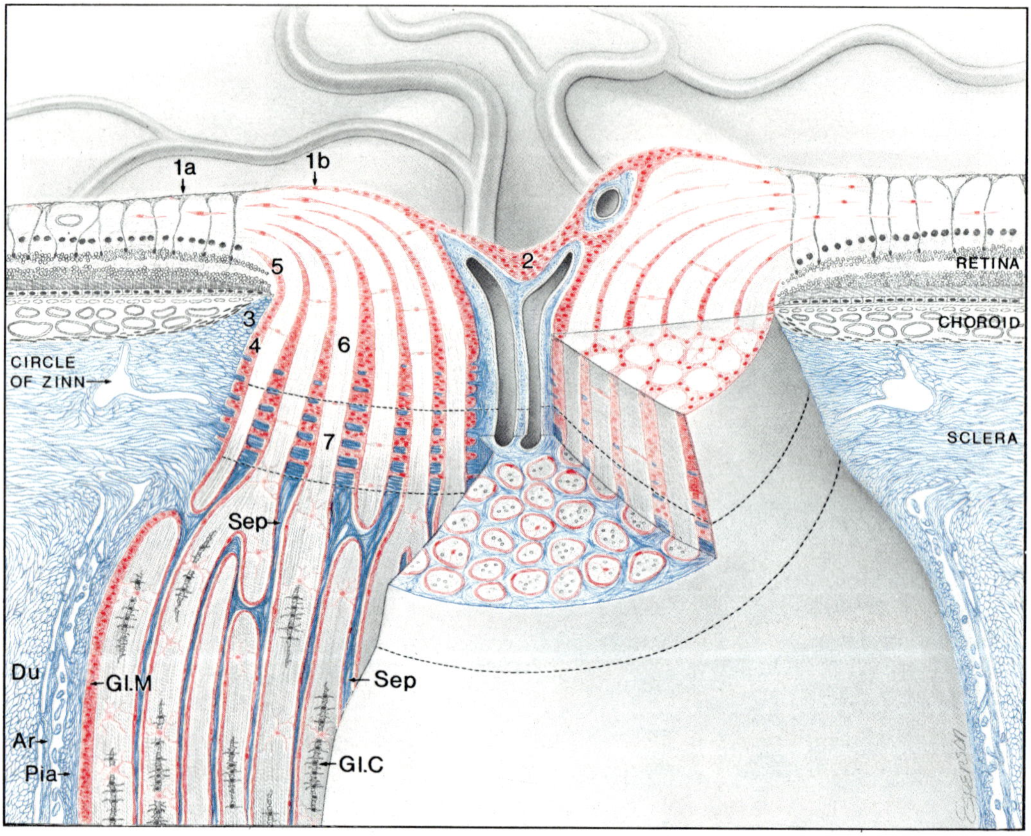

Plate 1. Schematic drawing of optic nerve within and adjoining the eyeball. Collagenous connective tissue is shown in blue, and astroglial structures are shown in red. Surrounding the intraorbital portion of the optic nerve is the dura mater *(Du)*, arachnoid mater *(Ar)*, and pia mater *(Pia)*. The pia mater is separated from the optic nerve itself by a glial mantle *(Gl. M)*, and connective tissue septal *(Sep)* are seen in the optic nerve behind the lamina cribrosa. Columns of glial cells *(Gl. C)* are seen within the bundles of myelinated nerve fibers. The numbered regions are as follows: *1a,* inner limiting membrane of retina; *1b,* inner limiting membrane of Elschnig; *2,* central meniscus of Kuhnt; *3,* border tissue of Elschnig; *4,* border tissue of Jacoby; *5,* intermediary tissue of Kuhnt; *6,* anterior portion of lamina cribrosa; and *7,* posterior portion of lamina cribrosa. (From Anderson, D. R., and Hoyt, W. F.: Arch. Ophthalmol. **82:**506, 1969.)

tissue found in the intraorbital portion of the optic nerve to the arrangement in the retina, which is more typical of the central nervous system in general.

The sclera, a mesodermal structure, has an opening, called the scleral canal, through which the optic nerve passes. At the margin of the scleral canal, the sclera is continuous with the meninges and with the collagenous portion of the lamina cribrosa. Sometimes, particularly on the temporal side of the optic nerve head, a flange of collagen extends anteriorly from the sclera to separate the choroid from the optic nerve. This lining tissue is called the border tissue of Elschnig. Perforated sheets, or trabeculae, of dense connective tissue extend as a continuation of the sclera across the scleral canal. This connective tissue has a cribriform structure and constitutes the posterior portion of the lamina cribrosa,* or *lamina cribrosa scleralis.* The posterior portion of the lamina cribrosa is continuous with the anterior termination of the longitudinal pial septa of the intraorbital portion of the optic nerve.

In the scleral portion of the optic nerve head, blood vessels, mostly capillaries, are contained within the collagenous sheets (Plate 2). More anteriorly in the optic nerve head, they are in the anterior glial continuation of the lamina cribrosa. The blood vessels are the type seen throughout the central nervous system, with nonfenestrated endothelium and tight junctions between adjacent endothelial cells.

The central connective tissue core containing the central retinal vessels projects forward through the lamina cribrosa into the optic nerve head and constitutes the adventitia of the central retinal vessels. The connective tissue core divides so that a sleeve of connective tissue extends along each branch or tributary of the central retinal vessels, tapering as it recedes from the disc in accordance with the smaller size of the vessels.

The vascular tree

Intraorbital portion of optic nerve. The intraorbital portion of the optic nerve derives much if not all of its arterial blood supply from a plexus of vessels in the pia mater. The pial network originates from a small number of arterial branches that perforate the leptomeninges from the orbit. Most of these perforating branches are posterior to the site at which the central retinal vessels cross the subarachnoid space. Other arterial branches to the pial network originate from the central retinal artery as it penetrates the optic nerve. In addition, recurrent branches to the pia mater originate from the short posterior ciliary arteries in the region of the optic nerve head.

The existence of an axial arterial supply in the optic nerve and its nature

*In everyday conversation and writing, the term *lamina cribrosa* is usually used to refer to the perforated sheets of collagen that bridge the scleral canal. In strict anatomic terminology, this is only the posterior, or scleral, portion of the lamina cribrosa. The lamina cribrosa also has an anterior portion, which is made up almost entirely of astrocytes. This is discussed later in this chapter.

plasmic tonofilaments. Between the meningothelial cells, particularly in the inner layers, are bundles of collagen from which originate the subarachnoid trabeculae. The arachnoid mater, like the dura mata, is essentially avascular, except for the perforating vessels to and from the pia mater that pass through it.

The subarachnoid trabeculae traverse the subarachnoid space, extending between the inner surface of the arachnoid mater and the outer surface of the pia mater. The core of each trabecula is a compact bundle of collagen. The surface of each trabecula is coated by a single layer of meningothelial cells.

The pia mater is the innermost of the meningeal sheaths of the optic nerve. The outer surface of the pia mater is lined by a mesothelial layer of meningothelial cells. Beneath this lining is a dense connective tissue of varying thickness. The pia mater, unlike the dura mater and arachnoid mater, contains a rich network of blood vessels derived from the orbital vessels by means of branches that perforate the dura and arachnoid mater.

From the undersurface of the pia mater, longitudinal septa delve into the optic nerve itself and separate the neuroectodermal compartment into longitudinal bundles. The separation is incomplete, however, and adjacent bundles of neuroectoderm are frequently in direct contact with one another. In addition to providing support, the septa act as a conduit for all the blood vessels that supply the optic nerve, most of which are capillaries. The capillaries thus stay within the mesodermal compartment and never enter directly into the neuroectodermal compartment. In the center of the optic nerve near the eye is a central connective tissue core that contains the central retinal vessels. This connective tissue core is basically only an expansion of the system of pial septa to accommodate these larger vessels. The connective tissue of this core constitutes the adventitia of the central retinal vessels.

This kind of connective tissue septum is not found elsewhere in the central nervous system (CNS). In other parts of the CNS, capillaries enter from the surface of the brain and are invested only by a thin sleeve of connective tissue around each vessel, this sleeve usually consisting of only a basement membrane. In the optic nerve this connective tissue investment, in the form of pial septa, is considerably more extensive and contains collagen as well as fibroblasts. These septa occur only in the intraorbital portion of the optic nerve, disappearing anteriorly at the region of the lamina cribrosa and posteriorly at the optic canal. Thus the intracranial portion of the optic nerve, the optic chiasm, and the optic tract do not have such septa.

Intraocular portion of the optic nerve

The intraocular portion of the optic nerve, also called the optic nerve head, is regarded as having three parts—scleral, choroidal, and retinal—as it passes, respectively, through the sclera, choroid, and outer retina (Plate 1). In this region there is a transition from the extensive mesodermal support